Digital Technologies for Psychiatric Mental Health Disorders

Digital Technologies for Psychiatric Mental Health Disorders

Editor: John Dalvi

AMERICAN
MEDICAL PUBLISHERS
www.americanmedicalpublishers.com

AMERICAN
MEDICAL PUBLISHERS
www.americanmedicalpublishers.com

Cataloging-in-Publication Data

Digital technologies for psychiatric mental health disorders / edited by John Dalvi.
p. cm.
Includes bibliographical references and index.
ISBN 979-8-88740-062-4
1. Mental illness--Treatment--Technological innovations. 2. Psychotherapy--Technological innovations.
3. Mental health services--Technological innovations. 4. Mental illness. 5. Mental health. 6. Psychiatry.
I. Dalvi, John.
RC480.5 .D54 2023
616.891 4--dc23

American Medical Publishers,
41 Flatbush Avenue,
1st Floor, New York,
NY 11217, USA

ISBN 979-8-88740-062-4 (Hardback)

Contents

Preface

This book has been an outcome of determined endeavour from a group of educationists in the field. The primary objective was to involve a broad spectrum of professionals from diverse cultural background involved in the field for developing new researches. The book not only targets students but also scholars pursuing higher research for further enhancement of the theoretical and practical applications of the subject.

Psychiatry is the branch of medical science concerned with the diagnosis, treatment, and prevention of mental health disorders. These disorders are conventionally divided into three general categories, namely, mental illnesses, severe learning disabilities, and personality disorders. There are various sub-specialties of psychiatry including addiction psychiatry, child and adolescent psychiatry, clinical neurophysiology, geriatric psychiatry, and sleep medicine. Psychiatrists use a variety of treatments for managing mental health disorders depending on the needs of each patient. Some of the treatment methods are psychotherapy, and medications such as antipsychotics, mood stabilizers, and antidepressants. Psychotherapy is a type of treatment that involves a talking relationship between a therapist and a patient. Cognitive behavior therapy, and family therapy or group counselling are some forms of psychotherapy. Digital technologies such as mobile devices, telepsychiatry applications, and web-enabled interventions delivered through online platforms are also used for diagnosing, screening, treating, and providing education or facilitating self-management of mental disorders. The book aims to shed light on some of the unexplored aspects of the application of digital technologies for the management of mental health disorders. It will prove to be immensely beneficial to medical students and practitioners of psychiatry.

It was an honour to edit such a profound book and also a challenging task to compile and examine all the relevant data for accuracy and originality. I wish to acknowledge the efforts of the contributors for submitting such brilliant and diverse chapters in the field and for endlessly working for the completion of the book. Last, but not the least; I thank my family for being a constant source of support in all my research endeavours.

Editor

1

Feasibility and Clinical Usefulness of the Unified Protocol in Online Group Format for Bariatric Surgery Candidates: Study Protocol for a Multiple Baseline Experimental Design

Alba Quilez-Orden [1,2], Vanesa Ferreres-Galán [3] and Jorge Osma [1,2,*]

1 Department of Psychology and Sociology, University of Zaragoza, 44003 Teruel, Spain; aquilez@iisaragon.es
2 Health Research Institute of Aragón, 50009 Zaragoza, Spain
3 Mental Health Unit of the Regional Hospital of Vinaròs, 12500 Castellón, Spain; ferreres_van@gva.es
* Correspondence: osma@unizar.es

Abstract: Obesity is currently becoming a serious global public health problem due to its high prevalence and continuous increase. This condition is associated with different physical and mental health problems. The presence of emotional disorders (anxiety, depression and related disorders) among candidates for bariatric surgery is very high and predicts worse physical and psychological results. The present study aims to explore the feasibility and clinical usefulness of the Unified Protocol, a transdiagnostic emotion regulation-based intervention, delivered in an online group format to patients with emotional disorder diagnosis or symptoms, who are waiting for bariatric surgery. We will conduct a pilot study with a repeated single-case experimental design (multiple baseline design) in a public mental health service. The sample will consist of 60 participants, who will be randomized to three baseline conditions: 8, 12 or 15 evaluation days before the intervention. Diagnostic criteria, symptomatology and body mass index are the primary outcome measures, and we will include affectivity, personality, quality of life, body image, eating behavior and surgical complications like secondary measures. An analysis of treatment satisfaction will be also performed. Assessment points will include pre-treatment, baseline, treatment, post-treatment, and follow-ups every three months until two years after post-treatment. The results obtained in this study may have important clinical, social and economic implications for public mental health.

Keywords: emotional disorders; transdiagnostic; online group format; unified protocol; bariatric surgery; obesity

---

1. Introduction

Obesity is a chronic disease characterised by an increase in body fatness, which is usually estimated by body mass index (BMI) calculated as measured body weight (kg) divided by measured height squared (m^2) [1]. Obesity is currently becoming a serious global public health problem due to its high prevalence and increase in recent years [2]. In Spain alone, 25% of the population is obese or overweight, and the expectations are alarming. It is expected that in 2030, up to 80% of Spanish men and 55% of women will be obese or overweight, exceeding 27.2 million of people [3].

The causes of obesity are complex and multifactorial [1], and this condition is associated with different health problems, such as myocardial infarction, hypertension, stroke, dyslipidemia, diabetes mellitus, or obstructive sleep apnea [4–6]. All these alterations affect the quality of life and can disturb important areas of functioning (e.g., physical function, vitality, social functioning and emotional role) [7,8]. In addition to all of these complications, people with obesity experience significant psychological difficulties [7]. Due to all of these health implications, obesity represents a challenge to the countries' economies [9]. As of 2016 in Spain, the obesity cost meant almost two billion euros of extra expenses for the National Health System [3].

For all these reasons (high prevalence and associated costs), many efforts have been made to find treatments for obesity and weight loss, which include lifestyle interventions, pharmacological interventions, surgical interventions, and endoscopic bariatric procedures [7]. Bariatric surgery (BS) is the most commonly performed procedure worldwide [10] and the most effective intervention for individuals with severe obesity (BMI greater than 40 kg/m^2) [11], and includes a group of surgical procedures performed to facilitate weight loss, such as open or laparoscopic roux-en-Y gastric bypass, sleeve gastrectomy, and adjustable gastric banding. The most obvious and studied benefits of BS refer to physical issues, specifically weight loss and improvement of obesity-related physical comorbidities; however, between 10% and 25% of patients who undergo BS show suboptimal weight loss, and it is estimated that they regain approximately 10% of their weight during the first decade after the intervention [12]. Regarding the psychological benefits of BS, limited and inconclusive results have been found [13]. Some systematic reviews have reported improvements after BS, especially in depressive symptoms, but also limited only to the first months after the intervention, and they tend to reappear after the first two years [10].

Some studies have questioned whether previous psychopathology history could influence the results obtained by BS [2]. This topic is especially relevant because the percentage of psychopathology among people waiting for BS (between 20.9% and 55.5%) [12] is much higher than in the general population (between 12.53% and 13.87%) [14]. Specifically, the group of emotional disorders (ED), which includes anxiety and mood disorders, eating disorders, and related disorders ([15]; Supplementary Materials), are the most prevalent disorders among BS candidates: eating disorders (50%), mood disorders (31.5%), anxiety disorders (24%), and substance use related disorders (10%) [12]. It has been concluded that the presence of EDs among candidates for BS predicts worse results in the long term [11], furthermore, a meta-analysis states that the prevalence of suicide mortality is up to 1.8%, and the prevalence of suicide is up to 0.3% after bariatric surgery [16].

As we can observe, psychological evaluation and intervention play a fundamental role in the multidisciplinary work performed with these patients before and after BS although, until now, it has not received much attention [12]. Improvements in eating psychopathology (e.g., binge eating, emotional eating, body image dissatisfaction) have been reported from psychological interventions using psychoeducation, goal setting, self-monitoring, normalized eating, stimulus control, cognitive restructuring, and relapse prevention [11]. Cognitive–behavioral therapy (CBT) is the one that accumulates the most evidence of the improvement of eating behaviors (e.g., binge eating and emotional eating) and psychological functioning (e.g., quality of life, depression, and anxiety symptoms) [11]. Despite the good outcomes achieved, these CBT interventions have been developed to treat specific disorders (e.g., eating disorders or anxiety disorders), and this fact raises some limitations. First, clinicians' great effort to specialize in a range of different interventions; second, the increased costs for health systems and clinicians in training, and as a consequence, the difficulties in dissemination and implementation of the CBT interventions [17]. Furthermore, if we consider that the most prevalent disorders among patients with obesity are EDs [12], there are additional limitations to specific CBT interventions. This is because in the case of these disorders, comorbidity is very high, and subclinical symptoms or unspecified disorders usually arise [18]. These comorbid conditions make it even more difficult to choose the best specific CBT treatment in each case [19].

To address all the limitations of the specific CBT treatments previously discussed, in recent years, different CBT interventions from a transdiagnostic approach have been developed and tested. In this sense, the Unified Protocol for the transdiagnostic treatment of EDs (UP) is a CBT emotion-based intervention designed to treat the etiological and maintenance mechanisms shared by all EDs [20]. This intervention focuses on a wide range of emotional psychopathology, considering comorbid disorders and subclinical or unspecified symptoms, reducing treatment times and costs, and improving response to treatment [17].

The UP is made up of eight treatment modules, five of which are considered core modules because they are focused on training different specific emotion-regulation skills [21]. Despite that the UP is a protocolized intervention, it is also flexible and versatile, allowing clinicians to use some of the modules or to change modules' order to personalize the UP to their patients [22]. Its main objective is to enhance emotion-regulation strategies to all people presenting emotional dysregulation problems [15]. To date, the UP has shown a significant improvement in pre-treatment symptoms and has obtained effect sizes that are at least comparable to existing specific CBT interventions, in on-site and online formats [23]. Beyond the mood or anxiety disorders per se, the UP has been applied to different health problems, such as cancer [24], HIV [25], or irritable bowel syndrome [26]. Despite the positive data on the effectiveness of the UP for the treatment of EDs in different health conditions, we have found no studies about its clinical utility to improve anxiety and depressive symptoms or EDs in patients with obesity who are waiting for BS.

As mentioned, the UP can be applied in various formats, such as onsite or online (both individual and group). Regarding online interventions in mental health (e-Health), there is an important amount of evidence over the last 15 years informing that online treatments are effective to treat a wide range of mental health disorders and that they can be as effective as onsite treatments [27]. We also know that online interventions do not negatively affect the therapeutic relationship [28] and that the users generally show high levels of acceptance and satisfaction with this delivery format [29]. The use of Information and Communication Technologies (ICTs) reduces the burden on health professionals and users, facilitating data collection and accessibility to Treatment [30]. In fact, different studies have shown the need to develop technology-based interventions to increase accessibility to treatment for BS candidates because their obesity condition significantly affects their mobility, and that makes it difficult for them to attend weekly sessions on-site [31]. Another practical benefit of delivering online psychological interventions is related to the current situation caused by the Covid-19 pandemic because the online format (e.g., emails, videoconference, etc.) will allow phycologists to continue their interventions and/or the follow-up assessments in case of new mobility restrictions [32]. Finally, the online group format can offer additional advantages to the online format itself, as it facilitates social support among the participants in the therapy and also allows them to share experiences and learn from each other [33].

Therefore, the general objective of this study is to analyze the feasibility and clinical usefulness of the UP, applied in an online group format, in a mental health setting of the National Health System to candidates for BS who have at least one diagnosis of ED or emotional symptoms.

The specific objectives pursued are: to evaluate adherence to treatment and clinical improvement in the primary and secondary measures after applying the UP and to study its long term clinical usefulness until two years after the intervention. Thus, the main hypotheses proposed for this study are: (1) statistically significant differences (reliable change index; RCI) will be obtained between the scores obtained at the pre-treatment, baseline, and post-treatment on the primary and secondary measures; (2) the improvements obtained after the application of the UP will be maintained in the long term (follow-ups of up to two years); (3) participants in the pilot study will report high adherence rates and high satisfaction scores regarding the treatment delivery format and its components.

2. Materials and Methods

This is a pilot study using a repeated single-case experimental design (multiple baseline design) to explore the feasibility and clinical usefulness of a transdiagnostic emotion-based online group intervention (UP) for BS candidates with EDs or subclinical anxious or depressive symptoms attended to in a public mental health service. We have chosen this design for three reasons: (1) the unit of intervention and unit of data analysis is an individual case, specifically a cluster of participants; (2) the case provides its own control for comparison purposes because a number of variables are measured before the intervention and compared with measures during and after the intervention and (3) the variable is repeatedly measured within and across different conditions or levels of the independent variable. Furthermore, and because our main objective is to answer the question "Is the Unified Protocol able to improve the emotional state of people waiting for BS?", we chose a multiple baseline design to improve experimental control throughout replication, introducing the independent variable at different points in time. The fundamental idea of choosing this type of design is that each of the participants can be their own control group [34].

The multiple baseline design involves the application of the treatment variable in a staggered way over time, through different observational units. This design is suitable for health services research interventions that are focused on changing patient behavior. This methodology facilitates a systematic comparison of pre-intervention and post-intervention measures [35], and conducting a preliminary assessment of a novel intervention [36]. Like randomized controlled trials (RCTs), the multiple baseline design can demonstrate that a significant change in behaviour has occurred and that is result of the intervention. One of the main limitations is that each participant must show changes only when the intervention is applied, and this issue, at a practical level is complicated, can make it difficult for the researcher to draw clear conclusions about the impact of the intervention. In order to reduce this limitation and improve the internal validity, researchers start treatment at different times across settings, behaviors, or people [37]. The multiple baseline design has advantages over the RCTs because this design requires fewer population groups and communities and they may act as their own controls [35]. In this sense, researchers often use this design with several people at once addressing the issue of external validity [37].

In the present investigation, all consecutive patients who are selected to undergo BS and who present anxiety or depressive symptoms or at least one diagnosis of ED, will be asked to participate. Once inclusion criteria are met (see "Inclusion and exclusion criteria" section), each patient will be randomly assigned to one of the multiple baseline conditions: 8, 12, or 15 evaluation days before the intervention. These multiple baseline conditions have been chosen following the current guides for single-case designs [34,38].

A random assignment will be carried out to reduce the threat of selection, and the fact of choosing three conditions is one of the established standards for this type of designs in order to reduce the threat of ambiguous temporal precedence and maturation [38]. Furthermore, the fact that all three conditions involve evaluation periods of 8, 12 and 15 days is due to the established standard of having a minimum of five data points in each phase to reduce the threat of attrition [38]. By choosing at least eight, we make sure to meet it even considering the probability that participants will forget to fill out the assessment one day. Actually, the reason for choosing those days is the temporal stability of the variables that we measured through the study.

In addition, the intervention will begin in a staggered manner with individual sessions (to reduce the threat of the history) and to reduce the threat of testing, a pre-treatment assessment will be performed prior to starting the baseline, to consider that the assessment process itself can have therapeutic effects on participants [38].

The study includes five assessment moments (pre-treatment, baseline, treatment, post-treatment, and follow-up, one every three months until two years after treatment completion). The flow chart of the study design is shown in Figure 1.

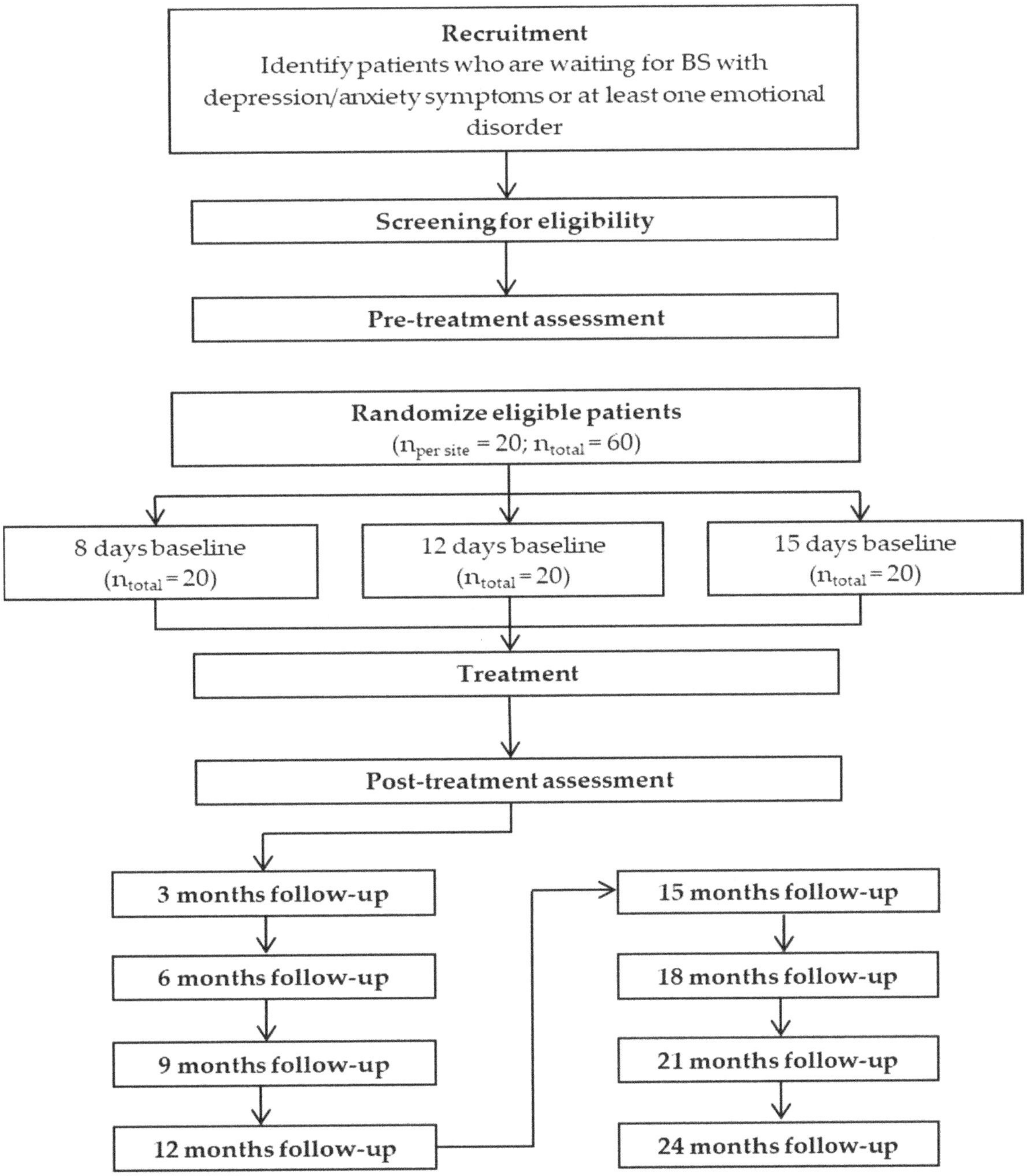

Figure 1. Study flow chart. BS: Bariatric surgery.

2.1. Sample and Recruitment

The study recruitment will start in September 2020 until December 2024. The study will be conducted in a public mental health center in Spain (Mental Health Unit of the Regional Hospital of Vinaròs, Castellón). Participants will be people over 18 years of age who have anxious or depressive symptoms, or at least one diagnosis of EDs according to Diagnostic and Statistical Manual of Mental Disorders five edition criteria [39] and who have been selected for a subsequent BS.

To calculate the sample size, we drew on a study that proposed stepwise rules of thumb for pilot studies based on the target effect size and the size of the future trial [40]. Previous works that study the efficacy of CBT procedures either in person or online have shown large variations in effect sizes, obtaining mainly medium to large effect sizes [41,42]. Taking these data into account, and expecting a 90% powered main trial and assuming a sample loss of 35% [43] we established a sample size of 20 participants per experimental condition for the present study, that is, a total sample of 60 participants.

2.2. Procedure

The participants who are referred to the mental health unit for having fulfilled the requirements to be candidates for BS, will be evaluated to see if they meet the rest of the inclusion criteria for this study. In Table 1, it can be seen the selection criteria used to choose the appropriate candidates to receive the BS. These criteria are based on the European Guidelines for Obesity Management in Adults, which indicates that a comprehensive obesity management can only be accomplished by a multidisciplinary obesity management team [44].

Table 1. Inclusion criteria and main contraindications for BS.

Inclusion Criteria
- BMI >40 or 35 with associated major comorbidities - Age between 18 and 65 years - Long-standing obesity (3–5 years) - Failure in dietary attempts and treatments under control - Absence of anesthetic contraindication and acceptable surgical risk - Not having endocrine causes of obesity - Understanding of the weight loss process, associated problems and the stated objective - Commitment to adhere to the monitoring standards
Contraindications
Relative - Clearly unfavorable family environment - Personality disorder - Psychogenic vomiting - Hyperphagia in other psychological disorders or other eating disorders - Mild intellectual disability - Psychotic disorders without positive symptoms - Any psychiatric illness that significantly hinders the good follow-up and completion of the guidelines and medical indications for this process and may worsen the patient's state of health Absolute - Drug dependency - Moderate or severe intellectual disability - Psychotic disorder with positive symptoms - Bulimia nervosa

Participants' evaluation and selection will be carried out by the clinical psychologists and psychiatrists of the mental health unit of the Regional Hospital of Vinaròs (Castellón). The clinical psychologists who will participate in this trial will be in charge of collecting all the information from the participants (alphanumeric codes assigned to the participants will be entered to safeguard their anonymity). The coded information will be given to the author J.O. to introduce it in the database and then, returned to the center.

Participants who have received the approval for BS by the multidisciplinary health team and also have met the inclusion criteria by the clinician (see "Eligibility criteria" section), will be invited to participate in the study through an informative document. They will also be provided with confidentiality and informed consent documents. After accepting to participate, an email will be sent to participants with a link through which they will be able to complete the pre-treatment evaluation on the Qualtrics survey platform [45]. Then, they will be informed by phone of the experimental condition to which they will have been randomly assigned, which may be 8, 12, or 15 days baseline assessment, and they will then complete online the baseline assessment protocol on the same platform [45]. Randomization to the different baselines will be done with randomizer software (www.randomizer.org). Randomization will be performed by a researcher unrelated to the study using the computer-generated sequence mentioned. In the program, the researcher will generate one set of 60 numbers, which will have a one to three range. Participants will be randomly assigned to the 8, 12 or 15 baseline days.

The baseline and psychological intervention will be conducted between the period of acceptance for BS and the BS implementation, that last approximately one year in public health settings. The intervention will be carried out in an online group format through the Cisco Webex platform. The UP will be applied in twelve weekly 2-h online group sessions. To comply with the experimental design of the multiple baseline, when each participant completes the baseline evaluation, they will receive the first online session in individual format (to receive the first session in stages), then they will continue with the second session and the rest of the treatment in group format. The content of each session is shown in Table 2. Participants will receive the therapy support manual [11]. The online group will consist of five to eight participants, one therapist (V.F.-G.), and one co-therapist (A.Q.-O.). For ethical reasons, if any of the patients feel uncomfortable during the study with the online group format, they may leave the group and receive individual onsite attention (treatment as usual). In this case, the content and estimated number of sessions will be the same, although the frequency will be stipulated by the mental health unit depending on its possibilities.

Table 2. Treatment content split by session.

Session Number	Content
Session 1	Setting Goals and Maintaining Motivation
Session 2	Understanding your Emotions: What is an Emotion?
Session 3	Understanding your Emotions: Following the ARC (Antecedent, Response, Consequence)
Session 4	Mindful Emotion Awareness—I
Session 5	Mindful Emotion Awareness—II
Session 6	Cognitive Flexibility—I
Session 7	Cognitive Flexibility—II
Session 8	Countering Emotional Behaviors
Session 9	Understanding and Confronting Physical Sensations
Session 10	Putting it into Practice: Emotion Exposures—I
Session 11	Putting it into Practice: Emotion Exposures—II
Session 12	Recognizing Accomplishments and Looking to the Future

The study plans to conduct a follow-up assessment every three months until two years after treatment completion. All follow-ups will be conducted online. Considering the time interval of the baseline, the psychological intervention and the BS procedure, the two first follow-ups (three and six months after intervention) will be conducted before BS, and the rest will be conducted after BS. In addition, at the baseline and during treatment, the participants must fill out an online survey made up of 14 questions that will ask about the intensity of the emotions of happiness, sadness, anxiety, other emotions, difficulties in emotion regulation, body image, and emotional eating. Through this weekly evaluation, we expect to observe how the participants evolve in the different variables throughout the different treatment modules.

2.3. *Eligibility Criteria*

The inclusion criteria for participation in the project will be: (1) being over 18 years of age; (2) being a BS candidate; (3) presenting anxious or depressive symptomatology (moderate scores on the Beck Depression Inventory-II [46,47] and/or Beck Anxiety Inventory [48,49]) or meeting the criteria for at least one ED (anxiety, mood, and related disorders) on the International Neuropsychiatric Interview (MINI; [50]); (4) speaking Spanish or Catalan fluently; (5) committing to attend the sessions; (6) understanding and accepting the contents of the informed consent, expressed by signing it; (7) having Internet to fulfill the protocol assessments and to participate in the online intervention and (8) agreeing to maintain the prescribed medication (including dosage) if any, during the evaluation period and treatment. If medication stability is not possible, the participant's data will be treated separately in the analyses.

and treatment. If medication stability is not possible, the participant's data will be treated separately in the analyses.

The protocol also includes one exclusion criteria that may interfere: (1) having a severe condition that would require being prioritized for treatment, so that an interaction between the two interventions cannot be ruled out. These include a severe mental disorder (bipolar disorder, personality disorder, schizophrenia, or an organic mental disorder), suicide risk at the time of assessment, or substance use in the last three months (excluding cannabis, coffee, and/or nicotine).

2.4. Ethics

All participants who meet the inclusion criteria will sign the personal data protection document before randomization so that they have a notion of whom and for what purpose this study's results will be used. Participants will be also informed of what the treatment consists of before starting it, as well as the duration and phases of the study (informed consent). Direct participation in the study will be voluntary. Participants will not obtain any financial or material compensation, and their participation will not imply any risk for them. The UP has already demonstrated its efficacy in previous experimental and quasi-experimental studies with different health problems (see "Introduction" section).

Data management will be carried out following the Spanish Royal Decree 1720/2008, of 19 January, which approves the Regulations for the development of the Organic Law 15/1999, of 13 December, on the protection of personal data [51]. The treatment, communication, and transfer of personal data will follow the provisions of the Declaration of Helsinki [52] in Law 14/2007 on biomedical research. As of 25 May 2018, the new legislation on personal data in the EU is fully applicable, specifically Regulation (EU) 2016/679 of the European Parliament and of the Council of 27 April 2016, on Data Protection (GDRP; General Data Protection Regulation). Under the aforementioned legislation, participants can exercise their rights of access, modification, opposition, and cancellation of data, for which they must contact their health professional of reference.

The data collected for the study will be identified by an alphanumeric code, and only the health professionals collaborating in the study will be able to relate these data to the participants and their corresponding medical records. Therefore, the identity of the participants in the study will not be revealed to any person, with exceptions in case of a medical emergency or legal requirement.

The study already has the approval by the Ethical Research Committee of the General University Hospital of Castellón (CEIm; CI/HIP version 1.0 de 20/07/2019). In addition, the protocol study has been registered at https://clinicaltrials.gov/ (6 March 2020; NCT04421443).

2.5. Measures

The evaluation protocol will be administered online by Qualtrics survey [45] at five different moments: pre-treatment, baseline, treatment, post-treatment, and follow-ups every three months until two years after the intervention. Assessment instruments will include demographic characteristics (age, sex, education, marital status, and employment status), a diagnostic interview, and well-established questionnaires for both primary and secondary outcomes. Next, the primary and secondary outcomes that will be evaluated at the pre, post-treatment, and follow-up periods will be described, and later the specific measures that will be used for the baseline evaluation and during the treatment will be specified. Table 3 shows the distribution of the measures that will be administered during the study.

Table 3. Distribution of the variables administered throughout the intervention.

Measures	Pre-Treatment	Baseline	Treatment	Post-Treatment	Follow-Ups [1]
Demographic characteristics	X				
MINI	X			X	X
BDI-II	X			X	X
BAI	X			X	X
BMI	X	X	X	X	X
PANAS	X			X	X
NEO-FFI	X			X	X
QLI	X			X	X
EuroQol	X			X	X
MI	X			X	X
DERS	X			X	X
BEAQ	X			X	X
PHLMS	X			X	X
ERQ	X			X	X
Surgical Complications	X				
BITE	X			X	X
BSQ	X			X	X
EES	X			X	X
OASIS			X		
ODSIS			X		
OESIS			X		
PESIS			X		
STQ				X	X
Baseline assessment battery [2]		X			
Assessment battery during treatment [3]			X		

Note: MINI: International Neuropsychiatric Interview; BDI-II: Beck Depression Inventory-II; BAI: Beck Anxiety Inventory; BMI: Body Mass Index; PANAS: Positive and Negative Affect Scale; NEO-FFI: NEO Five-Factor Inventory; QLI: Quality of Life Index; MI: Maladjustment Inventory; DERS: Difficulties in Emotion Regulation Scale; BEAQ: Brief Experiential Avoidance Questionnaire; PHLMS: Philadelphia Mindfulness Scale; ERQ: Emotion Regulation Questionnaire; BITE: Bulimic Investigatory Test; BSQ: Body Satisfaction Questionnaire; EES: Emotional Eating Scale; OASIS: Overall Anxiety Severity and Impairment Scales; ODSIS: Overall Depression Severity and Impairment Scales; OESIS: Other Emotions Severity and Impairment Scale; PESIS: Positive Emotion Severity and Impairment Scale; STQ: Satisfaction with Treatment Questionnaire. [1] Quarterly follow-ups up to two years after treatment; [2] For more information about the specific items that make up the baseline assessment battery see section "Baseline assessment"; [3] For more information about the specific items that make up the assessment during treatment battery see section "Assessment during treatment".

2.5.1. Primary Outcomes

Primary and secondary diagnosis according to the DSM-5 criteria will be evaluated with the International Neuropsychiatric Interview (MINI [50]). Subclinical symptoms of anxiety and depression will be evaluated through the Beck Depression Inventory-II (BDI-II [46,47]) and the Beck Anxiety Inventory (BAI [48,49]). The weight gain or loss of the participants will be evaluated through the Body Mass Index (BMI).

2.5.2. Secondary Outcomes

Secondary outcomes can be grouped around: affectivity, personality traits, quality of life and interference, emotion regulation, aspects related to surgical complications, eating behaviors and body image, and satisfaction with and evaluation of the treatment received.

To assess affectivity, the Positive and Negative Affect Scale (PANAS [53,54]) will be administered to evaluate positive and negative affect. Personality will be measured with the NEO Five-Factor Inventory (NEO-FFI [55]), which offers a rapid and general measure of the Big Five personality traits of which we will only assess Neuroticism and Extraversion. The Quality of Life Index (QLI [56]) will be used to evaluate several aspects related to quality of life (i.e., physical disability, emotional well-being, self-care and independent functioning, occupational functioning, interpersonal functioning, social–emotional support, community and services support, personal fulfillment, spiritual fulfillment, and overall quality of life). EuroQol [57,58] is a generic instrument that will be used to measure health-related quality of life. It has five dimensions (mobility, personal care, daily activities, pain, and anxiety/depression), and a general state of health perceived through a visual analog scale. Similarly, the Maladjustment Inventory (MI [59]) will be used to evaluate the extent to which the subject's current problems impact negatively on different areas of daily life, namely, work, social life, leisure time, relationship with the partner, family life, and overall adjustment in daily activities.

Regarding emotion regulation, it will be assessed using the Difficulties in Emotion Regulation Scale (DERS [60,61]), which presents five dysregulation dimensions: emotional lack of control, emotional rejection, life interference, lack of emotional attention, and emotional confusion. In addition, to assess the different emotion regulation skills that will be trained through the UP, we will use the Brief Experiential Avoidance Questionnaire (BEAQ [62,63]), which is a self-report questionnaire with 15 items that measure experiential avoidance; the Philadelphia Mindfulness Scale (PHLMS [64,65]), which is a 20-item questionnaire that assesses two mindfulness constructs: awareness and acceptance and the Emotion Regulation Questionnaire (ERQ [66,67]), which is a self-report questionnaire commonly used to assess two emotion-regulation strategies: cognitive reappraisal (six items) and expressive suppression (four items).

To assess surgical complications, the professional will be asked to refer the participant to the mental health unit a report describing the course of the operation and the recovery from it. Specific measures related to eating disorders will also be used, such as the Bulimic Investigatory Test (BITE [68,69]), which is a self-report questionnaire used to evaluate the presence and severity of bulimic symptomatology, and cognitive and emotional signs and symptoms associated with binge eating; the Body Satisfaction Questionnaire (BSQ [70,71]), which is a self-applied scale used to evaluate the fear of gaining weight, feelings of low self-esteem because of one's appearance, the desire to lose weight, and body dissatisfaction, and Emotional Eating Scale (EES [72]), which is a 25-item self-report assessing a person's tendency to cope with negative affect through eating. Participants' weight will be checked monthly to calculate their body mass index (BMI).

Additionally, we created an ad hoc questionnaire to evaluate the participants' evaluation of and satisfaction with the treatment received, the Satisfaction with Treatment Questionnaire (STQ). The Evaluation of the UP Components section consists of nine items that evaluate the extent to which the participants consider that the UP in general, and each of its components in particular, were useful to help them to regulate their emotions adaptively; the Satisfaction with Treatment section presents seven items that evaluate participants' overall satisfaction with the treatment received. In both sections, higher scores show higher levels of positive evaluation and satisfaction. A total of 12 items will also be added to assess the participants' opinion of the online evaluation through Qualtrics and of the Cisco Webex platform used to carry out the online evaluation. At the end of the questionnaire, six open-ended questions appear in which the participants can qualitatively express their opinion of different aspects of the treatment received and the delivery format.

All measures used in the study have been standardized in Spanish. Administration time is between 30 and 40 min for the MINI and approximately 90 min for the primary and secondary outcomes conjointly.

2.5.3. Baseline Assessment

To facilitate the daily baseline assessment, we have summarized in one item the variable we want to evaluate, for example, the emotion regulation strategies. For this purpose, we have chosen the item with the greatest factor load for each variable [73]. Specifically, participants will answer a battery of 19 questions: six questions about the presence and intensity of specific emotions (e.g., happiness, sadness, anxiety); five questions to assess the five subscales of the Difficulties in Emotion Regulation Scale (DERS [60,61]), which are emotional lack of control, emotional rejection, life interference, lack of emotional attention, and emotional confusion (e.g., "During this day, to what extent have you paid attention to your feelings?"); two questions that refer to the two subscales of the Emotion Regulation Questionnaire (ERQ [66,67]), which are reappraisal and suppression (e.g.," During this day, to what extent have you been able to control your emotions by changing the way you think about the situation you were in?"); two questions that refer to the two subscales of the Philadelphia Mindfulness Scale (PHLMS [64,65]), which are acceptance and awareness (e.g., "During this day, when your emotions have changed, to what extent have you been aware of it immediately?"); one question to assess experiential avoidance based on the Brief Experiential Avoidance Questionnaire (BEAQ [62,63]) ("During this day, would you say that one of your biggest goals has been to be free of any painful emotion?"); one question from the Emotional Eating Scale (EES [72]) regarding the impulse to eat as a consequence of having experienced an intense emotion ("During this day, to what extent have you felt the urge to eat as a result of experiencing intense emotions?") and one last question from the Body Satisfaction Questionnaire (BSQ [70,71]), which asks about the extent to which the participant has been satisfied with their body image ("During this day, how satisfied have you been with your body image?").

2.5.4. Assessment during Treatment

The assessment during treatment battery involves continuing to fill in the same baseline questions once a week. In addition, before starting each online session, participants will be asked to fill in an emotional scale to assess its presence, intensity, and interference during the last week. Participants can choose the emotion or emotions that should be assessed. The UP offers four different emotional rating scales: The Overall Anxiety and Depression Severity and Impairment Scales (OASIS; ODSIS [74–76]), Other Emotions Severity and Impairment Scale (e.g., guilt, shame, or anger) (OESIS [77]), and a Positive Emotion Severity and Impairment Scale (e.g., happiness) (PESIS [77]; Supplementary Materials). All of them are used in the UP to help patients to continuously monitor the scores throughout the sessions and their progress over the treatment.

2.6. Data Analysis

The analyses will be carried out with the statistical package IBM SPSS Statistics version 22.0 for Windows [78]. First, the sociodemographic characteristics of the sample will be analyzed with descriptive statistics, calculating the mean and standard deviation of the scores in the different questionnaires administered. Next, a missing-value analysis and the Little Missing Completely At Random (MCAR) test will be performed to determine whether or not the distribution of missing values is random, and therefore whether the last observation made (LOCF) can be used. Internal consistency will be explored using Cronbach's alpha.

As the sample size is expected to be less than 50, the normal distribution of the variables will be verified with the Shapiro–Wilk normality test. Depending on the result of this test, parametric or non-parametric repeated measures analysis will be carried out to verify whether or not the differences in the scores of the variables measured at different times are statistically significant. In case the variables follow a normal distribution, parametric repeated measures analysis will be carried out, specifically the Multivariate Analysis of Variance (ANOVA), and in case the variables do not follow a normal distribution, non-parametric repeated measures analysis will be carried out, specifically the Friedman test. If the repeated measures analysis show statistically significant differences between the evaluation time points, post-hoc comparisons will be carried out to correct the level of significance to avoid increasing the type I error. Thus, regarding adjustment for multiple comparisons, the Bonferroni correction will be carried out in case of having performed parametric analysis, and the Wilcoxon signed rank test in case of having performed non-parametric analysis in the comparison of means. More detailed information on this has been added in the data analysis section, explaining step by step which statistical analyzes will be carried out.

Finally, the Reliable Change Index (RCI), which assesses the clinically significant change obtained to determine in which variables the scores have approached those of the normative sample, will be calculated. A clinically significant change will be considered if the RCI score obtained is equal to or greater than 1.96 [79].

Another aspect that we consider important to analyze is how the participants change their scores in each of the variables evaluated based on the content addressed each module. For this purpose, a visual analysis of the changes in the scores will be carried out, to see how the slopes change in the different phases of the study (evaluation and treatment), and in the different modules within the treatment. This visual analysis has been used in previous studies [21]. To carry out this visual analysis, the data from 19 questions that the participants will fill in weekly will be used.

Attendance at sessions will also be recorded to calculate the attendance rate, which will be used as an indicator of viability and acceptance of treatment by users. For the same purpose, quantitative and qualitative analyses will be carried out. At the quantitative level, the participants' evaluation of and satisfaction with the treatment received will be evaluated using an ad hoc designed questionnaire (see "Measures" section). Qualitatively, participants will be asked to answer six main questions about treatment, and their answers will be analyzed by selecting and classifying the information through a segmentation process, identifying key themes and categories of analysis [80].

3. Expected Results

Based on the reviewed bibliography, the type of design of the present study, the proposed objectives and the characteristics of the intervention that will be carried out, we hope that the results will reveal the feasibility and clinical usefulness of the UP applied in an online group format, in a mental health setting of the national health system for candidates of BS who have at least one diagnosis of ED or emotional symptoms. The concrete results that are expected to reach this conclusion are shown in more detail in Table 4.

Table 4. Main expected outcomes. UP: Unified Protocol for the transdiagnostic Treatment of Eds.

Clinical Usefulness of the UP for Bariatric Surgery Candidates
Group Results: - Depending on the characteristics of the sample obtained (we will check if the parametric assumptions are met), the results of the parametric/non-parametric tests that allow comparing the group scores between the different time points are expected to show statistically significant differences in the desired direction.
Individual Results: - To obtains statistically significant differences (Reliable Change Index; RCI) between the scores obtained at the pre-treatment, baseline, and post-treatment on the primary and secondary measures. - A maintaining of improvements obtained after the application of the UP in the long term (follow-ups of up to two years), with statistically significant differences (Reliable Change Index; RCI) between the scores obtained at the pre-treatment/post-treatment and follow-ups on the primary and secondary measures.
In both cases, the expected directions for the different variables are: - An increase for the variables positive affect, extraversion, quality of life and health-related quality of life. - A decrease for the variables negative affect, neuroticism, interference of symptoms, emotional dysregulation, bulimic symptomatology, dissatisfaction with body image and emotional eating. Feasibility of the UP for Bariatric Surgery Candidates - High session attendance rates. - High scores on the STQ both in the questions that refer to the treatment itself and its different modules, and in the questions that refer to the group and online format.

Reporting of results will follow the Consolidated Standards of Reporting Trials (CONSORT) recommendations, specifically its extension for designs N-of-one Trials [81].

4. Discussion

Obesity and being overweight have become a serious public health problem due to their high prevalence and associated costs [2,9]. EDs are highly present in people with obesity [7], and this can interfere with a commitment to voluntary weight loss [82] and it is also associated with worse post-intervention outcomes [11]. An intervention based on emotion-regulation training could help those patients to achieve both aims, to lose weight before the BS to prevent surgery problems and the emergence of emotional symptoms after the BS, maintaining their emotional and physical achievements over time. In addition to the clinical implications, the results derived from this study may also have an important economic impact. Thus, health policies and the managing of this health condition in public health settings could be also influenced.

To prove this, longitudinal studies are needed and some limitations regarding the interventions (specific CBT versus transdiagnostic intervention) and the delivery formats (onsite versus online) must be considered. The use of the UP in an online group intervention format in a public mental health setting with people waiting for BS has the following benefits:

1. It can allow clinicians to use a single treatment for those candidates who present different EDs, with comorbidity, and also with subclinical symptoms or unspecified disorders [15].
2. In other public health systems similar to the Spanish one, where onsite specific CBT is the most common delivery format, and therapy sessions occur at long intervals (e.g., more than a month) due to waiting lists, a UP online group intervention can help to increase the frequency of sessions and reduce costs because there are more patients treated simultaneously (five to eight patients in the same group), which can facilitate better patient care.
3. Thanks to the online format, this intervention will facilitate access to psychological interventions in those candidates who face mobility challenges due to their obesity condition [31]. This innovative approach would be in line with the goals of the World Health Organization proposed in the mental health action plan to use electronic technologies to expand the delivery of mental health care [83].
4. The fact of receiving quarterly follow-ups up to two years after treatment allows guaranteeing the prevention of relapses and maintaining the results, especially beyond the year and a half or two years, which is the moment in which the literature recognizes that pre-BS problems tend to reappear [42].
5. Furthermore, this advantage offered by long term relapse prevention follow-ups leads to a condition of reduced healthcare costs that are associated with the care of comorbid health problems in this type of patients [3].
6. And finally, it is known that group therapy provides benefits to the patient that are not obtained with individual treatment, such as reducing isolation, facilitating social support, and learning from the experiences of others [33], which could improve its efficiency.

Our study also has some limitations. First, some people who are going to undergo BS will prefer individual treatment, which could be a barrier to enroll those participants in our study (e.g., abandonment or decrease in UP satisfaction and effectiveness). In this case, it could be explained to the patient that group treatment resulted in greater weight losses than individual treatment, even for those clients with a preference for individual therapy and that matching clients with their preferences for individual or group therapy did not enhance treatment outcome either in terms of weight loss or improvements in psychological functioning [84]. Furthermore, a study in a sample of people with EDs diagnosis attended to in public mental health settings in Spain found that the majority of participants preferred receiving psychological treatment in an individual format, followed by group format, and, rarely, in an online format, so it will be necessary to explain to patients the advantages and disadvantages of receiving psychotherapy through individual, group, or online format to help them to decide whether or not to participate in this study [85]. In this sense, the arguments that must be strengthened to justify a group application, in addition to those mentioned previously, are the possibility of sharing experiences, the opportunity to learn from others and receive comments and support and for the online format, convenience [85]. The second main limitation, is that, due to this being a pilot study, the results must be interpreted with caution, as further RCT studies with greater rigor will be required. In this sense, it should be noted that this kind of study is an advisable cost-effective method to preliminarily examine the efficacy, feasibility and/or implementation of recent intervention programs or applications with different samples [86].

Despite the aforementioned limitations, the present study may have different implications. At the research level, it will be the first pilot study aimed at evaluating the feasibility and clinical utility of an online group format of a transdiagnostic intervention for the treatment of ED in public settings in Spain with people waiting for BS, allowing us to increase the evidence on UP's effectiveness, flexibility, and versatility. At a clinical level, the results of the study will reveal whether UP can improve emotional symptoms in candidates and, therefore, improve the effects of BS in the long term. This would have important implications for patients, as it could achieve much more notable improvements after the intervention, and would serve to prevent relapses that generally appear in the long term around two years after BS.

5. Conclusions

In sum, the present study supports the idea of the need to test new forms of psychological interventions with patients waiting for BS [12]. This would allow us to improve the previous psychopathology, and, therefore, to potentiate the effects of BS in the short and long term [2].

The UP may be a good treatment option, considering that it is directed at EDs (which are the most prevalent in people with obesity problems) [12], and that it allows addressing comorbidity, subclinical symptoms, and unspecified disorders [15].

In addition, its application through an online group format can provide extra advantages, as it allows access to treatment for people with mobility problems, something very common among candidates for BS [31], and also fosters social support among the members of the group [33].

Based on all this, the results of the development of this study may have important implications for the National Health System, which will be able to meet the psychological needs of patients with obesity problems, improving their quality of life before the intervention, and enhancing its results in the long term, which will mean a reduction in costs to the system and more specialized and multidisciplinary care for patients who are in this situation.

Author Contributions: Conceptualization, J.O.; methodology, J.O. and A.Q.-O.; description of the analysis, A.Q.-O.; resources, J.O. and V.F.-G.; writing—original draft preparation, A.Q.-O.; writing—review and editing, J.O., A.Q.-O. and V.F.-G.; supervision, J.O.; funding acquisition, J.O. All authors have read and agreed to the published version of the manuscript.

Acknowledgments: We would like to thank all mental health professionals working at the General University Hospital of Vinaròs in Castellón (Spain) for its commitment to ongoing scientific research in clinical and health psychology.

References

1. Yumuk, V.; Tsigos, C.; Fried, M.; Schindler, K.; Busetto, L.; Micic, D.; Toplak, H. European Guidelines for Obesity Management in Adults. *Obes. Facts* **2015**, *8*, 402–424. [CrossRef] [PubMed]
2. Oltmanns, J.R.; Rivera, J.; Cole, J.; Merchant, A.; Steiner, J.P. Personality psychopathology: Longitudinal prediction of change in body mass index and weight post-bariatric surgery. *Health Psychol.* **2020**, *39*, 245–254. [CrossRef] [PubMed]
3. Hernáez, A.; Zomeño, M.D.; Dégano, I.R.; Pérez-Fernández, S.; Goday, A.; Vila, J.; Civeira, F.; Moure, R.; Marrugat, J. Exceso de peso en España: Situacioón actual, proyecciones para 2030 y sobrecoste directo estimado para el Sistema Nacional de Salud [Excess Weight in Spain: Current Situation, Projections for 2030, and Estimated Direct Extra Cost for the Spanish Health Sy. *Span. J. Cardiol.* **2019**, *72*, 916–924. [CrossRef]
4. Castaneda, D.; Popov, V.B.; Wander, P.; Thompson, C.C. Risk of Suicide and Self-harm Is Increased After Bariatric Surgery—A Systematic Review and Meta-analysis. *Obes. Surg.* **2019**, *29*, 322–333. [CrossRef]
5. De Luca, M.; Angrisani, L.; Himpens, J.; Busetto, L.; Scopinaro, N.; Weiner, R.; Sartori, A.; Stier, C.; Lakdawala, M.; Bhasker, A.G.; et al. Indications for Surgery for Obesity and Weight-Related Diseases: Position Statements from the International Federation for the Surgery of Obesity and Metabolic Disorders (IFSO). *Obes. Surg.* **2016**, *26*, 1659–1696. [CrossRef]

6. OECD/European Union. *Health at a Glance: Europe 2018: State of Health in the EU Cycle*; OECD Publishing, Paris/European Union: Brussels, Belgium, 2018. [CrossRef]
7. Spirou, D.; Raman, J.; Smith, E. Psychological outcomes following surgical and endoscopic bariatric procedures: A systematic review. *Obes. Rev.* **2020**, e12998. [CrossRef]
8. Dixon, J.B.; Dixon, M.E.; O'Brien, P.E. Depression in Association With Severe Obesity. *Arch. Intern. Med.* **2003**, *163*, 2058. [CrossRef]
9. OECD. *The Heavy Burden of Obesity: The Economics of Prevention, OECD Health Policy Studies 2019*; OECD: Paris, France, 2019. [CrossRef]
10. Jumbe, S.; Hamlet, C.; Meyrick, J. Psychological Aspects of Bariatric Surgery as a Treatment for Obesity. *Curr. Obes. Rep.* **2017**, *6*, 71–78. [CrossRef]
11. Lauren, A.D.; Sijercic, I.; Cassin, S.E. Preoperative and post-operative psychosocial interventions for bariatric surgery patients: A systematic review. *Obes. Rev.* **2020**, e12926. [CrossRef]
12. Sarwer, D.B.; Heinberg, L.J. A Review of the Psychosocial Aspects of Clinically Severe Obesity and Bariatric Surgery. *Am. Psychol. Assoc.* **2020**, *75*, 252–264. [CrossRef]
13. Geller, S.; Dahan, S.; Levy, S.; Goldzweig, G.; Hamdan, S.; Abu-Abeid, S. Body Image and Emotional Eating as Predictors of Psychological Distress Following Bariatric Surgery. *Obes. Surg.* **2019**. [CrossRef] [PubMed]
14. Institute for Health Metrics and Evaluation. Global Health Data Exchange. Available online: http://ghdx.healthdata.org/gbd-results-tool (accessed on 5 May 2020).
15. Barlow, D.H.; Farchione, T.J.; Sauer-Zavala, S.; Murray-Latin, H.; Ellard, K.K.; Bullis, J.R.; Bentley, K.H.; Boettcher, H.T.; Cassiello-Robbins, C. *Unified Protocol for Transdiagnostic Treatment of Emotional Disorders: Therapist Guide*, 2nd ed.; Oxford University Press: New York, NY, USA, 2018.
16. Lim, R.B.C.; Zhang, M.W.B.; Ho, R.C.M. Prevalence of all-cause mortality and suicide among bariatric surgery cohorts: A meta-analysis. *Int. J. Environ. Res. Public Health* **2018**, *15*, 1519. [CrossRef] [PubMed]
17. Barlow, D.H.; Farchione, T.J.; Bullis, J.R.; Gallagher, M.W.; Murray-Latin, H.; Sauer-Zavala, S.; Bentley, K.H.; Thompson-Hollands, J.; Conklin, L.R.; Boswell, J.F.; et al. The unified protocol for transdiagnostic treatment of Emotional Disorders compared with diagnosis-specific protocols for anxiety disorders: A randomized clinical trial. *JAMA Psychiatry* **2017**, *74*, 875–884. [CrossRef] [PubMed]
18. Brown, T.; Campbell, L.; Lehman, C.; Grisham, J.; Mancill, R. Current and Lifetime Comorbidity of the DSM-IV Anxiety and Mood Disorders in a Large Clinical Sample. *J. Abnorm. Psychol.* **2001**, *110*, 585–599. [CrossRef] [PubMed]
19. McManus, F.; Shafran, R.; Cooper, Z. What does a 'transdiagnostic approach have to offer the treatment of anxiety disorders? *Br. J. Clin. Psychol.* **2010**, *49*, 491–505. [CrossRef] [PubMed]
20. Brown, T.A.; Barlow, D.H. A proposal for a dimensional classification system based on the shared features of the DSM-IV Anxiety and Mood Disorders: Implications for Assessment and Treatment. *Psychol. Assess.* **2009**, *21*, 256–271. [CrossRef]
21. Sauer-Zavala, S.; Cassiello-Robbins, C.; Conklin, L.R.; Bullis, J.R.; Thompson-Hollands, J.; Kennedy, K.A. Isolating the Unique Effects of the Unified Protocol Treatment Modules Using Single Case Experimental Design. *Behav. Modif.* **2017**, *41*, 286–307. [CrossRef]
22. Sauer-Zavala, S.; Cassiello-Robbins, C.; Ametaj, A.A.; Wilner, J.G.; Pagan, D. Transdiagnostic Treatment Personalization: The Feasibility of Ordering Unified Protocol Modules According to Patient Strengths and Weaknesses. *Behav. Modif.* **2019**, *43*, 518–543. [CrossRef]
23. Sakiris, N.; Berle, D. A systematic review and meta-analysis of the Unified Protocol as a transdiagnostic emotion regulation based intervention. *Clin. Psychol. Rev.* **2019**, *72*, 1017–1051. [CrossRef]
24. Weihs, K.L.; McConnell, M.H.; Wiley, J.F.; Crespi, C.M.; Sauer-Zavala, S.; Stanton, A.L. A Preventive Intervention to Modify Depression Risk Targets after Breast Cancer Diagnosis: Design and Single-Arm Pilot Study. *Psychooncology* **2019**, *28*, 880–887. [CrossRef]
25. Parsons, J.T.; Rendina, H.J.; Moody, R.L.; Gurung, S.; Starks, T.J.; Pachankis, J.E. Feasibility of an Emotion Regulation Intervention to Improve Mental Health and Reduce HIV Transmission Risk Behaviors for HIV-Positive Gay and Bisexual Men with Sexual Compulsivity. *Aids Behav.* **2017**, *21*, 1540–1549. [CrossRef] [PubMed]
26. Johari-Fard, R.; Ghafourpour, R. The effectiveness of Unified Treatment approach on quality of life and symptoms of patients with irritable bowel syndrome referred to gastrointestinal clinics. *Int. J. BodyMind Cult.* **2015**, *2*, 85–94.

27. Andersson, G. Internet-Delivered Psychological Treatments. *Annu. Rev. Clin. Psychol.* **2016**, *12*, 157–179. [CrossRef] [PubMed]
28. Andersson, G. Using the Internet to provide cognitive behaviour therapy. *Behav. Res. Ther.* **2009**, *47*, 175–180. [CrossRef]
29. Andrews, G.; Cuijpers, P.; Craske, M.G.; McEvoy, P.; Titov, N. Computer therapy for the anxiety and depressive disorders is effective, acceptable and practical health care: A meta-analysis. *PLoS ONE* **2010**, *5*. [CrossRef]
30. Andreu-pejó, L.; Martínez-borba, V.; Suso-ribera, C.; Osma, J. Can we predict the evolution of depressive symptoms, adjustment, and perceived social support of pregnant women from their personality characteristics? A technology-supported longitudinal study. *Int. J. Environ. Res. Public Health* **2020**, *17*, 3439. [CrossRef]
31. King, W.C.; Engel, S.G.; Elder, K.A.; Chapman, W.H.; Eid, G.M.; Wolfe, B.M.; Belle, S.H. Walking capacity of bariatric surgery candidates. *Surg. Obes. Relat. Dis.* **2012**, *8*, 48–59. [CrossRef]
32. Wind, T.R.; Rijkeboer, M.; Andersson, G.; Riper, H. The COVID-19 pandemic: The 'black swan' for mental health care and a turning point for e-health. *Internet Interv.* **2020**, *20*, 100317. [CrossRef]
33. Yalom, I.D.; Leszcz, M. *The Theory and Practice of Group Therapy*, 5th ed.; IUP: New York, NY, USA, 2005.
34. Kratochwill, T.R.; Hitchcock, J.H.; Horner, R.H.; Levin, J.R.; Odom, S.L.; Rindskopf, D.M.; Shadish, W.R. Single-Case Intervention Research Design Standards. *Remed. Spec. Educ.* **2012**, *34*, 26–38. [CrossRef]
35. Hawkins, N.G.; Sanson-Fisher, R.W.; Shakeshaft, A.; D'Este, C.; Green, L.W. The multiple baseline design for evaluating population-based research. *Am. J. Prev. Med.* **2007**, *33*, 162–168. [CrossRef]
36. Barlow, D.H.; Nock, M.K.; Hersen, M. *Single Case Experimental Designs: Strategies for Studying Behavior Change*, 3rd ed.; Allyn & Bacon: Boston, MA, USA, 2009.
37. Barlow, H.D.; Durand, V.M.; Hofmann, S.G. *Abnormal Psychology: An Integrative Approach*, 8th ed.; Cengage Learning: Boston, MA, USA, 2018.
38. Kratochwill, T.R.; Hitchcock, J.; Horner, R.H.; Levin, J.R.; Odom, S.L.; Rindskopf, D.M.; Shadish, W.R. Single-Case Design Technical Documentation. *What Work. Clear. House* **2010**. [CrossRef]
39. American Psychiatric Association. *Diagnostic and Statistical Manual of Mental Disorders*, 5th ed.; American Psychiatric Association: Arlington, VA, USA, 2013.
40. Bell, M.L.; Whitehead, A.L.; Julious, S.A. Guidance for using pilot studies to inform the design of intervention trials with continuous outcomes. *Clin. Epidemiol.* **2018**, *10*, 153–157. [CrossRef] [PubMed]
41. Cassin, S.; Sockalingam, S.; Du, C.; Wnuk, S.; Hawa, R.; Parikh, S.V. A pilot randomized controlled trial of telephone-based cognitive behavioural therapy for preoperative bariatric surgery patients. *Behav. Res. Ther.* **2016**, *80*, 17–22. [CrossRef] [PubMed]
42. Sockalingam, S.; Leung, S.E.; Hawa, R.; Wnuk, S.; Parikh, S.V.; Jackson, T.; Cassin, S.E. Telephone-based cognitive behavioural therapy for female patients 1-year post-bariatric surgery: A pilot study. *Obes. Res. Clin. Pract.* **2019**, *13*, 499–504. [CrossRef]
43. Andersson, G.; Cuijpers, P. Internet-based and other computerized psychological treatments for adult depression: A meta-analysis. *Cogn. Behav. Ther.* **2009**, *38*, 196–205. [CrossRef]
44. Martín, E.; Ruiz-Tovar, J.; Sánchez, R. *Vía Clínica de Cirugía Bariátrica 2017*; Im3mediA comunicación: Albacete, Spain, 2017.
45. *Qualtrics (Version 2.16)*; Qualtrics software: Provo, UT, USA, 2017.
46. Beck, A.T.; Steer, R.A.; Brown, G.K. *Manual for the Beck Depression Inventory-II*; Psychological Corporation: San Antonio, TX, USA, 1996.
47. Sanz, J.; Perdigón, A.L.; Vázquez, C. The Spanish adaptation of the Beck's Depression Inventory-II (BDI-II): Psychometric properties in the general population. *Clin. Salud* **2003**, *14*, 249–280.
48. Beck, A.T.; Steer, R. *Beck Anxiety Inventory Manual*; Psychological Corporation: San Antonio, TX, USA, 1993.
49. Magán, I.; Sanz, J.; García-Vera, M.P. Psychometric properties of a Spanish version of the Beck Anxiety Inventory (BAI) in general population. *Span. J. Psychol.* **2008**, *11*, 626–640. [CrossRef]
50. Sheehan, D.V. *Mini International Neuropsychiatric Interview 7.0. (MINI 7.0)*; Medical Outcomes Systems: Jacksonville, FL, USA, 2015.
51. Ministerio de Justicia. Real Decreto 1720/2008, de 19 de Enero, Para la Aprobación de la Ley Orgánica 15/1999 de Protección de Datos de Carácter Personal. *Boletín Oficial del Estado*, 19 January 2008; pp. 4103–4136.

52. Asociación Medica Mundial Declaración de Helsinki. Principios éticos Para las Investigaciones Con Seres Humanos. In Proceedings of the 59th Asamblea General, Seúl, Korea, 18 October 2008.
53. Watson, D.; Clark, L.A.; Tellegen, A. Development and validation of brief measures of positive and negative affect: The PANAS scales. *J. Personal. Soc. Psychol.* **1988**, *54*, 1063–1070. [CrossRef]
54. Sandín, B.; Chorot, P.; Lostao, L.; Joiner, T.E.; Santed, M.A.; Valiente, R.M. Escalas PANAS de Afecto Positivo y Negativo: Validación factorial y convergencia transcultural. *Psicothema* **1999**, *11*, 37–51.
55. Costa, P.T.; McCrae, R.R. *Revised NEO Personality Inventory (NEO-PI-R) and NEO Five-Factor Inventory (NEO-FFI)*; TEA Ediciones: Madrid, Spain, 1999.
56. Mezzich, J.E.; Ruipérez, M.A.; Pérez, C.; Yoon, G.; Liu, J.; Mahmud, S. The Spanish Version of the Quiality of Life Index. *J. Nerv. Ment. Dis.* **2000**, *188*, 301–305. [CrossRef]
57. Brooks, R. EuroQol: The current state of play. *Health Policy* **1996**, *37*, 53–72. [CrossRef]
58. Badia, X.; Roset, M.; Montserrat, S.; Herdman, M.; Segura, A. La versión española del EuroQol: Descripción y aplicaciones EuroQol Spanish Version: Description and Aplications. *Clin. Med.* **1999**, *112*, 79–86.
59. Echeburúa, E.; Corral, P.; Fernández-Montalvo, J. Maladjustment Inventory (MI): Psychometric properties in clinical contexts. *Análisis Modif. Conducta* **2000**, *26*, 325–340.
60. Gratz, K.L.; Roemer, L. Multidimensional assessment of emotion regulation and dysregulation: Development, factor structure, and initial validation of the difficulties in emotion regulation scale. *J. Psychopathol. Behav. Assess.* **2004**, *26*, 41–54. [CrossRef]
61. Hervás, G.; Jódar, R. The Spanish version of the Difficulties in Emotion Regulation Scale. *Clin. Salud* **2008**, *19*, 139–156.
62. Gámez, W.; Chmielewski, M.; Kotov, R.; Ruggero, C.; Suzuki, N.; Watson, D. The Brief Experiential Avoidance Questionnaire: Development and initial validation. *Psychol. Assess.* **2014**, *26*, 35–45. [CrossRef]
63. Vázquez-Morejón, R.; León, J.M.; Martín, A.; Vazquez, A.J. Validation of a spanish version of the brief experiential avoidance questionnaire (BEAQ) in clinical population. *Psicothema* **2019**, *31*, 335–340. [CrossRef]
64. Cardaciotto, L.; Herbert, J.D.; Forman, E.M.; Moitra, E.; Farrow, V. The assessment of present-moment awareness and acceptance: The Philadelphia Mindfulness Scale. *Assessment* **2008**, *15*, 204–223. [CrossRef]
65. Tejedor, R.; Feliu-Soler, A.; Pascual, J.C.; Cebolla, A.; Portella, M.J.; Trujols, J.; Soriano, J.; Pérez, V.; Soler, J. Psychometric properties of the Spanish version of the Philadelphia Mindfulness Scale. *Rev. Psiquiatr. Salud Ment.* **2014**, *7*, 157–165. [CrossRef]
66. Gross, J.J.; John, O.P. Individual differences in two emo- tion regulation processes: Implications for affect, relationships, and well-being. *J. Personal. Soc. Psychol.* **2003**, *85*, 348–362. [CrossRef]
67. Cabello, R.; Salguero, J.M.; Fernández-Berrocal, P.; Gross, J.J. A Spanish adaptation of the Emotion Regulation Questionnaire. *Eur. J. Psychol. Assess.* **2013**, *29*, 234–240. [CrossRef]
68. Henderson, M.; Freeman, C.P.L. A self-rating scale for bulimia the 'bite'. *Br. J. Psychiatry* **1987**, *150*, 18–24. [CrossRef] [PubMed]
69. Moya, T.R.; Bersabé, R.; Jiménez, M. Fiabilidad y validez del test de investigación bulímica de Edimburgo (BITE) en una muestra de adolescentes españoles; Reliability and validity of the Bulimic Investigatory Test Edinburgh (BITE) in a sample of Spanish adolescents. *Psicol. Conduct.* **2004**, *12*, 447–461.
70. Cooper, P.J.; Taylor, M.J.; Cooper, Z.; Fairburn, C.G. The development and validation of the Body Shape Questionnaire. *Int. J. Eat. Disord.* **1987**, *6*, 485–494. [CrossRef]
71. Raich, R.M.; Mora, M.; Soler, A.; Avila, C.; Clos, I.; Zapater, L. Adaptación de un instrumento de evaluación de la insatisfacción corporal; Adaptation of a body dissatisfaction assessment instrument. *Clin. Health* **1996**, *7*, 51–66.
72. Arnow, B.; Kenardy, J.; Agras, W. The Emotional Eating Scale: The development of a measure to assess coping with negative affect by eating. *Int. J. Eat. Disord.* **1995**, *18*, 79–90. [CrossRef]
73. Suso-Ribera, C.; Castilla, D.; Zaragozá, I.; Ribera-Canudas, M.V.; Botella, C.; García-Palacios, A. Validity, Reliability, Feasibility, and Usefulness of Pain Monitor, a Multidimensional Smartphone App for Daily Monitoring of Adults with Heterogeneous Chronic Pain. *Clin. J. Pain* **2018**, *34*, 900–908. [CrossRef]
74. Norman, S.B.; Cissel, S.H.; Means-Christensen, A.J.; Stein, M.B. Development and validation of an Overall Anxiety Severity and Impairment Scale. *Depress. Anxiety* **2006**, *23*, 245–249. [CrossRef]
75. Bentley, K.H.; Gallagher, M.W.; Carl, J.R.; Barlow, D.H. Development and validation of the Overall Depression Severity and Impairment Scale. *Psychol. Assess.* **2014**, *26*, 815–830. [CrossRef]
76. Osma, J.; Quilez-Orden, A.; Suso-Ribera, C.; Peris-Baquero, O.; Norman, S.B.; Bentley, K.H.; Sauer-Zavala, S.

Psychometric properties and validation of the Spanish versions of the overall anxiety and depression severity and impairment scales. *J. Affect. Disord.* **2019**, *252*, 9–18. [CrossRef]

77. Barlow, D.; Sauer-Zavala, S.; Farchione, T.; Murray, H.; Ellard, K.; Bullis, J.; Castellano-Robbins, C. *The Unified Protocol for Transdiagnostic Treatment of Emotional Disorders: Client Workbook*, 2nd ed.; Oxford University Press: New York, NY, USA, 2018.
78. IBM Corp. *IBM SPSS Statistics for Windows*; Version 22.0 2013; IBM: Armonk, NY, USA, 2013.
79. Jacobson, N.S.; Truax, P. Clinical significance: A statistical approach to defining meaningful change in psychotherapy research. *J. Consult. Clin. Psychol.* **1991**, *59*, 12–19. [CrossRef]
80. De Andrés Pizarro, J. El análisis de estudios cualitativo. *Aten. Primaria* **2000**, *25*, 42–46. [CrossRef]
81. Shamseer, L.; Sampson, M.; Bukutu, C.; Schmid, C.H.; Nikles, J.; Tate, R.; Johnston, B.C.; Zucker, D.; Shadish, W.R.; Kravitz, R.; et al. Consort extension for reporting N-of-1 trials (CENT) 2015: Explanation and elaboration. *J. Clin. Epidemiol.* **2016**, *76*, 18–46. [CrossRef]
82. Welbourn, R.; Dixon, J.; Barth, J.H.; Finer, N.; Hughes, C.A.; le Roux, C.W.; Wass, J. NICE-Accredited Commissioning Guidance for Weight Assessment and Management Clinics: A Model for a Specialist Multidisciplinary Team Approach for People with Severe Obesity. *Obes. Surg.* **2016**, *26*, 649–659. [CrossRef] [PubMed]
83. World Health Organization. *Mental Health Action Plan 2013–2020*; World Health Organization: Geneva, Switzerland, 2013.
84. Renjilian, D.A.; Perri, M.G.; Nezu, A.M.; McKelvey, W.F.; Shermer, R.L.; Anton, S.D. Individual versus group therapy for obesity: Effects of matching participants to their treatment preferences. *J. Consult. Clin. Psychol.* **2001**, *69*, 717–721. [CrossRef] [PubMed]
85. Osma, J.; Suso-Ribera, C.; Peris-Baquero, O.; Gil-Lacruz, M.; Pérez-Ayerra, L.; Ferreres-Galan, V.; Torres-Alfosea, M.A.; López-Escriche, M.; Domínguez, O. What format of treatment do patients with emotional disorders prefer and why? Implications for public mental health settings and policies. *PLoS ONE* **2019**, *14*, e0218117. [CrossRef] [PubMed]
86. Osma, J.; Sánchez-Gómez, A.; Peris-Baquero, O. Applying the unified protocol to a single case of major depression with schizoid and depressive personality traits. *Psicothema* **2018**, *30*, 364–369. [CrossRef]

2

Clinical Utility of an Internet-Delivered Version of the Unified Protocol for Transdiagnostic Treatment of Emotional Disorders in Adolescents (iUP-A)

Bonifacio Sandín, Julia García-Escalera, Rosa M. Valiente *, Victoria Espinosa and Paloma Chorot

Facultad de Psicología, Universidad Nacional de Educación a Distancia (UNED), 20040 Madrid, Spain; bsandin@psi.uned.es (B.S.); jgarciaescalera@psi.uned.es (J.G.-E.); vespinosa36@alumno.uned.es (V.E.); pchorot@psi.uned.es (P.C.)

* Correspondence: rmvalien@psi.uned.es

Abstract: The Unified Protocol for Transdiagnostic Treatment of Emotional Disorders in Adolescents (UP-A) has been shown to be effective for reducing symptoms of anxiety and depression in adolescents with emotional disorders. Internet-delivered psychological treatments have great potential to improve access to evidence-based psychological therapy since they are associated with reduced human and economic costs and less social stigma. Recently, our group developed an online version of the UP-A (the iUP-A) for the treatment of emotional disorders in adolescents. The aim of this pilot trial was to test the clinical utility of the iUP-A in a small sample (n = 12) of adolescents with elevated anxiety and/or depressive symptoms. Intention-to-treat and completer analyses revealed pre- to post-intervention self-reported decreases of anxiety and depressive symptoms, anxiety sensitivity, emotional avoidance, panic disorder symptoms, panic disorder severity, generalized anxiety disorder symptoms, pathological worry, and major depressive disorder symptoms. We found high feasibility and acceptability of the program with all participants and responsible parents reporting an improvement in the adolescents' ability to cope with emotions. Results suggest that the iUP-A may provide a new approach to improve access to treatment for anxious and depressive adolescents in Spain; however, further research must be conducted before firm conclusions can be drawn.

Keywords: transdiagnostic; iUP-A; i-CBT; AMTE; anxiety; depression; adolescents; online therapy

---

1. Introduction

Anxiety and depression in youth represent a growing public health concern. Epidemiological studies indicate that as many as 32.4% and 10.6% of adolescents have lifetime prevalence rates of anxiety and depressive disorders, respectively [1]. Anxiety and depression have been associated with severe impairment and increased risk for future psychopathological problems [2]. Subclinical symptoms of anxiety and depression are also very prevalent (32% and 29.2%, respectively) and have been related to functional impairment and suicidality [3]. In addition to the high prevalence of these emotional disorders, anxiety and depression are overlapping conditions throughout the lifespan, with rates of comorbidity as high as 75% in clinical samples [4]. Children and adolescents with anxiety and mood disorders also share a number of underlying vulnerability and maintenance factors, such as temperament (e.g., negative affect), difficulty regulating affect across emotions (e.g., behavioral avoidance), and clinical dispositions to experiment negative reactions to emotions (e.g., anxiety sensitivity) [5,6].

Evidence-based cognitive-behavioral therapy (CBT) for anxiety and depressive disorders has traditionally been disorder-specific, i.e., focused on treating one disorder at a time without paying therapeutic attention to comorbid conditions. In contrast, the transdiagnostic approach tries to address this limitation by focusing on the shared features of anxiety and depressive disorders rather than on the symptoms specific to each of these disorders [7]. In line with this perspective, transdiagnostic CBT (T-CBT) for emotional disorders has emerged as a new therapeutic approach that targets psychopathological processes common to both anxiety and depression. Addressing emotional disorders' risk and maintenance factors during adolescence may also help prevent the development of anxiety and depression later in life. The efficacy of T-CBT for emotional disorders has been found to be high and comparable to disorder-specific CBT treatments' efficacy in recent meta-analyses [8–10].

The Unified Protocols for Transdiagnostic Treatment of Emotional Disorders in Children (UP-C) and Adolescents (UP-A) are recent manualized treatments developed by Ehrenreich-May et al. [11] to address a broad array of emotional disorders' symptoms in children and adolescents. Both protocols take a transdiagnostic approach by focusing on a set of core change principles including prevention of emotional avoidance (effortful engagement in experiencing intense emotions), enhancement of cognitive flexibility (evaluation of potentially problematic cognitions), and change of maladaptive action tendencies (encouraging youth to alter problematic behavioral patterns related to their emotional symptoms). These protocols place particular emphasis on emotion regulation since a goal of these treatments is to help patients to learn how to experience uncomfortable emotions and how to respond to them in more adaptive and non-avoidant ways. The UP-C and UP-A are flexible administered treatment protocols designed to improve emotion reactivity and emotion regulation and to ameliorate anxiety and depressive symptoms by means of an array of evidence-based treatment techniques (e.g., psychoeducation, behavioral activation, cognitive restructuring, etc.) that are applied to a range of emotions including fear, anxiety, sadness, and anger.

The UP-A has a growing body of data supporting its efficacy in treating anxiety and depressive disorders and symptoms in adolescent samples [8–15]. In a multiple-baseline trial with three adolescents, all participants experienced a reduction in the severity of their principal anxiety or depression diagnosis at post-treatment [12]. The study of Trosper et al. [15], an open trial with 12 adolescents, found significant reductions in the principal disorders' severity from pre- to post-treatment, as well as improvements in adolescents' emotion regulation according to parent ratings. In a most recent study, Ehrenreich et al. [13] demonstrated the efficacy of the UP-A in a randomized, waitlist-controlled trial including 51 adolescents with a primary diagnosis of an anxiety or depressive disorder. According to the authors, the UP-A outperformed the waitlist condition since significant treatment effects were found in favor of the UP-A on all outcome measures. Additionally, at post-treatment participants in the UP-A condition showed lower diagnostic severity and greater improvements according to clinician-rated measures compared to those in the waitlist condition.

Recently, our group has reported data concerning the Spanish validation of the UP-A adapted as a universal school-based prevention program of anxiety and depression [16,17]. In an open-trial including 28 adolescents, significant self-reported decreases from pre- to post-intervention were found in anxiety outcome measures [17]; in addition, this study also provided support for the acceptability and feasibility of the Spanish version of the UP-A. In a more recent publication using the Spanish UP-A, results of a randomized waitlist-controlled trial including 151 school adolescents revealed that those participants with greater baseline emotional symptoms in the UP-A group trended toward significantly greater decreases in depression symptoms compared to the control group [16].

Internet-delivered psychological treatments represent an emerging model of service delivery with the potential to improve access to evidence-based treatments for anxiety and depressive disorders [18]. It has been suggested that internet-based treatments have several advantages compared with traditional face-to-face interventions, including improved access to evidence-based treatments and cost-effectiveness [19]. As these authors suggested, the fact that patients can return to the program at their convenience to access treatment information may facilitate learning and retention. Additionally, patients in internet interventions may receive therapist support faster than they would in traditional face-to-face treatments and may feel less stigma than when attending traditional psychological therapy. Several reviews and meta-analyses have shown comparable reductions in anxiety and depression symptoms from internet-based CBT (iCBT) and face-to-face CBT in adults [18,20,21], children, and adolescents [22].

A transdiagnostic iCBT treatment (T-iCBT) was recently developed by Titov's group to treat anxiety and depression [18]. In a similar vein, Botella's group developed a T-iCBT protocol based on Barlow's UP [23] designed to treat emotional disorders in adults [24]. Several meta-analyses have shown that T-iCBT protocols could be effective in the reduction of anxious and depressive symptomatology [9,25]. Recently, our group has developed an internet-based version of the UP-A (i.e., the iUP-A) [26]. As far as we know, this is the first T-iCBT treatment that targets anxiety and depression in adolescents, as well as the first adaptation of the UP-A into a web-based or online format.

The aim of this pilot trial was to test the clinical utility, feasibility, and acceptability of the iUP-A in a small sample of adolescents living in Spain. We hypothesized to find a significant change from pre- to post-treatment in: (a) primary outcome measures (general levels of anxiety and depression), (b) transdiagnostic variables (positive and negative affect, anxiety sensitivity, and emotional avoidance), and (c) disorder-specific measures (symptoms of anxiety and depressive disorders, panic disorder severity, pathological worry, and symptoms of social anxiety). Specifically, we hypothesized that participants would evidence a significant reduction in all outcome measures at posttreatment compared to pretreatment levels, except for positive affect where we expected to find a significant increase. A second aim of the study was to examine the feasibility and acceptability of the iUP-A and of the web platform that implements it, called Learn to Manage your Emotions (Aprende a Manejar tus Emociones; AMTE).

2. Materials and Methods

2.1. Participants

Families were recruited through information posted by the Universidad Nacional de Educación a Distancia (UNED) on Twitter and on the UNED's website as well as through school counselors' referrals. The inclusion criteria for the adolescents were: (a) 12 to 18 years of age; (b) meeting diagnostic criteria for any anxiety and/or depressive disorder or having subthreshold anxiety and/or depression symptoms based on the Mini International Neuropsychiatric Interview (MINI) [27,28] at assessment; (c) having an e-mail address and daily access to the internet through a computer or electronic tablet; (d) stability of psychotropic medications (if any) for at least three months; (e) Spanish proficiency.

Exclusion criteria were: (a) a diagnosis of a severe psychopathology such as psychotic disorder, bipolar disorder, severe depressive disorder, intellectual disability, severe learning disability, autism spectrum disorder, or substance dependence; (b) being at moderate or severe risk for suicide (based on the MINI); (c) on-going psychological treatment; (d) no informed consent.

A total of 23 families were screened by telephone for eligibility. Participant flow through the study is presented in Figure 1. Post-treatment data were available for eight participants, all of whom completed the eight modules of the iUP-A. A total of four adolescents dropped out of the study, three reported being dissatisfied with the program whereas one reported a lack of time for the intervention. Of these four adolescents, two finished the first module, one finished the first four modules and one finished the first five modules.

A total of 12 adolescents met the inclusion criteria and were included in the study. There were eight girls (67%) and four boys (M age = 15.58 years old; SD = 1.73; range = 13 to 18). All adolescents were Spanish residents. Regarding the living situation, 10 adolescents (83.3%) were living with both of their parents whereas two were living with their mother and siblings due to parents' divorce. In all cases (100%), the gender of the parent responsible for treatment was female.

None of the enrolled participants were taking psychotropic medication and only one had previously received psychological treatment (for a total of 10 sessions). Lastly, five adolescents (41.7%) were waiting for an appointment in the mental health department of the Spanish public healthcare system after being referred by their general practitioner or family doctor.

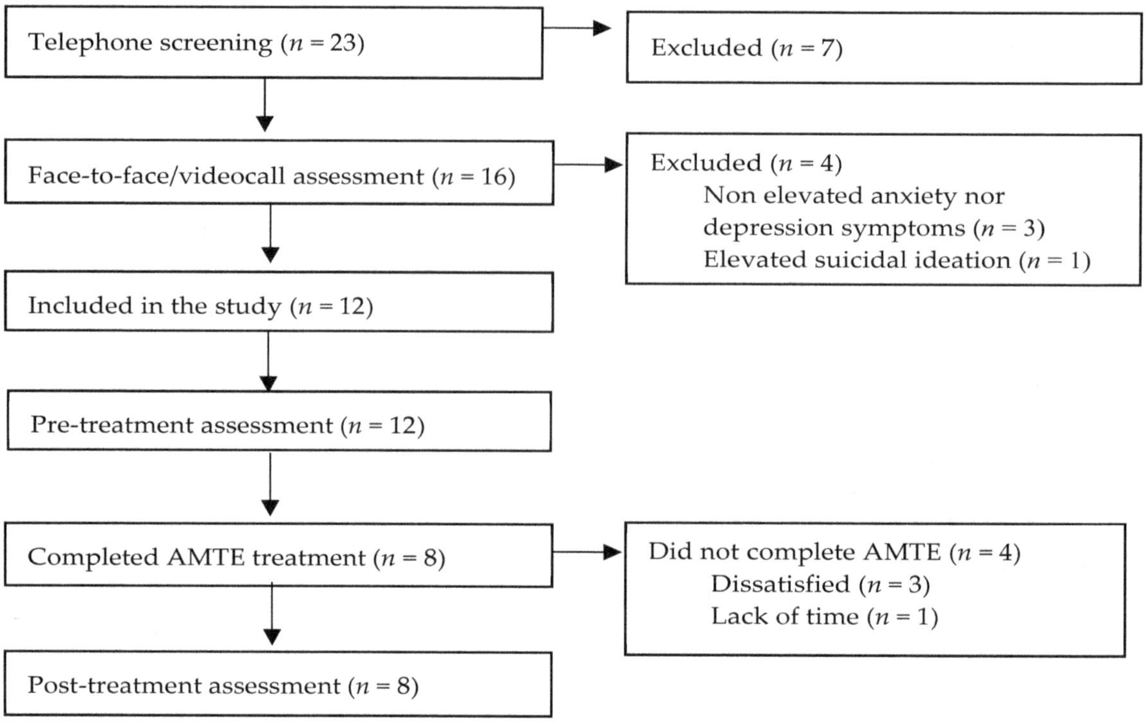

Figure 1. Participant flow through the study.

Regarding participants' diagnoses, nine participants (75%) were diagnosed with some clinical disorder whereas three showed subthreshold anxiety and/or depressive symptoms (see Table 1).

Table 1. Diagnoses or symptoms of the 12 participants.

Principal Diagnosis/Symptoms	Comorbid Diagnoses/Symptoms
Social phobia	Depressive symptoms
Bulimia	Major depressive disorder
Anxiety and depressive symptoms	—
Social phobia	—
Major depressive disorder	Generalized anxiety disorder
Panic disorder with agoraphobia	Obsessive-compulsive disorder
Anxiety symptoms	—
Hypomanic episode–current and past	Separation anxiety disorder; Obsessive-compulsive disorder; Oppositional defiant disorder
Depressive symptoms	—
Panic disorder without agoraphobia	—
Major depressive disorder	Posttraumatic stress disorder
Posttraumatic stress disorder	Agoraphobia; Social phobia; Obsessive-compulsive disorder; Transient TIC Disorder

2.2. Procedure and Design

This study employed an uncontrolled pre-post open trial design. It was granted ethical approval from the Research Ethics Committee of the UNED and was registered on Clinicaltrials.gov (Identifier NCT04182061). The TREND Statement guidelines for nonrandomized interventions [29] were followed when reporting the trial. No incentives were provided to the adolescents or parents for participating in this trial.

Recruitment was carried out in two steps: a telephone screening with the responsible parent and a face-to-face or video call assessment. Once the telephone screening had been made and the informed consent had been signed and returned, potential participants and their parents were invited to an assessment session that was conducted either face-to-face or through video call. In this session, a clinical psychologist conducted a full diagnostic interview with the adolescent and briefly talked with the parent(s) to gain insight regarding their concerns about the adolescents' main problems and symptoms.

Following the assessment session, the adolescents meeting inclusion criteria were included in the study and both the responsible parent and the adolescent received an e-mail to register on the web platform Aprende a Manejar tus Emociones (AMTE) (Learn to Manage your Emotions). Then, one week before the intervention started, the adolescents were invited to fill in the self-report measures (see the Instruments section) on the AMTE platform. A week after the intervention ended, the adolescents were also invited to fill in the same self-report measures on the AMTE platform.

2.3. *Intervention*

The internet UP-A (iUP-A) was delivered by means of the AMTE platform. The iUP-A was adapted from the Unified Protocol for Transdiagnostic Treatment of Emotional Disorders in Adolescents (UP-A) [30].

As does the UP-A, the iUP-A uses evidence-based treatment techniques that cut across disorder-specific CBT treatment manuals for adolescent anxiety and depression (e.g., psychoeducation, cognitive restructuring, exposure, behavioral activation, relapse prevention, etc.). It also includes motivational enhancement as well as mindfulness-based techniques. The AMTE program includes the same eight core modules of the UP-A and participants are advised to complete one module per week (except for module seven, which usually takes one more week to complete). Table 2 provides an overview of the structure and specific topics address in the eight treatment modules.

Table 2. Descriptions of the modules (M) included in the AMTE platform.

Module Title	Main Contents
[M1] Building motivation	Obtain three top problems, severity ratings, and a goal for each problem. Discover what motivates the adolescent to change.
[M2] Getting to know your emotions	Psychoeducation about emotions and their function. Understand the three parts of emotional experiences. Learn about emotional behaviors and the cycle of avoidance.
[M3] Enjoy positive activities	Psychoeducation about opposite action and behavioral experiments. Come up with a list of enjoyed activities. Engage the adolescent in behavioral experiments (behavioral activation) for sadness.
[M4] Awareness of your emotional experiences	Introduce the rationale for present-moment awareness and non-judgmental awareness. Practice body scanning. Practice awareness skills when exposed to non-emotional and emotional triggers.
[M5] Learn to be flexible in your thinking	Learn about the concept of "thinking traps" (i.e., cognitive distortions), automatic thoughts, and alternative thoughts. Learn detective thinking and problem-solving skills.
[M6] Cope with your body sensations	Psychoeducation about body sensations, their relationship with intense emotions, and their harmlessness. Conduct exposures to body sensations to learn to tolerate uncomfortable physical feelings.
[M7] Cope with emotional situations	Review the cycle of avoidance and introduce situational emotion exposures. Create an Emotional Behaviors Form to identify relevant exposures. Assign exposures for home learning.
[M8] Maintain your gains	Review skills that have been most useful for each adolescent and make an individualized relapse prevention plan.

The intervention can be used on (laptop) computers and tablets. Parents log in to a separate section of the program and have access to a summary of each module as well as to information regarding the progress of their adolescent in treatment. The therapists log in to a therapists' section of the AMTE platform where they can monitor the progression of each adolescent in the treatment (last access to the platform, progression in the treatment modules, time spent on the platform, etc.) and see the adolescent's answers to the home learning assignments.

The treatment platform was designed with an age-appropriate appearance. The first time the adolescents log in, they personalize an avatar (virtual human) by changing its hair, skin color, clothing, and gender. The platform AMTE uses a narrator (called "Doctor") that presents treatment contents through written messages whereas the avatar presents encouraging written messages to the participant. The AMTE platform uses an island overarching theme (see Figure 2).

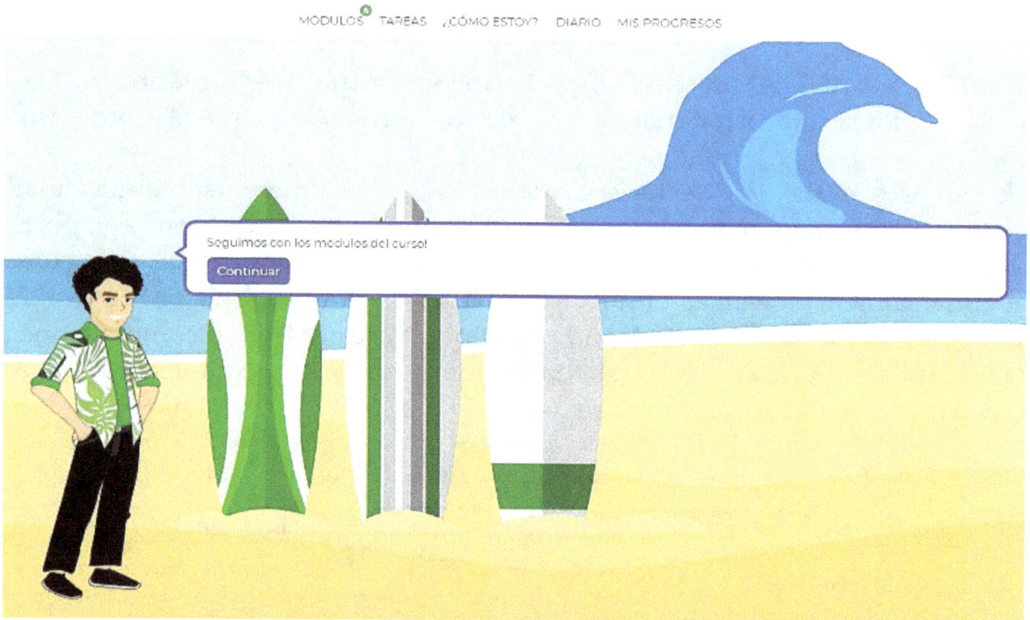

Figure 2. Screenshot of the AMTE homepage.

Each module contains written texts presented by the Doctor or the avatar, explanatory videos, exercises, home learning assignments, and downloadable PDFs (with the exercises, the home learning assignments, and summaries of each module). The expected time to complete each module (contents, exercises, and home learning assignments) is approximately 50 min. The AMTE platform is interactive with responses to home learning assignments being directly entered into the program and saved so that the therapist can immediately review the adolescent's progress. Participants may also initiate contact with the therapists by sending messages via the AMTE platform whenever they have questions or want to discuss any aspects of the treatment.

During the treatment period, both the adolescent and the treatment responsible parent had weekly telephone contact with their assigned clinical psychologist, the same one that did the face-to-face or videocall assessment. The psychologist called the responsible parent's cell phone, spoke for about 10 min with the parent (to check on the parent's main concerns regarding the adolescent and address any problems that may have arisen) and for another 10 min or so with the adolescent (to review the participant's responses to the home learning assignments and support the adolescent in using the program).

2.4. Instruments

The clinical diagnoses were conducted by means of the MINI [27,28]. The questionnaires EAN [31], CDN [31], and the total score on the RCADS-30 [32] were used as primary outcome measures. To assess transdiagnostic constructs the questionnaires PANASN [33], CASI [34,35], and EASI-A [36,37] were used. Disorder-specific symptoms of anxiety and depressive disorders were assessed through the RCADS-30 subscales [32], and the questionnaires PSWQ-11 [38], SASC-R [39,40], and PDSS-SR [39–42].

Finally, the Feasibility and Acceptability Questionnaire (FAQ) was used to assess the experiences of the adolescents and parents with the program.

Mini International Neuropsychiatric Interview for Children and Adolescents (MINI-KID) [27,28]. The MINI-KID is a structured diagnostic interview for people aged 6 to 17 years. It is based on DSM-IV and ICD-10 criteria for psychiatric disorders. The reliability and validity of MINI-KID has been demonstrated [43].

Revised Child Anxiety and Depression Scale–30 (RCADS-30) [32]. The RCADS-30 is a 30-item self-report scale comprised of the following subscales derived from the Diagnostic and Statistical Manual of Mental Disorders (DSM-IV/5) criteria: (1) social phobia (Soc.P), (2) generalized anxiety disorder (GAD), (3) obsessive-compulsive disorder (OCD), (4) panic disorder (PD), (5) separation anxiety disorder (SAD), and (6) major depressive disorder (MDD). This scale has previously demonstrated good psychometric properties [7]. Each item is scored from zero ("never") to three ("always"), with higher scores representing more severe symptoms.

Anxiety Scale for Children (Escala de Ansiedad para Niños, EAN) [31]. The EAN is a 10-item self-report scale that assesses anxiety symptoms in children and adolescents. It has shown good psychometric properties [16]. The participants are instructed to indicate how frequently they have experienced general anxiety symptoms (cognitive, physiological, etc.) on a four-point, Likert-type scale, ranging from zero ("never or almost never") to three ("always or almost always").

Depression Questionnaire for Children (Cuestionario de Depresión para Niños; CDN) [31]. The CDN scale is a 16-item, self-report questionnaire designed to assess symptoms of major depressive disorder and dysthymic disorder (according to DSM-IV/5 criteria) in children and adolescents. Participants rate each item on a four-point, Likert-type scale, ranging from zero ("never or almost never") to three ("always or almost always"). The CDN has demonstrated good psychometric properties [16,32].

Positive and Negative Affect Schedule for Children and Adolescents (Escalas PANAS de Afecto Positivo y Negativo para Niños y Adolescentes; PANASN) [33]. The PANASN provides scores for two subscales of 10 items each measuring positive and negative affect. Participants are asked to rate items according to how they usually feel from one ("never or almost never") to three ("a lot of the time"). This self-report scale has demonstrated adequate psychometric properties [32].

Childhood Anxiety Sensitivity Index (CASI) [34,35]. The CASI is an 18-item self-report questionnaire measuring anxiety sensitivity in children and adolescents, that is, distress reactions to symptoms of anxiety. Participants rate the frequency with which they experience each item using a three-point, Likert-type scale from one ("never") to three ("a lot of the time"). The Spanish adaptation of the CASI used in the present study has demonstrated good psychometric properties in previous studies [44].

Emotional Avoidance Strategy Inventory for Adolescents (EASI-A) [36,37]. The EASI-A is a 17-item self-report questionnaire in which respondents are instructed to indicate the degree to which each statement is true using a five-point, Likert-type scale ranging from zero ("never or almost never") to four ("always or almost always").

PSWQ-11 questionnaire for children and adolescents (PSWQN-11) [38]. It is an age-downward version of the 11-item Penn State Worry Questionnaire [45]. This 11-item self-report questionnaire assesses pathological worry. Respondents are instructed to indicate the degree to which they agree with each statement using a five-point Likert-type scale from one ("Totally disagree") to five ("totally agree").

Social Anxiety Scale for Children-Revised (SASC-R) [39,40]. The SASC-R is an 18-item self-report questionnaire in which respondents are instructed to indicate the frequency with which they experience each symptom of social anxiety using a four-point Likert-type scale from one ("never") to three ("a lot of the time").

Panic Disorder Severity Scale—Self-Report (PDSS—SR) [41]. The abbreviated adapted version by Sandin (2010) [42] was used. The PDSS—SR is a seven-item self-report questionnaire that assesses the severity of the panic disorder in the last month. Using a five-point Likert-type scale from zero ("not at all") to four ("very much"), participants rate the distress associated with panic attacks, anticipatory anxiety regarding new attacks, and interoceptive and situational avoidance. This scale has demonstrated adequate psychometric properties in adult samples [46].

Feasibility and Acceptability Questionnaire (FAQ) [47]. This questionnaire includes a version for the adolescents and a version for the parents. Both versions include three separate sections (subscales) each comprised of six items: (1) experience with the online platform, (2) satisfaction with the program, and (3) therapeutic alliance. All items are assessed on an 11-point scale from 0 ("totally disagree") to 10 ("totally agree"). The parents' version includes an additional section that assesses the experience of the treatment responsible parent with the parents' section of the online platform. This section includes two items. The satisfaction with the program section of the FAQ includes the six questions from the satisfaction questionnaire of Rapee et al. (2006) [48].

2.5. Statistical Analysis

All statistical analyses were done with the SPSS v.24 software program (IBM Corp., Armonk, NY, USA). For the completer sample ($n = 8$), changes in the outcome scores between pre- and post-treatment were examined using the Wilcoxon signed-rank test, a nonparametric alternative to paired samples t-test. In addition to the completer analyses, calculations were repeated with the total sample ($n = 12$) after replacing missing values for the dropout cases with their last observation carried forward (LOCF). To gain further insight into the statistical significance of the improvements, effect sizes were calculated for all outcome measures using Cohen's d (meanpre-meanpost/pooled SD) [49]. Before the statistical analysis of the data, we computed the statistical power (with an alpha error of 0.05, one-tailed) of the Wilcoxon signed-rank test (matched pairs) using the G*Power 3.1.9.7 [50]. The statistical power ranged from 75% to 100% (average = 96.7%) for the statistically significant outcome measures (described in Tables 3 and 4); the power was 57% for the two marginally significant variables (SAD subscale of the RCADAS-30) and 87% PANASN-Positive Affect.

Table 3. Means (M), standard deviations (SD), Wilcoxon tests, and effect sizes (Cohen's d) for primary (CDN, EAN, and RCADS-30 total score) and disorder-specific (subscales of the RCADS-30) outcome measures.

Measures	Pre-Treatment $n = 12$		Post-Treatment $n = 8$		Completer Sample Analyses $n = 8$		Intention-to-Treat Analyses [b] $n = 12$
	M	SD	M	SD	Z [a]	d	d
CDN	19.17	11.50	15.25	8.92	1.47	1.14	0.66
EAN	14.50	8.58	10.88	5.82	2.38 **	2.36	1.43
RCADS-30							
Total	32.58	18.43	24.25	9.68	2.38 **	4.14	2.58
MDD	6.42	4.08	4.88	3.23	2.05 *	0.96	0.58
PD	4.83	5.11	1.75	1.98	1.99 *	2.54	1.75
Soc.P	8.58	4.40	8.25	3.49	1.06	0.88	0.52
SAD	1.25	1.54	0.88	1.13	1.84 +	0.74	0.52
GAD	7.33	3.80	5.88	2.10	2.21 *	2.27	1.25
OCD	4.17	4.59	2.63	1.85	1.10	1.32	0.93

Note. [a] Z Wilcoxon test based on positive ranks (exact signification, one-tailed). [b] Z values are identical to those of the completer sample. CDN = Depression Questionnaire for Children; EAN = Anxiety Scale for Children; GAD = generalized anxiety disorder; MDD = major depressive disorder; OCD = obsessive compulsive disorder; PD = panic disorder; RCADS-30 = Revised Child Anxiety and Depression Scale-30; SAD = separation anxiety disorder; Soc.P = social phobia. $^{+}$ $p < 0.10$; * $p < 0.05$; ** $p < 0.01$.

Table 4. Means (M), standard deviations (SD), Wilcoxon test and effect sizes (Cohen's d) for transdiagnostic (PANAS, CASI and EASI) and disorder-specific (PDSS-SR, PSWQ-N, and SASC-R) outcome measures.

Measures	Pre-Treatment $n = 12$		Post-Treatment $n = 8$		Completer Sample Analyses $n = 8$		Intention-to-Treat Analyses [b] $n = 12$
	M	SD	M	SD	Z [a]	d	d
PANASN-NA	21.08	2.91	20.75	2.66	0.50	0.53	0.35
PANASN-PA	20.50	3.80	23.38	4.27	1.47 +	−1.13	−0.73
CASI	31.92	8.52	29.00	4.66	2.22 *	2.87	1.74
EASI-A	37.25	16.24	32.13	12.91	1.82 *	2.97	1.19
PDSS-SR	10.58	8.03	2.75	3.49	2.52 **	4.82	2.59
PSWQ-N	32.92	12.92	27.25	5.42	2.39 **	3.40	2.30
SASC-R	37.67	10.82	40.88	5.79	0.42	0.67	0.37

Note. [a] Z Wilcoxon test based on positive ranks (exact signification, 1-tailed) (for PANAS-PA, the Z score was based on negative ranks). [b] Z values are identical to those of the completer sample. CASI = Childhood Anxiety Sensitivity Index; EASI-A = Emotional Avoidance Strategy Inventory for Adolescents; FNE = Fear of Negative Evaluation; PANASN-NA = Negative Affect scale of the Positive and Negative Affect Schedule for Children and Adolescents; PANASN-PA = Positive Affect scale of the Positive and Negative Affect Schedule for Children and Adolescents; PDSS-SR = Panic Disorder Severity Scale—Self-Report; PSWQ-N = PSWQ-11 questionnaire for children and adolescents; SASC-R = Social Anxiety Scale for Children—Revised. $^{+}$ $p < 0.10$; * $p < 0.05$; ** $p < 0.01$.

3. Results

3.1. *Intervention Effects*

A Wilcoxon matched-pairs signed-rank test including the completer sample, i.e., all the adolescents that finished the intervention ($n = 8$), showed a significant decrease in anxiety symptoms (EAN, $p = 0.008$) associated with a large effect size. Likewise, there were significant reductions in the RCADS-30 total score ($p = 0.008$), associated with a very large effect size. There were also significant reductions associated to several subscales of the RCADS-30: major depressive disorder ($p = 0.031$), panic disorder ($p = 0.031$), and generalized anxiety disorder ($p = 0.016$). Due to the small sample size, we also took into account marginally significant results ($p < 0.10$), which were found for the separation anxiety disorder subscale of the RCADS-30 ($p = 0.063$). Identical results were obtained including the intent-to-treat sample ($n = 12$); see Table 3.

Wilcoxon tests including the adolescents that finished the intervention ($n = 8$) showed significant reductions on the transdiagnostic outcome measures of anxiety sensitivity (CASI; $p = 0.016$) and emotional avoidance (EASI-A; $p = 0.039$), both associated with large effect sizes. Also, there were significant reductions in panic disorder severity (PDDSS-SR; $p = 0.004$) and pathological worry (PSWQ-N; $p = 0.008$), both associated with large within-group effect sizes. We also found that an increase in PANASN-PA from pre- to post-treatment was marginally significant ($p = 0.094$). Identical results were obtained including the intent-to-treat sample ($n = 12$); see Table 4.

3.2. *Feasibility and Acceptability*

3.2.1. Adolescent Report

The FAQ was completed by eight adolescents (66.66% of those who participated in the program) on a scale from 0 to 10 (see Table 5). In relation to the questions assessing experience with the program, mean ratings ranged between 7.25 and 9.38. Regarding the satisfaction with the program, the mean ratings of the first four questions ranged between 8.50 and 9.38. In addition, all adolescents reported that their ability to cope with emotions had improved significantly (mean improvement from 4.13 to 8.25). Finally, ratings on the therapeutic alliance were high with mean ratings ranging from 8.88 to 9.88.

Table 5. Descriptive statistics for the items of the FAQ (adolescent version) (n = 8).

Experience with the Online Platform (Range: 0–10)	M	SD
How easy has it been for you to use the AMTE online platform?	9.00	1.20
How easy has it been for you to understand what the videos and Dr. AMTE were telling you?	8.50	1.77
How useful has it been for you what Dr. AMTE and the different videos were teaching you?	9.38	0.92
How easy has it been for you to include the AMTE program in your daily routine?	8.50	1.60
To what degree have you been able to do the exercises and home learning assignments without technical or computer problems?	7.25	1.58
To what extent have you applied what you have learned with AMTE to your real life?	8.50	0.93
Satisfaction with the Program (Range: 0–10)	**M**	**SD**
How much did you learn in this program?	8.75	1.58
How effective was this program in helping you cope with your problems?	8.86	1.07
How much did you enjoy doing this program?	8.50	1.20
To what extent would you recommend the program to other adolescents?	9.38	0.74
What was your ability to cope with emotions before the program?	4.13	1.64
What was your ability to cope with emotions after the program?	8.25	1.39
Ability to cope with emotions after the program minus ability before	4.13	1.96
Therapeutic Alliance (Range: 0–10)	**M**	**SD**
How much has your therapist helped you deal with your top problems?	8.88	1.46
How appreciated by your therapist have you felt?	9.50	0.76
To what extent have you felt that you and your therapist respected each other?	9.88	0.35
To what extent have you agreed with your therapist on what things were important for you to work to overcome?	9.50	1.07
To what extent have you felt that your therapist cared about you?	9.38	0.92
How correct do you think the way you and your therapist have worked to solve your problems has been?	9.38	0.92

3.2.2. Parents Report

The FAQ (parent version) was also completed by eight mothers (the mothers of the eight adolescents that finished the intervention) on a scale from 0 to 10 (see Table 6). In relation to the questions assessing the experience of the adolescent with the program according to the perception of the parent, mean ratings ranged between 8.38 and 9.25. Likewise, seven mothers (out of eight) reported having logged in to the family section of the platform at least once with the mean satisfaction with the platform being 7.29. Regarding the parent perception of satisfaction of the adolescents with the program, the mean ratings of the first four questions ranged between 8 and 9.75. Also, all mothers reported that the ability of their child to cope with emotions had significantly improved (mean improvement from 4.63 to 8.00). Finally, ratings on the therapeutic alliance were very high with mean ratings ranging from 9.38 to 9.88.

Table 6. Descriptive statistics for the items of the FAQ (parent version) (n = 8).

Experience of the Adolescent with the Online Platform (Range: 0–10)	M	SD
How easy has it been for your son/daughter to use the AMTE online platform?	8.50	1.31
How easy has it been for your child to understand what the videos and Dr. AMTE were telling them?	9.25	1.04
How useful has it been for your child what Dr. AMTE and the different videos were teaching them?	8.88	1.36
How easy has it been for your child to include the AMTE program in their daily routine?	8.63	1.41
To what degree has your child been able to do the exercises and home learning assignments without technical or computer problems?	8.63	1.06
To what extent has your child applied what he/she has learned with AMTE to their real life?	8.38	1.60
Experience with the Parent's Section of the Online Platform	***n* (%) [yes]**	
Have you ever logged in to the parent's section of the AMTE platform?	7 (87.50%)	
To what extent has the parent's section of the platform helped you to help your son/daughter during treatment? (range: 0–10)	7.29	2.81

Table 6. *Cont.*

Satisfaction with the Program (Range: 0–10)	M	SD
How much has your child learned in this program?	9.14	0.69
How effective was this program in helping your child cope with their problems?	9.14	1.07
How much has your child enjoyed doing this program?	8.00	2.27
To what extent would you recommend the program to other adolescents?	9.75	0.71
What was the ability of your child to cope with emotions before the program?	4.63	2.00
What was the ability of your child to cope with their emotions after the program?	8.00	1.51
Ability to cope with emotions after the program minus ability before	3.38	1.51
Therapeutic Alliance (Range: 0–10)	**M**	**SD**
How much has the therapist helped your child deal with their top problems?	9.38	0.92
How appreciated by the therapist has your child felt?	9.88	0.35
To what extent have you felt that you and the therapist respected each other?	9.88	0.35
To what extent have you agreed with the therapist on what things were important for your son/daughter to work to overcome?	9.75	0.46
To what extent have you felt that the therapist cared about your child?	9.88	0.35
How correct do you think the AMTE's approach to solving your child problems has been?	9.75	0.46

4. Discussion

The purpose of the current study was to examine the clinical utility of the UP-A adapted to an internet-delivered program (i.e., the iUP-A). We explored whether the iUP-A would significantly decrease, from pretreatment to posttreatment, the levels of (a) general measures of anxiety and depression, (b) transdiagnostic constructs (positive and negative affect, anxiety sensitivity, and emotional avoidance), and (c) disorder-specific measures (anxiety and depressive disorder symptoms, panic disorder severity, pathological worry, and social anxiety). We also examined the acceptability and feasibility of the iUP-A. As far as we know, this is the first study that examines the clinical utility of an online T-CBT program for the treatment of anxiety and depression in adolescents; thus, this is also the first evaluation of the UP-A implemented as a web-based intervention.

Consistent with our hypotheses, the participants of this study reported improvements in general symptoms of anxiety and depression, transdiagnostic measures, and disorder-specific symptomatology. According to the effect sizes' estimates, the magnitude of the changes were medium (for positive affect and symptoms of MDD, social phobia, and separation anxiety disorder), large (for anxiety sensitivity, emotional avoidance and symptoms of general anxiety, panic disorder, GAD, and OCD), and very large (for panic disorder severity, pathological worry, and general symptomatology of anxiety and depression measured by RCADS-total score). Overall, we found significant or marginally significant improvements in all variables except for general symptoms of depression (questionnaire CDN), negative affect, social anxiety, and symptoms of OCD and social phobia. One surprising finding was the lack of significant effects on positive and negative affect. Although, according to the descriptive statistics, these temperamental variables changed from pretreatment to posttreatment as expected (the positive affect increased whereas the negative affect decreased), such changes did not reach the level of statistical significance.

The findings of this open trial are particularly noteworthy because the iUP-A appears to be effective at managing the three kinds of main variables examined (general symptoms of anxiety and depression, transdiagnostic measures, and specific symptoms of several anxiety and depressive disorders). Most of these positive effects were associated with large and very large effect sizes, which is consistent with results of the UP-A reported by Ehrenreich-May's group [12,13,15], as well as with findings of our group related to the Spanish version of the UP-A [16,17]. These data are also consistent with the results reported by authors who administered Super Skills for Life, a T-CBT protocol that has been applied as an indicated prevention program for adolescents [51] and children [52] at risk of developing anxiety disorders.

The fact that the iUP-A was able to modify two major transdiagnostic variables (i.e., anxiety sensitivity and emotional avoidance) is an important strength of the present study. The core treatment modules of the UP-A, like the UP's core modules [23], were designed to explicitly target aversive reactions to emotions (e.g., anxiety sensitivity) and the subsequent emotional avoidance. These are core transdiagnostic underlying processes related to the vulnerability and maintenance of emotional disorders and, therefore, processes shared by individuals with anxiety and depression. Surprisingly, there is a lack of evidence in the literature concerning the efficacy and clinical utility of the UP and UP-A reducing the levels of these main transdiagnostic mechanisms [10]. To our knowledge, this is the first study that provides empirical evidence of the UP-A's ability to modify high levels of anxiety sensitivity and emotional avoidance in youth. The study of Calear et al. [53] used the same scale we used to measure anxiety sensitivity (i.e., the CASI) but did not obtain significant results. Concerning affectivity, although some studies have shown the ability of the UP to produce changes in negative affect (or neuroticism) and positive affect (or extraversion) [10,54] we did not find such an effect.

This is the first trial that examines the feasibility and acceptability of an internet-based version of the UP-A. Regarding feasibility, the attrition rate in this study was 33.33%, a percentage comparable to studies that have evaluated face-to-face transdiagnostic treatments for anxiety and depressive disorders in adults [55], children [56], and adolescents [13]. Other authors have reported lower rates of adherence in studies based on computerized treatments. For example, Stallard et al. [57] reported an adherence rate of 60% for a computerized CBT intervention for anxiety and depression in a sample of children and adolescents. In addition, eight participants in our study completed the post-treatment assessment and had also finished all treatment modules, whereas in other studies with adolescent samples, e.g., Tillfors et al. [58], the average number of completed modules was only 2.9 out of a total of 10 modules. The good adherence shown by participants of the present study may be related to the fact that our treatment included a weekly call from the therapist; the study of Carlbring et al. [59] found that weekly calls increased by 93% the number of participants who finished all modules.

The second aspect of feasibility is the usability, which is the degree to which the participants had a positive experience with the web platform. This was assessed by means of the subscale "experience with the online platform". Both the adolescents and parents reported a very positive experience with the platform (e.g., mean ratings ranged from 7.25 to 9.38 on a 0 to 10 Likert scale). The third indicator of feasibility is the alliance with the therapist. This was highly rated both by the adolescents (mean ratings ranged from 8.88 to 9.88) and by the parents (mean ratings ranged from 9.38 to 9.88). The levels of therapeutic alliance found in the present study are rather higher than the ones reported by other studies of internet-CBT [60].

Regarding acceptability, the iUP-A and AMTE platform were very positively evaluated by the adolescents and their parents. Users' satisfaction scores ranged from 8.50 to 9.38 (Likert scale 0 to 10) whereas parents' satisfaction with the program was also very high, with mean scores ranging from 8 to 9.75 (strong endorsement). These ratings were higher than the ones of similar studies [48]. The participants reported an increase in their coping skills, enjoyment of the program, and reported that they would recommend the program to other adolescents. It is worth noting that a good acceptability is an important issue because expectations about the treatment may affect treatment outcomes.

5. Limitations and Future Research

The strengths of this study include performing a comprehensive assessment of feasibility and acceptability, as well as including relevant outcomes in several important domains (general symptoms of anxiety and depression, transdiagnostic constructs, and disorder-specific anxiety and depression symptoms). However, as a preliminary investigation of the iUP-A, it also has several limitations. The first limitation is that the sample size of the current study was too small and may have limited our ability to detect effects of the treatment; however, most of the outcome measures' effect sizes were large. A second limitation is the lack of a control group since this limits the possibility of establishing causal inferences between the treatment and the changes in the dependent variables. Due to this, it is difficult to determine whether the large effects associated with the treatment may partially reflect a spontaneous improvement over time. Thirdly, the present study did not include follow-up assessments, thereby reducing our ability to draw firm conclusions about the long-term efficacy of the iUP-A. Finally, the current investigation relied on self-report outcome measures.

Although the results are promising, they are very preliminary. These limitations preclude from drawing firm conclusions concerning the efficacy of the iUP-A in the treatment of anxiety and depressive disorders in adolescents. Future research on the efficacy of the iUP-A should address these shortcomings including (a) larger sample size and control conditions in order to be able to establish causal inferences regarding the effect of the intervention vs. the effect due to the passage of time, (b) follow-up assessments to examine if the effect of the treatment is sustained over time, and (c) clinical-rated outcome measures in addition to self-report measures. New research on the efficacy of the iUP-A has important implications for clinical psychology related to the treatment and prevention of anxiety and depression in youth since the UP-A is a consolidated transdiagnostic program for the treatment of emotional disorders. On the other hand, the iUP-A has the advantages of an internet-delivered intervention, thus being a particularly promising intervention program to be applied in the current situation of social isolation linked to COVID-19.

6. Conclusions

Overall, the results of the present study suggest that the UP-A delivered via the internet (i.e., the iUP-A) is a promising transdiagnostic CBT program for the treatment of anxiety and depressive disorders in adolescents. Importantly, the iUP-A was not only potentially efficacious but also feasible and acceptable to the participants and their parents. The present study provides preliminary empirical evidence in support of the clinical utility of a Spanish, web-based version of the UP-A (i.e., the iUP-A). This is the first study that provides empirical evidence of the clinical utility of an internet-based version of the UP-A. We found improvements in outcomes associated with several important domains (i.e., anxiety and depression symptoms, as well as vulnerability transdiagnostic constructs), suggesting that the iUP-A is an efficacious treatment reducing general comorbidity of anxiety and depression across emotional disorders (anxiety and depressive disorders). This study also provides empirical evidence concerning the ability of the iUP-A to ameliorate the disorder-specific symptomatology related to anxiety disorders. An innovative contribution of this investigation was to empirically test the effect of the iUP-A on core mechanisms underlying emotional disorders (positive and negative affectivity, anxiety sensitivity, and emotional avoidance). We found that the iUP-A was able to significantly reduce the levels of anxiety sensitivity and emotional avoidance (effect sizes = 1.74 and 1.19, respectively). Finally, the data concerning adherence, usability, therapeutic alliance, and satisfaction with the web platform suggest that the adolescents perceived the treatment as feasible and were highly satisfied with it. We conclude that the iUP-A is feasible and acceptable, as well as potentially efficacious in reducing symptoms (comorbid and disorder-specific) of anxiety and depression as well as underlying vulnerability and maintenance processes.

Author Contributions: B.S., R.M.V. and P.C. development of the iUP-A protocol and the web platform, conceptualization and design of the study, study coordination, preparation of the pre-posttreatment assessment protocol, original draft preparation, writing review and editing, and interpretation of data. B.S. statistical analysis. J.G.-E. data collection, diagnostic interviews, initial screening, clinical support, preparation of database, statistical analysis, interpretation of data, original draft preparation, writing review and editing, and study coordination. V.E. data collection, diagnostic interviews, and clinical support. All authors have read and agreed to the published version of the manuscript.

References

1. Kessler, R.C.; Petukhova, M.; Sampson, N.A.; Zaslavsky, A.M.; Wittchen, H. Twelve-month and lifetime prevalence and lifetime morbid risk of anxiety and mood disorders in the United States. *Int. J. Methods Psychiatry. Res.* **2012**, *21*, 169–184. [CrossRef]

2. Ahlen, J.; Lenhard, F.; Ghaderi, A. Universal prevention for anxiety and depressive symptoms in children: A meta-analysis of randomized and cluster-randomized trials. *J. Prim. Prev.* **2015**, *36*, 387–403. [CrossRef]
3. Balázs, J.; Miklósi, M.; Keresztény, Á.; Hoven, C.W.; Carli, V.; Wasserman, C.; Apter, A.; Bobes, J.; Brunner, R.; Cosman, D. Adolescent subthreshold-depression and anxiety: Psychopathology, functional impairment and increased suicide risk. *J. Child. Psychol. Psychiatry* **2013**, *54*, 670–677. [CrossRef]
4. Weersing, V.R.; Gonzalez, A.; Campo, J.V.; Lucas, A.N. Brief behavioral therapy for pediatric anxiety and depression: Piloting an integrated treatment approach. *Cogn. Behav. Pract.* **2008**, *15*, 126–139. [CrossRef]
5. Ehrenreich-May, J.; Bilek, E.L.; Queen, A.H.; Hernandez Rodriguez, J. A unified protocol for the group treatment of childhood anxiety and depression. *Rev. Psicopatol. Psicol. Clin.* **2012**, *17*, 219–236. [CrossRef]
6. Sandín, B.; Chorot, P.; Valiente, R.M. Psicopatología de la ansiedad y trastornos de ansiedad: Hacia un enfoque transdiagnóstico [*Psychopathology of anxiety and the anxiety disorders: Towards a transdignostic perspective*]. In *Manual de Psicopatología*, 3rd ed.; Belloch, A., Sandín, B., Ramos, F., Eds.; McGraw-Hill: Madrid, Spain, 2020; Volume 2, pp. 3–34.
7. Sandín, B.; Chorot, P.; Valiente, R.M. Transdiagnóstico: Nueva frontera en psicología clínica [*Transdiagnostic: A new frontier in clinical psychology*]. *Rev. Psicopatol. Psicol. Clin.* **2012**, *17*, 185–203. [CrossRef]
8. Andersen, P.; Toner, P.; Bland, M.; McMillan, D. Effectiveness of transdiagnostic cognitive behaviour therapy for anxiety and depression in adults: A systematic review and meta-analysis. *Behav. Cogn. Psychother.* **2016**, *44*, 673–690. [CrossRef] [PubMed]
9. García-Escalera, J.; Chorot, P.; Valiente, R.M.; Reales, J.M.; Sandín, B. Efficacy of transdiagnostic cognitive-behavioral therapy for anxiety and depression in adults, children and adolescents: A meta-analysis. *Rev. Psicopatol. Psicol. Clin.* **2016**, *21*, 147–175. [CrossRef]
10. Sakiris, N.; Berle, D. A systematic review and meta-analysis of the unified protocol as a transdiagnostic emotion regulation based intervention. *Clin. Psychol. Rev.* **2019**, *72*, 1–13. [CrossRef]
11. Ehrenreich-May, J.; Kennedy, S.M.; Sherman, J.A.; Bilek, L.B.; Buzzella, B.A.; Bennett, S.M.; Barlow, D.H. *Unified Protocols for Transdiagnostic Treatment of Emotional Disorders in Children and Adolescents*; Oxford University Press: New York, NY, USA, 2018.
12. Ehrenreich, J.T.; Goldstein, C.R.; Wright, L.R.; Barlow, D.H. Development of a unified protocol for the treatment of emotional disorders in youth. *Child. Fam. Behav. Ther.* **2009**, *31*, 20–37. [CrossRef]
13. Ehrenreich-May, J.; Rosenfield, D.; Queen, A.H.; Kennedy, S.M.; Remmes, C.S.; Barlow, D.H. An initial waitlist-controlled trial of the unified protocol for the treatment of emotional disorders in adolescents. *J. Anxiety Disord.* **2017**, *46*, 46–55. [CrossRef] [PubMed]
14. Osma, J. *Aplicaciones del Protocolo Unificado Para el Tratamiento Transdiagnóstico de la Disregulación Emocional*; Alianza Editorial: Madrid, Spain, 2019.
15. Trosper, S.E.; Buzzella, B.A.; Bennett, S.M.; Ehrenreich, J.T. Emotion regulation in youth with emotional disorders: Implications for a unified treatment approach. *Clin. Child. Fam. Psychol. Rev.* **2009**, *12*, 234–254. [CrossRef] [PubMed]
16. García-Escalera, J.; Valiente, R.M.; Sandín, B.; Ehrenreich-May, J.; Prieto, A.; Chorot, P. The unified protocol for transdiagnostic treatment of emotional disorders in adolescents (UP-A) adapted as a school-based anxiety and depression prevention program: An initial cluster randomized wait-list-controlled trial. *Behav. Ther.* **2020**, *51*, 461–473. [CrossRef] [PubMed]
17. García-Escalera, J.; Chorot, P.; Sandín, B.; Ehrenreich-May, J.; Prieto, A.; Valiente, R.M. An open trial applying the unified protocol for transdiagnostic treatment of emotional disorders in adolescents (UP-A) adapted as a school-based prevention program. *Child. Youth Care Forum* **2019**, *48*, 29–53. [CrossRef]
18. Titov, N.; Dear, B.F.; Johnston, L.; Terides, M. Transdiagnostic internet treatment for anxiety and depression. *Rev. Psicopatol. Psicol. Clin.* **2012**, *17*, 237–260. [CrossRef]
19. Andersson, G.; Titov, N. Advantages and limitations of internet-based interventions for common mental disorders. *World Psychiatry* **2014**, *13*, 4–11. [CrossRef]
20. Carlbring, P.; Andersson, G.; Cuijpers, P.; Riper, H.; Hedman-Lagerlöf, E. Internet-based vs. face-to-face cognitive behavior therapy for psychiatric and somatic disorders: An updated systematic review and meta-analysis. *Cogn. Behav. Ther.* **2018**, *47*, 1–18. [CrossRef]
21. Etzelmueller, A.; Vis, C.; Karyotaki, E.; Baumeister, H.; Titov, N.; Berking, M.; Cuijpers, P.; Riper, H.; Ebert, D.D. Effects of internet-based cognitive behavioral therapy in routine care for adults in treatment for depression and anxiety: Systematic review and meta-analysis. *JMIR* **2020**, *22*, 1–27. [CrossRef]

22. Vigerland, S.; Lenhard, F.; Bonnert, M.; Lalouni, M.; Hedman, E.; Ahlen, J.; Olén, O.; Serlachius, E.; Ljótsson, B. Internet-delivered cognitive behavior therapy for children and adolescents: A systematic review and meta-analysis. *Clin. Psychol. Rev.* **2016**, *50*, 1–10. [CrossRef]
23. Barlow, D.H.; Farchione, T.J.; Sauer-Zavala, S.; Latin, H.M.; Ellard, K.K.; Bullis, J.R.; Bentley, K.H.; Boettcher, H.T.; Cassiello-Robbins, C. *Unified Protocol for Transdiagnostic Treatment of Emotional Disorders: Therapist Guide*; Oxford University Press: New York, NY, USA, 2018.
24. Gonzalez-Robles, A.; Garcia-Palacios, A.; Baños, R.; Riera, A.; Llorca, G.; Traver, F.; Haro, G.; Palop, V.; Lera, G.; Romeu, J.E.; et al. Effectiveness of a transdiagnostic internet-based protocol for the treatment of emotional disorders versus treatment as usual in specialized care: Study protocol for a randomized controlled trial. *Trials* **2015**, *16*, 488–493. [CrossRef]
25. Păsărelu, C.R.; Andersson, G.; Bergman Nordgren, L.; Dobrean, A. Internet-delivered transdiagnostic and tailored cognitive behavioral therapy for anxiety and depression: A systematic review and meta-analysis of randomized controlled trials. *Cogn. Behav. Ther.* **2017**, *46*, 1–28. [CrossRef] [PubMed]
26. Sandín, B.; Valiente, R.M.; García-Escalera, J.; Pineda, D.; Espinosa, V.; Magaz, A.M.; Chorot, P. Protocolo unificado para el tratamiento transdiagnóstico de los trastornos emocionales en adolescentes a través de internet (iUP-A): Aplicación web y protocolo de un ensayo controlado aleatorizado [*Internet-delivered unified protocol for transdiagnostic treatment of emotional disorders in adolescents (iUP-A): Web application and study protocol for a randomized controlled trial*]. *Rev. Psicopatol. Psicol. Clin.* **2019**, *24*, 197–215. [CrossRef]
27. Sheehan, D.V.; Lecrubier, Y.; Sheehan, K.H.; Amorim, P.; Janavs, J.; Weiller, E.; Hergueta, T.; Baker, R.; Dunbar, G.C. The Mini-International Neuropsychiatric Interview (MINI): The development and validation of a structured diagnostic psychiatric interview for DSM-IV and ICD-10. *J. Clin. Psychiatry* **1998**, *59*, 22–33. [CrossRef] [PubMed]
28. Colón-Soto, M.; Díaz, V.; Soto, O.; Santana, C. *Mini International Neuropsychiatric Interview Para Niños y Adolescentes (MINI-KID) Versión en Español*; Medical Outcome Symptoms: Tampa, FL, USA, 2005.
29. Des Jarlais, D.C.; Lyles, C.; Crepaz, N. TREND Group Improving the reporting quality of nonrandomized evaluations of behavioral and public health interventions: The TREND statement. *Am. J. Public Health* **2004**, *94*, 361–366. [CrossRef] [PubMed]
30. Ehrenreich-May, J.; Queen, A.H.; Bilek, E.L.; Remmes, C.S.; Kristen, K.M. The Unified Protocols for the Treatment of Emotional Disorders in Children and Adolescents. In *Transdiagnostic Treatments for Children and Adolescents: Principles and Practice*; Ehrenreich-May, J., Chu, B.C., Eds.; Guilford Press: New York, NY, USA, 2014; pp. 267–292.
31. Sandín, B.; Chorot, P.; Valiente, R.M. *TCC de los Trastornos de Ansiedad: Innovaciones en Niños y Adolescentes [CBT for Anxiety Disorders: Innovations for Children and Adolescents]*; Klinik: Madrid, Spain, 2016.
32. Sandín, B.; Chorot, P.; Valiente, R.M.; Chorpita, B.F. Development of a 30-item version of the Revised Child Anxiety and Depression Scale. *Rev. Psicopatol. Psicol. Clin.* **2010**, *15*, 165–178. [CrossRef]
33. Sandín, B. Escalas PANAS de afecto positivo y negativo para niños y adolescentes (PANASN) *[The PANAS scales of positive and negative affect for children and adolescents (PANASN)]. Rev. Psicopatol. Psicol. Clin.* **2003**, *8*, 173–182. [CrossRef]
34. Silverman, W.K.; Fleisig, W.; Rabian, B.; Peterson, R.A. Childhood anxiety sensitivity index. *J. Clin. Child. Adolesc. Psychol.* **1991**, *20*, 162–168. [CrossRef]
35. Sandín, B.; Chorot, P.; Santed, M.A.; Valiente, R.M. Análisis factorial confirmatorio del Índice de Sensibilidad a la Ansiedad para Niños *[A confirmatory factor analysis of the Childhood Anxiety Sensitivity Index]. Psicothema* **2002**, *14*, 333–339.
36. Kennedy, S.M.; Ehrenreich-May, J. Assessment of emotional avoidance in adolescents: Psychometric properties of a new multidimensional measure. *J. Psychopathol. Behav. Assess.* **2016**, *39*, 279–290. [CrossRef]
37. García-Escalera, J.; Chorot, P.; Valiente, R.; Sandín, B.; Tonarely, N.; Ehrenreich-May, J. *Spanish Version of the Emotional Avoidance Strategy Inventory for Adolescents (EASI-A)*; Universidad Nacional de Educación a Distancia: Madrid, Spain, 2016; Unpublished.
38. Sandín, B.; Chorot, P.; Valiente, R.M. *Cuestionario PSWQ para Niños y Adolescentes (PSWQN-11) [Questionnaire PSWQ for Children and Adolescents (PSWQ-11)]*; Universidad Nacional de Educación a Distancia: Madrid, Spain, 2010; Unpublished.
39. La Greca, A.M.; Stone, W.L. Social anxiety scale for children-revised: Factor structure and concurrent validity. *J. Clin. Child. Psychol.* **1993**, *22*, 17–27. [CrossRef]

40. Sandín, B. *Ansiedad, Miedos y Fobias en Niños y Adolescentes [Anxiety, Fears and Phobias in Children and Adolescents]*; Dykinson: Madrid, Spain, 1997.
41. Houck, P.R.; Spiegel, D.A.; Shear, M.K.; Rucci, P. Reliability of the self-report version of the panic disorder severity scale. *Depress. Anxiety* **2002**, *15*, 183–185. [CrossRef] [PubMed]
42. Sandín, B. Panic Disorder Severity Scale–Self Report (PDSS-SR) (Spanish version). In *Trastorno de Pánico*; Sandín, B., Ed.; UNED: Madrid, Spain, 2010.
43. Sheehan, D.V.; Sheehan, K.H.; Shytle, R.D.; Janavs, J.; Bannon, Y.; Rogers, J.E.; Milo, K.M.; Stock, S.L.; Wilkinson, B. Reliability and validity of the mini international neuropsychiatric interview for children and adolescents (MINI-KID). *J. Clin. Psychiatry* **2010**, *71*, 313–326. [CrossRef] [PubMed]
44. Valiente, R.M.; Sandín, B.; Chorot, P. Miedos comunes en niños y adolescentes: Relación con la sensibilidad a la ansiedad, el rasgo de ansiedad, la afectividad negativa y la depresión *[Common fears in children and adolescents: Their relationship to anxiety sensitivity, trait anxiety, negative affectivity, and depression]*. *Rev. Psicopatol. Psicol. Clin.* **2002**, *7*, 61–70. [CrossRef]
45. Sandín, B.; Chorot, P.; Valiente, R.M.; Lostao, L. Validación española del cuestionario de preocupación PSWQ: Estructura factorial y propiedades psicométricas *[Spanish validation of the PSWQ: Factor structure and psychometric properties]*. *Rev. Psicopatol. Psicol. Clin.* **2009**, *14*, 107–122. [CrossRef]
46. Sánchez-Arribas, C.; Chorot, P.; Valiente, R.M.; Sandín, B. Evaluación de factores cognitivos positivos y negativos relacionadas con el trastorno de pánico: Validación del CATP *[Assessment of positive and negative cognitive factors related to panic disorder: Validation of the CATP]*. *Rev. Psicopatol. Psicol. Clin.* **2015**, *20*, 85–100. [CrossRef]
47. Sandín, B.; Valiente, R.M.; García-Escalera, J.; Chorot, P. *Feasibility and Acceptability Questionnaire (FAQ)*; Universidad Nacional de Educación a Distancia: Madrid, Spain, 2020; Unpublished.
48. Rapee, R.M.; Wignall, A.; Sheffield, J.; Kowalenko, N.; Davis, A.; McLoone, J.; Spence, S.H. Adolescents' reactions to universal and indicated prevention programs for depression: Perceived stigma and consumer satisfaction. *Prevent. Sci.* **2006**, *7*, 167–177. [CrossRef]
49. Cohen, J. A power primer. *Psychol. Bull.* **1992**, *112*, 155. [CrossRef]
50. Faul, F.; Erdfelder, E.; Lang, A.-G.; Buchner, A. G*Power 3: A flexible statistical power analysis program for the social, behavioral, and biomedical sciences. *Behav. Res. Methods* **2007**, *39*, 175–191. [CrossRef]
51. De la Torre-Luque, A.; Fiol-Veny, A.; Essau, C.A.; Balle, M.; Bornas, X. Effects of a transdiagnostic cognitive behaviour therapy-based programme on the natural course of anxiety symptoms in adolescence. *J. Affect. Disord.* **2020**, *264*, 474–482. [CrossRef]
52. Fernández-Martínez, I.; Orgilés, M.; Morales, A.; Espada, J.P.; Essau, C.A. One-Year follow-up effects of a cognitive behavior therapy-based transdiagnostic program for emotional problems in young children: A school-based cluster-randomized controlled trial. *J. Affect. Disord.* **2020**, *262*, 258–266. [CrossRef]
53. Calear, A.L.; Batterham, P.J.; Poyser, C.T.; Mackinnon, A.J.; Griffiths, K.M.; Christensen, H. Cluster randomised controlled trial of the e-couch Anxiety and Worry program in schools. *J. Affect. Disord.* **2016**, *196*, 210–217. [CrossRef] [PubMed]
54. González-Robles, A.; Díaz-García, A.; García-Palacios, A.; Roca, P.; Ramos-Quiroga, J.A.; Botella, C. Effectiveness of a Transdiagnostic Guided Internet-Delivered Protocol for Emotional Disorders Versus Treatment as Usual in Specialized Care: Randomized Controlled Trial. *J. Med. Internet Res.* **2020**, *22*, 1–23. [CrossRef] [PubMed]
55. Ellard, K.K.; Bernstein, E.E.; Hearing, C.; Baek, J.H.; Sylvia, L.G.; Nierenberg, A.A.; Barlow, D.H.; Deckersbach, T. Transdiagnostic treatment of bipolar disorder and comorbid anxiety using the Unified Protocol for Emotional Disorders: A pilot feasibility and acceptability trial. *J. Affect. Disord.* **2017**, *219*, 209–221. [CrossRef] [PubMed]
56. Bilek, E.L.; Ehrenreich-May, J. An open trial investigation of a transdiagnostic group treatment for children with anxiety and depressive symptoms. *Behav. Ther.* **2012**, *43*, 887–897. [CrossRef]
57. Stallard, P.; Richardson, T.; Velleman, S.; Attwood, M. Computerized CBT (Think, Feel, Do) for depression and anxiety in children and adolescents: Outcomes and feedback from a pilot randomized controlled trial. *Behav. Cogn. Psychother.* **2011**, *39*, 273. [CrossRef]
58. Tillfors, M.; Andersson, G.; Ekselius, L.; Furmark, T.; Lewenhaupt, S.; Karlsson, A.; Carlbring, P. A randomized trial of internet-delivered treatment for social anxiety disorder in high school students. *Cogn. Behav. Ther.* **2011**, *40*, 147–157. [CrossRef] [PubMed]

59. Carlbring, P.; Gunnarsdóttir, M.; Hedensjö, L.; Andersson, G.; Ekselius, L.; Furmark, T. Treatment of social phobia: Randomised trial of internet-delivered cognitive-behavioural therapy with telephone support. *Br. J. Psychiatry* **2007**, *190*, 123–128. [CrossRef]
60. Andersson, G.; Paxling, B.; Wiwe, M.; Vernmark, K.; Felix, C.B.; Lundborg, L.; Furmark, T.; Cuijpers, P.; Carlbring, P. Therapeutic alliance in guided internet-delivered cognitive behavioural treatment of depression, generalized anxiety disorder and social anxiety disorder. *Behav. Res. Ther.* **2012**, *50*, 544–550. [CrossRef]

3

The Use of a Virtual Reality Platform for the Assessment of the Memory Decline and the Hippocampal Neural Injury in Subjects with Mild Cognitive Impairment: The Validity of Smart Aging Serious Game (SASG)

Monia Cabinio [1], Federica Rossetto [1], Sara Isernia [1], Francesca Lea Saibene [1], Monica Di Cesare [1], Francesca Borgnis [1], Stefania Pazzi [2], Tommaso Migliazza [2], Margherita Alberoni [1], Valeria Blasi [1,*] and Francesca Baglio [1]

1 IRCCS Fondazione Don Carlo Gnocchi ONLUS, via Capecelatro 66, 20148 Milan, Italy; mcabinio@dongnocchi.it (M.C.); frossetto@dongnocchi.it (F.R.); sisernia@dongnocchi.it (S.I.); fsaibene@dongnocchi.it (F.L.S.); mdicesare@dongnocchi.it (M.D.C.); fborgnis@dongnocchi.it (F.B.); malberoni@dongnocchi.it (M.A.); fbaglio@dongnocchi.it (F.B.)
2 Consorzio di Bioingegneria e Informatica medica (CBIM), 27100 Pavia, Italy; s.pazzi@cbim.it (S.P.); t.migliazza@cbim.it (T.M.)
* Correspondence: vblasi@dongnocchi.it

Abstract: Due to the lack of pharmacological treatment for dementia, timely detection of subjects at risk can be of seminal importance for preemptive rehabilitation interventions. The aim of the study was to determine the usability of the smart aging serious game (SASG), a virtual reality platform, in assessing the cognitive profile of an amnestic mild cognitive impairment (aMCI) population, its validity in discriminating aMCI from healthy controls (HC), and in detecting hippocampal degeneration, a biomarker of clinical progression towards dementia. Thirty-six aMCI and 107 HC subjects were recruited and administered the SASG together with a neuropsychological evaluation. All aMCI and 30 HC subjects performed also an MRI for hippocampal volume measurement. Results showed good usability of the SASG despite the low familiarity with technology in both groups. ROC curve analyses showed similar discriminating abilities for SASG and gold standard tests, and a greater discrimination ability compared to non-specific neuropsychological tests. Finally, linear regression analysis revealed that the SASG outperformed the Montreal cognitive assessment test (MoCA) in the ability to detect neuronal degeneration in the hippocampus on the right side. These data show that SASG is an ecological task, that can be considered a digital biomarker providing objective and clinically meaningful data about the cognitive profile of aMCI subjects.

Keywords: virtual reality; serious game; mild cognitive impairment; dementia; Alzheimer disease; digital biomarker; hippocampus; MRI; cognitive rehabilitation; computerized assessment

---

1. Introduction

Virtual reality (VR) has been defined as an application that allows users to navigate and interact with a three-dimensional computer-generated environment in real time [1]. Paralleling the advancements of information technology (IT) in the implementation of multi-dimensional platforms for the care of patients [2–4], VR gives the opportunity to improve cognitive assessment allowing more ecological and smart instruments of evaluation [5–10]. In particular, serious games (SGs), defined as "digital applications specialized for purposes other than entertaining" [11,12], with their capacity to implement

VR environments can represent an easily-accessible method to assess cognitive functions in a more ecological way, since they can host complex environments resembling real-life context with different levels of complexity [7,9,10,13].

Although the field of SGs is quite young, digital applications for clinical purposes are becoming more and more available, and some of them have been validly used in healthy subjects [10,14,15] as well as in clinical populations, particularly in Parkinson's disease [9,16] and in subjects with amnestic mild cognitive impairment (aMCI) and dementia [17–22]. Data from the literature confirm that SGs are not only appropriate but also recommended for the assessment and stimulation of elderly people with MCI and dementia [23].

Faced with the increasing number of new evaluation instruments, the need to implement scientifically valid, reliable and smart instruments to detect clinical and pre-clinical conditions in the early stages is of pivotal importance.

MCI is a "mild neurocognitive disorder" [24,25] lying on the continuum between normal aging and cognitive decline [26,27], affecting approximately 10% to 20% of adults over 65 years of age [26]. MCI is defined as a symptomatic pre-dementia stage in which the cognitive impairment does not affect the functional activities of daily living [26]. The incidence for the development of dementia in individuals with MCI older than 65 years of age is approximately 4.9% in two years [28]. Among the different forms of MCI, the amnestic form (aMCI) refers to a condition in which the memory dysfunction predominates [29] and that is associated with specific brain changes, such as reduction of hippocampal volume [30,31] and cortical thinning in medial temporal [30] and parietal [32,33] cortices. These abnormalities are specific for aMCI and represent biomarker of neuronal degeneration [34]. In particular, the reduction of the hippocampal volume is currently considered a biomarker to detect the subjects with aMCI at higher risk of cognitive decline [35,36]. Consequently, with their brain changes aMCI subjects have a higher risk of developing Alzheimer's disease (AD), when compared to non-amnestic MCI [37]. This strong association with dementia makes aMCI an important target for early pharmacological and rehabilitation interventions such as cognitive and physical exercise training [38,39]. In this line, at the beginning of 2018 the American Academy of Neurology published the new practice guidelines, underlying the importance to assess people in this pre-clinical condition using validated tools, detecting both functional impairment and cognitive status in a longitudinal way [28]. For large scale and timely screening for aMCI, more ecological tools, mimicking everyday activities, are becoming a cardinal issue. In this line, an ecological, virtual 3D environment-based tool named "smart aging" (smart aging serious game, SASG-http://www.cbim.it/en_new/serious-games-en/index.html [7,10]), aimed at evaluating multiple cognitive domains, was developed. The SASG integrates five cognitive tasks in a setting resembling a real house. Subjects are asked to play the tasks of the game following simple instructions while moving through the rooms, while the software evaluates performance accuracy and reaction times. When tested in a large cohort of aged cognitively-preserved subjects, SASG was demonstrated to be a valid tool for assessing cognitive functions [10]. The interface of SASG is specifically designed to be easily accessible to older or non-expert computer users by means of a touchscreen, a first-person perspective, and an automatic navigation system.

According to these premises, the present study had a three-fold aim: 1. to evaluate the usability of SASG in a cohort of aMCI patients and healthy controls (HC), taking into account the familiarity with the used technology; 2. to investigate the validity of SASG in discriminating between aMCI and healthy control subjects in comparison with gold standard pencil paper neuropsychological tests; and 3. to determine the validity of the SASG in detecting hippocampal degeneration as a neuroimaging marker of neuronal injury in comparison to gold standard pencil paper neuropsychological tests.

2. Materials and Methods

2.1. Recruited Sample

A total sample of 139 subjects participated in the study. Subjects with a diagnosis of aMCI ($n = 32$) were consecutively recruited from the outpatient memory clinic at the IRCCS Fondazione Don Carlo Gnocchi ONLUS (FDG, Milan, Italy). The inclusion criteria were: (1) aMCI diagnosis according to the recommendations of the National Institute on Aging [27] and the DSM 5 diagnostic criteria [24]; (2) presence of a mini-mental state examination [40] score ≥ 24, corrected for age and years of education according to Italian normative data [41]; (3) age ≥ 65 years and school attendance ≥3 years; (4) abnormal memory function confirmed by an informant and documented by the neuropsychological examination; (5) no impairment in functional activities of daily living as determined by a clinical interview with both the patient and the caregiver; (6) absence of psychiatric illnesses, with particular attention to depressive symptoms (Hamilton depression rating scale score ≤ 12 [42]) and severe behavioral disturbance; (7) absence of severe auditory/visual loss that can prevent from the use of technological device and from the execution of the serious game; (8) absence of major brain abnormalities at MRI scan or significant cerebral vascular diseases (Hachinski score above 4) [43].

A sample of age-, gender- and education-matched HC ($n = 107$) was also included. HC were obtained from the CBIM repository and from volunteers recruited from FDG. In more detail, HC were recruited from universities of the third age, social clubs and among volunteers working in the FDG and caregivers of outpatients. All the HC lived independently, had active social and cognitive lives and were native Italian speakers. They underwent an in-clinic neuropsychological evaluation including MMSE score and a neurological interview to exclude major neurological complaint. They fit the inclusion criteria number 3, 5, 6 and 7 of the above listing and presented a MMSE ≥ 28. The study was approved by the Ethics Committee of the Don Gnocchi Foundation and all subjects signed a written and informed consent.

2.2. Neuropsychological Evaluation

All subjects performed in a clinical setting and in close proximity with SASG completion, a neuropsychological evaluation. This was conducted by a trained neuropsychologist using conventional pencil–paper test including:

[i] the Montreal cognitive assessment test (MoCA): an established rapid cognitive screening tool able to differentiate MCI from normal aging and from AD patients, with a high sensitivity and specificity [44,45]. Raw data were corrected according to Italian normative data [46].

[ii] the immediate and delayed recall scores obtained from the free and cued selective reminding test (FCSRT, [47]), a widely used memory test that provides details on the encoding and retrieval phases of the memorization processes. Data were corrected according to [48].

[iii] the trail making test (TMT, [49]), versions A and B, for the assessment of executive functions and mental flexibility, as well as visual search, and processing speed. Data were corrected according to [50].

2.3. Serious Game Task: The Smart Aging Serious Game (SASG)

Each subject was asked to complete, in a clinical setting, a single SASG (http://www.cbim.it/en_new/serious-games-en/index.html) session, extensively described elsewhere [6,7,10]. Shortly, the SASG was administered in presence of a neuropsychologist and was performed using a touch-screen monitor, in a first-person perspective. SAGS is an ecological serious game based on a virtual house, in which subjects are asked to interact with the different parts of the scenario and to perform specific tasks. All the actions performed by the subjects within the SAGS are recorded and measured, allowing the assessment of memory, executive functions, working memory, and visual spatial processes [10] through the execution of five tasks. Task 1 (T1), named "Object search", investigates memory, spatial orientation and attention; task 2 (T2), called "Water the flowers while listening to the radio", assesses executive functions and divided attention; task 3 (T3), "Make a phone call", evaluates executive functions, selective attention, working and perspective memory; task 4 (T4), "Choose the right object", investigates memory and task 5 (T5), "Find the objects", assesses long-term memory (recall), spatial orientation and attention.

In order to familiarize with the virtual environment and the use of the touch screen before the actual evaluative session, subjects naïve in the use of ICT and touch screens, were presented with a 10-min interactive demo. Successively, no other feedback was provided while the subjects were performing the serious games.

In line with Bottiroli (2017) [10], we collected accuracy (accuracy index, AI) and time (time index, TI) measurements for each SAGS task. AI and TI were then converted into z-scores considering the mean and standard deviation of the HC sample. For each task a total score was computed (as the difference between AI and TI, in line with [10] and the sum of the total scores of all tasks was computed to calculate the Smart Aging Total Score (SASG-Total).

Computer familiarity measures were collected with an ad hoc questionnaire according to [51]. Specifically, each subject was asked to fill out a computer questionnaire concerning its familiarity with computers and touch-screen use, expressed in terms of frequency of use, before SASG session.

2.4. MRI Acquisition and Analysis

All of the aMCI performed a single brain MRI acquisition (1.5 T Siemens Magnetom Avanto, Erlangen, Germany) within two weeks from the neuropsychological evaluation, to collect a high-resolution 3D-T1 image (MPRAGE; TR/TE = 1900/3.37 ms, FoV = 192 mm × 256 mm, in-plane resolution 1 mm × 1 mm, slice thickness = 1 mm, number of axial slices = 176) in order to measure hippocampal volumes. The MRI protocol included a dual-echo turbo spin echo proton density PD/T2-weighted image (repetition time (TR) = 5550 ms, echo time (TE) = 23/103 ms, matrix size = 320 × 320 × 45, resolution 0.8 × 0.8 × 3 mm^3) for the evaluation of the white matter hyperintensities.

High-resolution T1 images have been analyzed using Freesurfer's recon-all pipeline (https://surfer.nmr.mgh.harvard.edu/, [52]) and total hippocampal volumes have been segmented using the hippocampal subfield segmentation tool of Freesurfer (v.6.0) [53], basing on a statistical postmortem atlas built primarily upon ultra-high resolution (~0.1 mm isotropic) MRI data. Quality checks were performed at each step of the pipeline, and at the end of the cortical parcellation according to ENIGMA guidelines (http://enigma.ini.usc.edu). Total intracranial volume (TIV) has been computed using Freesurfer automatic subcortical segmentation, on the basis of the probabilistic aseg atlas [54]. Hippocampal volumes were then normalized for the total intracranial volume obtaining a normalized value (n-Hipp), using a proportional approach [55].

2.5. Statistical Analyses

Statistical analyses have been performed using MedCalc 18.5 (http://www.medcalc.org). Descriptive statistics included relative and absolute frequencies for categorical variables, median and IQ range for non-normally distributed continuous measures and means and standard deviation (SD) for continuous measures. The normality of data distribution was assessed considering the skewness and kurtosis coefficients and an appropriate parametric/non-parametric test was used for statistical analyses. When appropriate, data were corrected for multiple comparison using the Bonferroni correction, dividing the α-value (0.05) by the number of statistical tests on dependent variables.

Direct comparisons (one-way ANOVA or Mann–Whitney) on age, gender and educational level were performed to assess the between-groups matching for these variables. In order to assess the presence of hippocampal degeneration, n-Hipp volume of aMCI group was compared to an internal dataset of 30 healthy subjects with comparable age, gender and education and with the same inclusion criteria defined in the Section 2.1.

For aim 1, i.e., evaluating the usability of SASG, a between-groups comparison was performed on the results of the computer and touch screen familiarity questionnaire with a chi-squared analysis.

The key performance indicator considered for the usability of the platform was the percentage of subjects that completed the SASG evaluation (all 5 tasks). Moreover, in order to test the influence of the familiarity with computers and the SASG score, a 2 × 2 ANOVA with clinical group (aMCI vs HC) and frequency of computer use factor (infrequent vs. frequent) on SASG total score data was performed.

For aim 2, that is, determining the validity of SASG in discriminating between aMCI and HC, we performed between groups direct comparisons (one-way ANOVA or Mann–Whitney) for SASG, for the conventional pencil–paper test used to detect aMCI (MoCA total score, FCSRT scores), and for pencil paper–tests not focused on mnemonic functions (TMT-A and B). To further investigate the validity of SASG, a ROC (Receiver Operating Characteristics) curve analysis was performed to determine differences in the sensitivity and specificity of SASG in comparison with MoCA, FCSRT, TMT A and B. On the basis of our ROC curves, the best cut-off score for SASG in discriminating between HC and MCI was also investigated (Youden J index).

Finally, for aim 3, i.e., determining the ability of SASG to detect the hippocampal neuronal loss, a partial correlation analysis was performed between SASG Task total score (SASG-Total) and n-Hipp and between MoCA test and n-Hipp. Age, gender and years of education were included as a covariate of no interest. Only tasks that resulted significantly correlated with n-Hipp volume were entered into a linear regression analysis.

3. Results

3.1. Demographics and SASG Usability

Demographics of the recruited sample are detailed in Table 1. No between-group differences in age, education and gender were found. As expected, the two groups differed in the MMSE score. Moreover, aMCI subjects showed significantly lower n-Hipp volume bilaterally compared to the HC group belonging to the MRI internal database (n = 27; mean age 73.59 ± 4.88 years; nine males, mean education 11.59 ± 3.81 years; MMSE 29.33 ± 0.89). Due to movement artifacts, two subjects with aMCI were excluded from MRI data analyses (n = 30; mean age 76.07 ± 4.73 years, 15 males, mean education 10.87 ± 3.80; MMSE 27.69 ± 1.76).

Table 1. Group comparison to compare healthy controls (HC) and amnestic mild cognitive impairment (aMCI) groups for demographic variables.

	aMCI	HC	*p*-Value [η2; Observed Power]
n	32	107	
Age, yrs (mean ± SD)	76.75 ± 5.31	76.47 ± 3.03	n.s.
Gender (M:F)	17:15	54:53	n.s. #
Education, yrs (mean ± SD)	10.75 ± 3.84	10.95 ± 4.09	n.s.
MMSE	27.65 ± 1.79	28.74 ± 1.27	0.0027
N-Hipp volume	n = 30	n = 27	
Left n-Hipp (mean ± SD)	0.001710 ± 0.0000	0.002055 ± 0.0000	<0.001 ** [0.22; 0.96]
Right n-Hipp (mean ± SD)	0.001783 ± 0.0000	0.002099 ± 0.0000	<0.001 ** [0.26; 0.99]

n: number of subjects; yrs: years; SD: standard deviation; M: male; F: female; MMSE: mini mental state examination; N-Hipp volume: normalized hippocampal volume; # Chi-squared Test; ** ANOVA = age and education as covariates and (η2 partial value; observed power).

Results from the computer familiarity scale (Table 2) shows no differences between groups in the frequency of computer use, with 53.12% of aMCI and 60.38% of HC subjects who never used a PC, while the remaining had a frequent use (at least weekly). The frequency of use of a touch screen was comparable between groups: 62.5% of aMCI and 72.65% of HC who had never used a touch screen before the participation in the study; 18.75% of aMCI and 20.75% of HC who used it unfrequently (not more than once a month); and 18.75% of aMCI and 6.60% of HC who had a frequent (at least weekly) use. All the subjects from both groups completed the five tasks of the SASG session indicating an appropriate level of usability of the digital tool also for a population of aMCI. Testing the influence of familiarity on SASG score our ANOVA 2 × 2 results shows significant group effect (F(1134) = 64.109,

$p < 0.001$), however, the effect of frequency of use factor was not significant ($F(1134) = 2.975$, $p = 0.087$) and no significant interactions were found ($F(1134) = 0.74$, $p = 0.391$), indicating that familiarity with the use of the PC did not influence SASG score.

Table 2. Frequency of use for technological devices in our sample.

	aMCI	HC	*p*-Value
n	32	106	
Frequency of computer use			
Infrequent % (*n*)	53.12% (17)	60.38% (64)	n.s. #
Frequent (at least once a week) % (*n*)	46.88% (15)	39.62% (42)	
Frequency of use of a touch screen (last year)			
Never % (*n*)	62.5% (20)	72.64% (77)	n.s. #
Infrequent % (*n*)	18.75% (6)	20.76% (22)	
Frequent (at least once a week) % (*n*)	18.75% (6)	6.60% (7)	

n: number of subjects; # Chi-squared test; n.s.: not significant.

3.2. Neuropsychological Assessment Results

Data relative to the neuropsychological evaluation (Table 3) reveal that for the MoCA test total score the aMCI group performance was within the normal range (see cut-off values in Table 3) but significantly worse than the HC. As for the memory performances, assessed with the FCSRT test, the aMCI group performed worse than controls and below the cut-off value in all four indices assessing immediate and delayed free and total recall memory. On the contrary, the performances at the TMT A and B test were in the normal range and comparable between groups.

Table 3. Neuropsychological evaluation. ES = Equivalent Score. ES = 0 pathological score; ES = 1 borderline range.

Test	aMCI	HC	Cut-off (ES = 0)	ES = 1	*p*-Value
n	32	107			
MoCA (mean ± SD)	22.26 ± 2.84	26.97 ± 2.35	≤15.50	15.51–18.28	**<0.001** *
FCSRT (median, IQ range)					
IFR adjusted	19.59 (15.79 to 23.80)	27.38 (25.38 to 29.42)	≤19.59	19.60–22.53	**<0.0001** §
ITR	36 (33.5 to 36.00)	36 (36.0 to 36)	<35	–	**0.0005** §
DFR adjusted	6.12 (2.67 to 10.16)	9.67 (8.67 to 10.89)	≤6.31	6.32–7.66	**<0.0001** §
DTR	12 (9.5 to 12.0)	12 (12 to 12)	<11	–	**<0.0001** §
TMT (median, IQ range)					
TMT-A	39 (21.5 to 64.0)	40 (28.0 to 59.0)	>93	93–69	n.s §
TMT-B	91 (55.0 to 182.75)	77.5 (49 to 115)	>282	282–178	n.s. §

n: number of subjects; MoCA: Montreal cognitive assessment—adjusted total scores [46]; FCSRT: free and cued selective reminding test [48]; IFR: immediate free recall; ITR: immediate total recall; DFR: delayed free recall; DTR: delayed total recall; TMT: trail making test [49]; in bold = *p*-values surviving Bonferroni's correction ($p < 0.007$) * One-Way ANOVA; § Mann–Whitney test.

3.3. SASG Results

Results of the SASG (Table 4) show significant differences between groups in the accuracy of all SASG tasks, with the exception of T2 and T3, and in the time indices of all subtests except the T4. SASG-total is significantly lower in the aMCI group.

ROC curves were computed to evaluate the diagnostic sensitivity and specificity of SASG-total and all the pencil–paper neuropsychological tests (Figure 1, Table 5). The results show high values for both parameters for all tests except the TMT A and B. Moreover, the ROC comparison analysis reveals that SASG-total is comparable to MoCA and FCSRT in the ability to discriminate between groups, while the comparison with TMT A and B reveals significantly higher ability for the SASG-total.

Table 4. Smart aging serious game (SASG) evaluation, expressed in z-scores. Mann–Whitney test. Effect size (d) and power are also included for each statistic.

Test	aMCI (Mean, IQ)	HC (Mean, IQ)	*p*-Value	Effect Size (d)	Power (1-β err prob)
SASG Accuracy Index (AI)					
Task 1	−0.96 (−1.60 to −0.31)	0.12 (−0.31 to 0.55)	**<0.0001**	1.04	0.99
Task 2	0.48 (0.10 to 0.74)	0.23 (−0.28 to 0.68)	0.040	0.33	0.36
Task 3	−0.78 (−0.78 to 0.83)	0.83 (−0.78 to 0.83)	0.026	0.45	0.59
Task 4	−0.99 (−2.39 to 0.15)	0.41 (−0.15 to 0.98)	**<0.0001**	0.94	0.99
Task 5	−1.75 (−2.51 to −0.63)	0.50 (−0.06 to 0.50)	**<0.0001**	1.28	0.99
SASG Time index (TI)					
Task 1	1.02 (0.72 to 1.53)	−0.06 (−0.70 to 0.65)	**<0.0001**	1.26	0.99
Task 2	0.63 (0.28 to 1.40)	−0.01 (−0.57 to 0.50)	**<0.0001**	0.90	0.99
Task 3	1.03 (0.69 to 1.46)	−0.19 (−0.78 to 0.77)	**<0.0001**	1.19	0.99
Task 4	0.45 (−0.20 to 0.69)	0.15 (−0.78 to 0.74)	n.s.	0.34	0.37
Task 5	1.33 (1.28 to 1.38)	−0.30 (−0.90 to 1.19)	**<0.0001**	1.81	0.99
SASG−Total	−8.29 (−12.04 to −4.90)	0.84 (−3.07 to 3.71)	**<0.0001**	1.61	0.99

SASG-total: smart aging serious game total score; in bold = *p*-values surviving Bonferroni correction ($p < 0.005$).

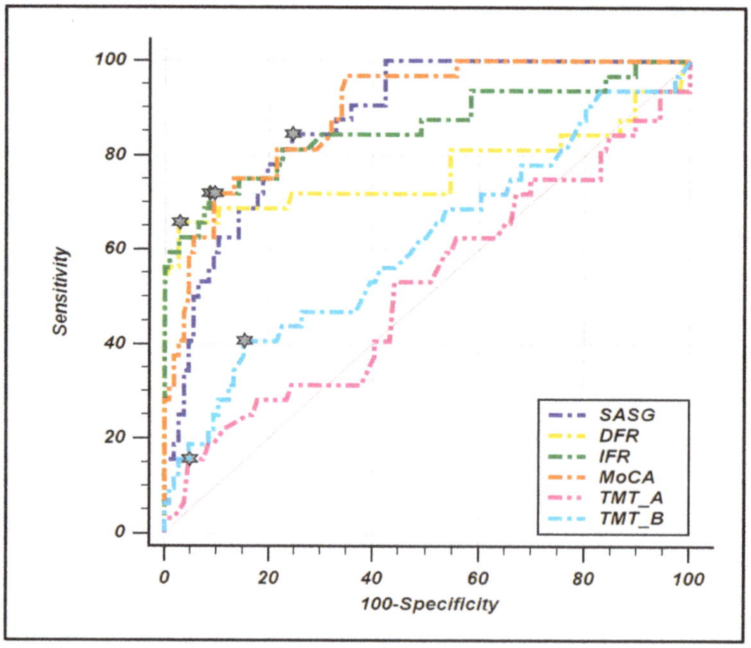

Figure 1. ROC curve comparison between smart aging total score and conventional paper-and-pencil test. Little stars indicate the criterion associated to Youden J statistic.

Table 5. Statistical comparison between the SASG ROC curve and other tests in terms of sensitivity, specificity, AUC, SE and confidence intervals.

Test	Sensitivity	Specificity	AUC	SE	95% CI	*p*-Value	Criterion Value (J Index)
SASG-Total	84.4	75.5	0.88	0.03	0.81 to 0.92	–	≤−3.28 (0.60)
MoCA (adj)	71.9	90.6	0.89	0.03	0.81 to 0.94	n.s.	≤23.44 (0.62)
FCSRT – DFR (adj)	65.6	97.2	0.76	0.06	0.67 to 0.83	n.s.	≤6.78 (0.63)
FCSRT – IFR (adj)	71.9	91.5	0.85	0.05	0.79 to 0.91	n.s.	≤22.35 (0.63)
TMT-A (adj)	15.6	95.3	0.52	0.06	0.43 to 0.60	<0.0001	≤14 (0.11)
TMT-B (adj)	40.63	84.91	0.61	0.06	0.53 to 0.70	0.0001	>130 (0.25)

Results have been considered as statistically significant when surviving Bonferroni corrected threshold, $p < 0.01$. *p*-value = comparison with SASG-Total. AOC: area under the curve; SE: standard error; CI: confidence interval; J: Youden J statistic; SASG-total: smart aging serious game total score; MoCA: Montreal cognitive assessment; FCSRT: free and cued selective reminding test; DFR: delayed free recall; IFR: immediate free recall; TMT: trail making test; adj: adjusted.

3.4. SASG, MoCA and Hippocampal Volume

When investigating the presence of neuronal degeneration through n-Hipp volume, we found a significant volumetric reduction in aMCI compared to HC subjects bilaterally (Table 1). Moreover, results of the partial correlations between SASG-total and neuropsychological variables (MoCA, FCSRT and TMT) with hippocampal volume reveal significant correlation between right n-Hipp volume and the serious game. No significant relation is present with MoCA score FCSRT and TMT after Bonferroni correction (Table 6).

Table 6. Partial correlations between test and normalized hippocampal volume. Age, gender and education have been included as covariates of no interest. Results have been considered as statistically significant when surviving Bonferroni-corrected threshold ($p < 0.008$).

		Left n-Hipp	Right n-Hipp
n		30	30
SASG-Total			
	Corr	0.28	0.50
	p-value	n.s.	0.0076
MoCA			
	Corr	−0.08	0.06
	p-value	n.s.	n.s.
FCSRT-IFR/DFR			
	Corr	0.30/0.4673	0.39/0.48
	p-value	n.s./0.0140	0.046/0.011
TMT-A/B			
	Corr	0.29/0.24	0.15/0.08
	p-value	n.s./n.s.	n.s./n.s.

n-Hipp: normalized hippocampal volume; SASG-total: smart aging serious game total score; Corr: correlation coefficient r; MoCA: Montreal cognitive assessment; FCSRT: free and cued selective reminding test; DFR: delayed free recall; IFR: immediate free recall; TMT: trail making test; n.s.: not significant.

Finally, a linear regression analysis to evaluate the predictive value of SASG to determine hippocampal volume reveals a significant relationship between right n-Hipp and SASG-total (R^2: 0.14; *p*-value: 0.042).

4. Discussion

The recent technological advancements in digital medicine have fostered the development of innovative tools for a better care of people's health and wellbeing [56]. In the last years, several lines of research have led to the development of innovative ICT solutions to perform cognitive evaluation with the use of SGs, virtually reality based instruments able to reproduce more ecological environments, in both healthy and neurological populations [5,7–10,16,23]. Recent data demonstrated the usability and efficacy of SG for the early detection and monitoring of cognitive impairment in neurodegenerative disorders [57].

The first aim of the present study was to test the usability of an innovative virtual reality tool, the smart aging serious game (SASG) platform, in a cohort of aMCI subjects.

In our sample, the majority of subjects (whether aMCI or HC) had never used a PC and a touch screen before performing the SASG session. Despite this finding, no effects of familiarity were found on the SASG score and all the participants were able to go through the whole SASG session in a clinical setting, indicating a good level of usability. This result confirms the good usability of the platform for our sample. Indeed, SASG interface was specifically implemented for older and non-expert users and did not necessitate skilled abilities [6,10]. All the aspects of the usability of the platform were considered in a previous work [6] and several technical precautions were considered. For instance, to overcome the difficulties in navigating through 3D scenarios, the touch screen was found to be more usable than the mouse. Moreover, these data suggest the possibility to also use the SASG platform remotely from the patient's home. This last use, though, will require a dedicated validation.

The second aim of the study was to determine the validity of the SASG in discriminating between a preclinical population with aMCI and successful aging subjects. Data on well-established pencil–paper tests confirmed the amnestic profile of the aMCI population that showed reduced scores in the MoCA test, and in the immediate and delayed FCSRT subtests and relative total scores [58]. On the contrary, as expected no differences between groups were found in the TMT tests, a task specifically targeted to measure visual–motor skills, mental flexibility, processing speed and sequencing [59]. This confirms the specificity of the amnestic impairment of the aMCI a preclinical condition with a high risk to develop AD type of dementia. The cognitive profile using SASG depicts a picture similar to the one observed with conventional paper-and-pencil tests. In detail, considering only the accuracy (i.e., independently from the time of execution), aMCI have a reduced performance in all tasks involving mnemonic functions (T1, T4 and T5) with preserved competences in tasks involving mainly executive functions and attention (T2 and T3). When considering the time of execution (i.e., independently from the accuracy), results show a slowdown in aMCI in all tasks except task 4, the only one presenting with a reduced visual complexity due to the bi-dimensional aspect of the scenario and thus not requesting an increased cognitive effort to deal with the greater graphical complexity of a 3D-environment [7,10]. Given the comparable unfamiliarity with technology in both groups, the reduced performances in the aMCI versus HC subjects can be reasonably interpreted as the result of the different neuropsychological profile. Taken together, these data highlight the validity of SASG in discriminating aMCI from HC.

To further investigate this issue, we calculated the specificity and sensitivity of SASG and compared them to those of gold standard tests for aMCI detection, the MoCA test and the immediate and delayed recall of the FCSRT. Results of these analyses show that SASG has a very good performance (AUC: 0.879) in discriminating between groups, and these are statistically comparable to immediate and delayed recall of the FCSRT and to MoCA test, as shown with the ROC analysis. This is in agreement with data demonstrating the validity of the FCSRT in detecting memory deficits in subjects at risk of AD, making the use of this test recommended by the International Working Group (IWG) [11]. Finally, SASG results in a significantly higher sensitivity and specificity when compared to the TMT. This result was expected due to lack of involvement of mnemonic abilities in the TMT. Taken together these data demonstrate the validity of SASG in detecting mild neurocognitive deficits involving the memory domain that do not impact the functionality of everyday life such as in the aMCI condition [26].

Finally, the third aim was to test the relationship between the SASG tasks and the hippocampal volumes. Results show that SGSA is comparable to FCSRT and outperforms MoCA in the ability to detect the reduction in the hippocampal volume. This datum is very important since pre-morbid hippocampal volume is predictive of a subsequent clinical progression towards AD and it is thus considered a biomarker [35,36]. In a previous study by Sarazin et al. [60], the FCSRT was proved to be correlated with left hippocampal volume, particularly in the CA1 region in AD patients [60]. In our study we found a significant relationship between SASG performance and right hippocampus volume. Interestingly, this asymmetric relationship can be due to the visual–spatial nature of the task. The right hippocampus has been indeed demonstrated to be involved in memory for locations within an environment, and this corresponds to some of the tasks involved in the SASG evaluation (see [61] for a review).

5. Conclusions

In conclusion, this virtual-based tool constitutes an ecological and clinically meaningful task, useful to assess the cognitive profile in subjects with subtle and selective memory complaints such as aMCI subjects. SASG has substantial advantages that make it useful even in a clinical context: it is user friendly, ecological and motivating for the users [10,62]. The integration of technology into cognitive assessment practices provides a new ground for a modern approach to neuropsychology, making it able to digitally collect and combine a higher number of variables in a better evaluation of the behavioral profile. This aspect is of seminal importance and, in this perspective, the SASG represents an ecological tool for the timely detection of the functional impairment of this clinical condition, as recommended in the practical guidelines on MCI of the American Academy of Neurology [28]. Moreover, the significant relationship of SASG performance with the right hippocampal volume demonstrates how results on this task hold the potential to offer a putative digital biomarker able to capture the aMCI condition. The herein presented data are relevant because they show the efficacy of SASG in recognition of patients at risk to develop AD in a pre-clinical stage. Considering the lack of pharmacological treatments for this condition, early detection of subjects at risk is decisive for the implementation of timely and effective rehabilitation interventions as the only opportunity to reduce the risk and the impact of the cognitive decline.

Author Contributions: Conceptualization, F.B. (Francesca Baglio) and V.B. Recruitment of subjects, M.A. and S.P. Software, S.P. and T.M. Data collection, F.R., S.I., F.L.S., M.D.C. and F.B. (Francesca Borgnis). Statistical analyses and data interpretation, M.C., V.B., and F.B. (Francesca Baglio). Writing first draft, M.C., V.B., F.B. (Francesca Baglio). Writing—review and editing, all authors. All authors have read and agreed to the published version of the manuscript.

Acknowledgments: In memoriam of Professor Massimo Musicco, an eminent scientist in the field of Dementia. The authors are grateful for his help in data analyses and interpretation.

References

1. Pratt, D.R.; Zyda, M.; Kelleher, K. Virtual reality: In the mind of the beholder. *IEEE Computer* **1995**, *7*, 17–19.
2. Realdon, O.; Rossetto, F.; Nalin, M.; Baroni, I.; Cabinio, M.; Fioravanti, R.; Saibene, F.L.; Alberoni, M.; Mantovani, F.; Romano, M.; et al. Technology-enhanced multi-domain at home continuum of care program with respect to usual care for people with cognitive impairment: The Ability-TelerehABILITation study protocol for a randomized controlled trial. *BMC Psychiatry* **2016**, *16*, 425. [CrossRef] [PubMed]
3. Wiederhold, B.K.; Riva, G. Virtual reality therapy: emerging topics and future challenges. *Cyberpsychol. Behav. Soc. Netw.* **2019**, *22*, 3–6. [CrossRef] [PubMed]
4. Colombo, D.; Fernandez-Alvarez, J.; Patane, A.; Semonella, M.; Kwiatkowska, M.; Garcia-Palacios, A.; Cipresso, P.; Riva, G.; Botella, C. Current state and future directions of technology-based ecological momentary assessment and intervention for major depressive disorder: A systematic review. *J. Clin. Med.* **2019**, *8*, 465. [CrossRef]
5. Realdon, O.; Serino, S.; Savazzi, F.; Rossetto, F.; Cipresso, P.; Parsons, T.D.; Cappellini, G.; Mantovani, F.; Mendozzi, L.; Nemni, R.; et al. An ecological measure to screen executive functioning in MS: The Picture interpretation test (PIT) 360 degrees. *Sci. Rep.* **2019**, *9*, 1–8. [CrossRef]
6. Zucchella, C.; Capone, A.; Codella, V.; Vecchione, C.; Buccino, G.; Sandrini, G.; Pierelli, F.; Bartolo, M. Assessing and restoring cognitive functions early after stroke. *Funct. Neurol.* **2014**, *29*, 255–262. [CrossRef]
7. Zucchella, C.; Sinforiani, E.; Tassorelli, C.; Cavallini, E.; Tost-Pardell, D.; Grau, S.; Pazzi, S.; Puricelli, S.; Bernini, S.; Bottiroli, S.; et al. Serious games for screening pre-dementia conditions: From virtuality to reality? A pilot project. *Funct. Neurol.* **2014**, *29*, 153–158.
8. Fabbri, L.; Mosca, I.E.; Gerli, F.; Martini, L.; Pancani, S.; Lucidi, G.; Savazzi, F.; Baglio, F.; Vannetti, F.; Macchi, C. GOAL working group the games for older adults active life (GOAL) project for people with mild cognitive impairment and vascular cognitive impairment: A study protocol for a randomized controlled trial. *Front. Neurol.* **2019**, *9*, 1040. [CrossRef]
9. Serino, S.; Baglio, F.; Rossetto, F.; Realdon, O.; Cipresso, P.; Parsons, T.D.; Cappellini, G.; Mantovani, F.; De Leo, G.; Nemni, R.; et al. Picture interpretation test (PIT) 360 degrees: An innovative measure of executive functions. *Sci. Rep.* **2017**, *7*, 1–10. [CrossRef]
10. Bottiroli, S.; Tassorelli, C.; Lamonica, M.; Zucchella, C.; Cavallini, E.; Bernini, S.; Sinforiani, E.; Pazzi, S.; Cristiani, P.; Vecchi, T.; et al. Smart aging platform for evaluating cognitive functions in aging: A comparison with the MoCA in a normal population. *Front. Aging Neurosci.* **2017**, *9*, 1–14. [CrossRef]
11. Dubois, B.; Feldman, H.H.; Jacova, C.; Hampel, H.; Molinuevo, J.L.; Blennow, K.; DeKosky, S.T.; Gauthier, S.; Selkoe, D.; Bateman, R.; et al. Advancing research diagnostic criteria for Alzheimer's disease: The IWG-2 criteria. *Lancet Neurol.* **2014**, *13*, 614–629. [CrossRef]
12. Robert, P.H.; Konig, A.; Amieva, H.; Andrieu, S.; Bremond, F.; Bullock, R.; Ceccaldi, M.; Dubois, B.; Gauthier, S.; Kenigsberg, P.A.; et al. Recommendations for the use of serious games in people with alzheimer's disease, related disorders and frailty. *Front. Aging Neurosci.* **2014**, *6*, 54. [CrossRef] [PubMed]

13. Valladares-Rodriguez, S.; Perez-Rodriguez, R.; Anido-Rifon, L.; Fernandez-Iglesias, M. Trends on the application of serious games to neuropsychological evaluation: A scoping review. *J. Biomed. Inform.* **2016**, *64*, 296–319. [CrossRef] [PubMed]
14. Savazzi, F.; Isernia, S.; Jonsdottir, J.; Di Tella, S.; Pazzi, S.; Baglio, F. Design and implementation of a serious game on neurorehabilitation: Data on modifications of functionalities along implementation releases. *Data Brief.* **2018**, *20*, 864–869. [CrossRef]
15. Savazzi, F.; Isernia, S.; Jonsdottir, J.; Di Tella, S.; Pazzi, S.; Baglio, F. Engaged in learning neurorehabilitation: Development and validation of a serious game with user-centered design. *Comput. Educ.* **2018**, *125*, 53–61. [CrossRef]
16. Cipresso, P.; Albani, G.; Serino, S.; Pedroli, E.; Pallavicini, F.; Mauro, A.; Riva, G. Virtual multiple errands test (VMET): A virtual reality-based tool to detect early executive functions deficit in Parkinson's disease. *Front. Behav. Neurosci.* **2014**, *8*, 405. [CrossRef]
17. Plancher, G.; Tirard, A.; Gyselinck, V.; Nicolas, S.; Piolino, P. Using virtual reality to characterize episodic memory profiles in amnestic mild cognitive impairment and Alzheimer's disease: Influence of active and passive encoding. *Neuropsychologia* **2012**, *50*, 592–602. [CrossRef]
18. Lee, J.Y.; Kho, S.; Yoo, H.B.; Park, S.; Choi, J.S.; Kwon, J.S.; Cha, K.R.; Jung, H.Y. Spatial memory impairments in amnestic mild cognitive impairment in a virtual radial arm maze. *Neuropsychiatr. Dis. Treat.* **2014**, *10*, 653–660. [CrossRef]
19. Manera, V.; Petit, P.D.; Derreumaux, A.; Orvieto, I.; Romagnoli, M.; Lyttle, G.; David, R.; Robert, P.H. 'Kitchen and cooking,' a serious game for mild cognitive impairment and Alzheimer's disease: A pilot study. *Front. Aging Neurosci.* **2015**, *7*, 24. [CrossRef]
20. Fukui, Y.; Yamashita, T.; Hishikawa, N.; Kurata, T.; Sato, K.; Omote, Y.; Kono, S.; Yunoki, T.; Kawahara, Y.; Hatanaka, N.; et al. Computerized touch-panel screening tests for detecting mild cognitive impairment and Alzheimer's disease. *Intern. Med.* **2015**, *54*, 895–902. [CrossRef]
21. Zygouris, S.; Giakoumis, D.; Votis, K.; Doumpoulakis, S.; Ntovas, K.; Segkouli, S.; Karagiannidis, C.; Tzovaras, D.; Tsolaki, M. Can a virtual reality cognitive training application fulfill a dual role? Using the virtual supermarket cognitive training application as a screening tool for mild cognitive impairment. *J. Alzheimers Dis.* **2015**, *44*, 1333–1347. [CrossRef] [PubMed]
22. Allain, P.; Foloppe, D.A.; Besnard, J.; Yamaguchi, T.; Etcharry-Bouyx, F.; Le Gall, D.; Nolin, P.; Richard, P. Detecting everyday action deficits in Alzheimer's disease using a nonimmersive virtual reality kitchen. *J. Int. Neuropsychol. Soc.* **2014**, *20*, 468–477. [CrossRef] [PubMed]
23. Manera, V.; Ben-Sadoun, G.; Aalbers, T.; Agopyan, H.; Askenazy, F.; Benoit, M.; Bensamoun, D.; Bourgeois, J.; Bredin, J.; Bremond, F.; et al. Recommendations for the use of serious games in neurodegenerative disorders: 2016 Delphi panel. *Front. Psychol.* **2017**, *8*, 1243. [CrossRef] [PubMed]
24. American Psychiatric Association (APA). *Diagnostic and Statistical Manual of Mental Disorders (DSM V)*; American Psychiatric: Washington, DC, USA, 2013.
25. Stokin, G.B.; Krell-Roesch, J.; Petersen, R.C.; Geda, Y.E. Mild neurocognitive disorder: An old wine in a new bottle. *Harv. Rev. Psychiatry* **2015**, *23*, 368–376. [CrossRef] [PubMed]
26. Langa, K.M.; Levine, D.A. The diagnosis and management of mild cognitive impairment: A clinical review. *JAMA* **2014**, *312*, 2551–2561. [CrossRef] [PubMed]
27. Albert, M.S.; DeKosky, S.T.; Dickson, D.; Dubois, B.; Feldman, H.H.; Fox, N.C.; Gamst, A.; Holtzman, D.M.; Jagust, W.J.; Petersen, R.C.; et al. The diagnosis of mild cognitive impairment due to Alzheimer's disease: Recommendations from the national institute on Aging-Alzheimer's association workgroups on diagnostic guidelines for Alzheimer's disease. *Alzheimers Dement.* **2011**, *7*, 270–279. [CrossRef]
28. Petersen, R.C.; Lopez, O.; Armstrong, M.J.; Getchius, T.S.D.; Ganguli, M.; Gloss, D.; Gronseth, G.S.; Marson, D.; Pringsheim, T.; Day, G.S.; et al. Author response: Practice guideline update summary: Mild cognitive impairment: Report of the guideline development, dissemination, and implementation subcommittee of the American academy of neurology. *Neurology* **2018**, *91*, 373–374. [CrossRef]
29. Petersen, R.C.; Lopez, O.; Armstrong, M.J.; Getchius, T.S.D.; Ganguli, M.; Gloss, D.; Gronseth, G.S.; Marson, D.; Pringsheim, T.; Day, G.S.; et al. Practice guideline update summary: Mild cognitive impairment: Report of the guideline development, dissemination, and implementation subcommittee of the American academy of neurology. *Neurology* **2018**, *90*, 126–135. [CrossRef]

30. Martin, S.B.; Smith, C.D.; Collins, H.R.; Schmitt, F.A.; Gold, B.T. Evidence that volume of anterior medial temporal lobe is reduced in seniors destined for mild cognitive impairment. *Neurobiol. Aging.* **2010**, *31*, 1099–1106. [CrossRef]
31. Apostolova, L.G.; Mosconi, L.; Thompson, P.M.; Green, A.E.; Hwang, K.S.; Ramirez, A.; Mistur, R.; Tsui, W.H.; de Leon, M.J. Subregional hippocampal atrophy predicts Alzheimer's dementia in the cognitively normal. *Neurobiol. Aging.* **2010**, *31*, 1077–1088. [CrossRef]
32. Smith, S.M.; Nichols, T.E. Threshold-free cluster enhancement: Addressing problems of smoothing, threshold dependence and localisation in cluster inference. *Neuroimage* **2009**, *44*, 83–98. [CrossRef] [PubMed]
33. Smith, C.D.; Chebrolu, H.; Wekstein, D.R.; Schmitt, F.A.; Jicha, G.A.; Cooper, G.; Markesbery, W.R. Brain structural alterations before mild cognitive impairment. *Neurology* **2007**, *68*, 1268–1273. [CrossRef] [PubMed]
34. Whitwell, J.L.; Petersen, R.C.; Negash, S.; Weigand, S.D.; Kantarci, K.; Ivnik, R.J.; Knopman, D.S.; Boeve, B.F.; Smith, G.E.; Jack, C.R., Jr. Patterns of atrophy differ among specific subtypes of mild cognitive impairment. *Arch. Neurol.* **2007**, *64*, 1130–1138. [CrossRef]
35. Devanand, D.P.; Pradhaban, G.; Liu, X.; Khandji, A.; De Santi, S.; Segal, S.; Rusinek, H.; Pelton, G.H.; Honig, L.S.; Mayeux, R.; et al. Hippocampal and entorhinal atrophy in mild cognitive impairment: Prediction of Alzheimer disease. *Neurology* **2007**, *68*, 828–836. [CrossRef]
36. Jack, C.R. Jr.; Petersen, R.C.; Xu, Y.C.; O'Brien, P.C.; Smith, G.E.; Ivnik, R.J.; Boeve, B.F.; Waring, S.C.; Tangalos, E.G.; Kokmen, E. Prediction of AD with MRI-based hippocampal volume in mild cognitive impairment. *Neurology* **1999**, *52*, 1397–1403. [CrossRef] [PubMed]
37. Michaud, T.L.; Su, D.; Siahpush, M.; Murman, D.L. The risk of incident mild cognitive impairment and progression to dementia considering mild cognitive impairment subtypes. *Dement. Geriatr. Cogn. Dis. Extra* **2017**, *7*, 15–29. [CrossRef]
38. Nagamatsu, L.S.; Handy, T.C.; Hsu, C.L.; Voss, M.; Liu-Ambrose, T. Resistance training promotes cognitive and functional brain plasticity in seniors with probable mild cognitive impairment. *Arch. Intern. Med.* **2012**, *172*, 666–668. [CrossRef]
39. Suzuki, T.; Shimada, H.; Makizako, H.; Doi, T.; Yoshida, D.; Ito, K.; Shimokata, H.; Washimi, Y.; Endo, H.; Kato, T. A randomized controlled trial of multicomponent exercise in older adults with mild cognitive impairment. *PLoS ONE* **2013**, *8*, e61483. [CrossRef]
40. Folstein, M.F.; Folstein, S.E.; McHugh, P.R. "Mini-mental state". A practical method for grading the cognitive state of patients for the clinician. *J. Psychiatr. Res.* **1975**, *12*, 189–198. [CrossRef]
41. Measso, G.; Cavarzeran, F.; Zappalà, G.; Lebowitz, B.D.; Crook, T.H.; Pirozzolo, F.J.; Amaducci, F.A.; Massari, D.; Grigoletto, F. The mini mental state examination: Normative study of an Italian random sample. *Dev. Neuropsychol.* **1993**, *9*, 77–85. [CrossRef]
42. Hamilton, M. A rating scale for depression. *J. Neurol. Neurosurg. Psychiatry* **1960**, *23*, 56–62. [CrossRef] [PubMed]
43. Rosen, W.G.; Terry, R.D.; Fuld, P.A.; Katzman, R.; Peck, A. Pathological verification of ischemic score in differentiation of dementias. *Ann. Neurol.* **1980**, *7*, 486–488. [CrossRef] [PubMed]
44. Nasreddine, Z.S.; Phillips, N.A.; Bedirian, V.; Charbonneau, S.; Whitehead, V.; Collin, I.; Cummings, J.L.; Chertkow, H. The montreal cognitive assessment, MoCA: A brief screening tool for mild cognitive impairment. *J. Am. Geriatr Soc.* **2005**, *53*, 695–699. [CrossRef] [PubMed]
45. Conti, S.; Bonazzi, S.; Laiacona, M.; Masina, M.; Coralli, M.V. Montreal cognitive assessment (MoCA)-Italian version: Regression based norms and equivalent scores. *Neurol. Sci.* **2015**, *36*, 209–214. [CrossRef] [PubMed]
46. Santangelo, G.; Siciliano, M.; Pedone, R.; Vitale, C.; Falco, F.; Bisogno, R.; Siano, P.; Barone, P.; Grossi, D.; Santangelo, F.; et al. Normative data for the montreal cognitive assessment in an Italian population sample. *Neurol. Sci.* **2015**, *36*, 585–591. [CrossRef]
47. Grober, E.; Buschke, H. Genuine memory deficits in dementia. *Dev. Neuropsychol.* **1987**, *3*, 13–16. [CrossRef]
48. Frasson, P.; Ghiretti, R.; Catricala, E.; Pomati, S.; Marcone, A.; Parisi, L.; Rossini, P.M.; Cappa, S.F.; Mariani, C.; Vanacore, N.; et al. Free and cued selective reminding test: An Italian normative study. *Neurol. Sci.* **2011**, *32*, 1057–1062. [CrossRef]
49. Reitan, R.M. Validity of the trail making test as an indicator of organic brain damage. *Percept. Mot. Skills* **1958**, *8*, 271–276. [CrossRef]
50. Giovagnoli, A.R.; Del Pesce, M.; Mascheroni, S.; Simoncelli, M.; Laiacona, M.; Capitani, E. Trail making test: Normative values from 287 normal adult controls. *Ital. J. Neurol. Sci.* **1996**, *17*, 305–309. [CrossRef]

51. Bottiroli, S.; Cavallini, E. Can computer familiarity regulate the benefits of computer-based memory training in normal aging? A study with an Italian sample of older adults. *Neuropsychol. Dev. Cogn. B Aging Neuropsychol. Cogn.* **2009**, *16*, 401–418. [CrossRef]
52. Dale, A.M.; Fischl, B.; Sereno, M.I. Cortical surface-based analysis. I. Segmentation and surface reconstruction. *Neuroimage* **1999**, *9*, 179–194. [CrossRef] [PubMed]
53. Iglesias, J.E.; Augustinack, J.C.; Nguyen, K.; Player, C.M.; Player, A.; Wright, M.; Roy, N.; Frosch, M.P.; McKee, A.C.; Wald, L.L.; et al. Alzheimer's disease neuroimaging initiative. A computational atlas of the hippocampal formation using ex vivo, ultra-high resolution MRI: Application to adaptive segmentation of in vivo MRI. *Neuroimage* **2015**, *115*, 117–137. [CrossRef] [PubMed]
54. Fischl, B.; Salat, D.H.; Busa, E.; Albert, M.; Dieterich, M.; Haselgrove, C.; van der Kouwe, A.; Killiany, R.; Kennedy, D.; Klaveness, S; et al. Whole brain segmentation: Automated labeling of neuroanatomical structures in the human brain. *Neuron* **2002**, *33*, 341–355. [CrossRef]
55. Voevodskaya, O.; Simmons, A.; Nordenskjold, R.; Kullberg, J.; Ahlstrom, H.; Lind, L.; Wahlund, L.O.; Larsson, E.M.; Westman, E. Alzheimer's disease neuroimaging initiative. The effects of intracranial volume adjustment approaches on multiple regional MRI volumes in healthy aging and Alzheimer's disease. *Front. Aging Neurosci.* **2014**, *6*, 264. [CrossRef]
56. Topol, E. *Preparing the Healthcare Workforce to Deliver the Digital Future the Topol Review: An Independent Report on Behalf of the Secretary of State for Health and Social Care*; NHS Health Education: London, UK, 2019.
57. Tarnanas, I.; Schlee, W.; Tsolaki, M.; Muri, R.; Mosimann, U.; Nef, T. Ecological validity of virtual reality daily living activities screening for early dementia: Longitudinal study. *JMIR Serious Games* **2013**, *1*, e1. [CrossRef]
58. Grober, E.; Sanders, A.E.; Hall, C.; Lipton, R.B. Free and cued selective reminding identifies very mild dementia in primary care. *Alzheimer Dis. Assoc. Disord.* **2010**, *24*, 284–290. [CrossRef]
59. Bowie, C.R.; Harvey, P.D. Administration and interpretation of the trail making test. *Nat. Protoc.* **2006**, *1*, 2277–2281. [CrossRef]
60. Sarazin, M.; Chauvire, V.; Gerardin, E.; Colliot, O.; Kinkingnehun, S.; de Souza, L.C.; Hugonot-Diener, L.; Garnero, L.; Lehericy, S.; Chupin, M.; et al. The amnestic syndrome of hippocampal type in Alzheimer's disease: An MRI study. *J. Alzheimers Dis.* **2010**, *22*, 285–294. [CrossRef]
61. Burgess, N.; Maguire, E.A.; O'Keefe, J. The human hippocampus and spatial and episodic memory. *Neuron* **2002**, *35*, 625–641. [CrossRef]
62. Matamala-Gomez, M.; Maisto, M.; Montana, J.; Mavrodiev, P.; Baglio, F.; Rossetto, F.; Mantovani, F.; Riva, G.; Realdon, O. The role of engagement in teleneurorehabilitation: A systematic review. *Front. Neurol.* **2020**. [CrossRef]

4

Assessing the Relationship between Sense of Agency, the Bodily-Self and Stress: Four Virtual-Reality Experiments in Healthy Individuals

Yonatan Stern [1,2,*], Danny Koren [1], Renana Moebus [2], Gabriella Panishev [2] and Roy Salomon [2]

1 Psychology Department, University of Haifa, Haifa 3498838, Israel; dkoren@psy.haifa.ac.il
2 Gonda Brain Research Center, Bar-Ilan University, Ramat Gan 5290002, Israel; moebusrenana@gmail.com (R.M.); gabyp97@gmail.com (G.P.); roy.salomon@biu.ac.il (R.S.)
* Correspondence: yoniastern@gmail.com

Abstract: The bodily-self, our experience of being a body, arises from the interaction of several processes. For example, embodied Sense of Agency (SoA), the feeling of controlling our body's actions, is a fundamental facet of the bodily-self. SoA is disturbed in psychosis, with stress promoting its inception. However, there is little knowledge regarding the relationship between SoA, stress, and other facets of the bodily-self. In four experiments manipulating embodied SoA using a virtual hand (VH), we examined (1) How is embodied SoA related to other facets of the bodily-self?; and (2) How is SoA impacted by stress? We found that increased alteration of the VH significantly decreased subjective ratings of SoA and body ownership (Exp. 1), supporting the close relation between SoA and body ownership. Interoceptive accuracy and SoA were positively correlated (Exp. 3), connecting awareness to one's actions and cardiac signals. Contrary to our expectations, SoA was not related to trait anxiety (Exp. 3), nor did induced stress impair SoA (Exp. 4). Finally, we found a negative correlation between self-reported prodromal symptoms and SoA. These results strongly support the connection between SoA and the bodily-self. Whereas, SoA was not impaired by stress, and weakly related to psychotic symptoms.

Keywords: sense of agency; metacognition; virtual reality; psychosis; stress; bodily-self

---

1. Introduction

1.1. *Sense of Agency and the Bodily-Self*

Experiencing one's self as a physical entity grounded in a body is termed the 'bodily-self' or 'minimal self', emphasizing the fundamental nature of this stratum of selfhood [1–4]. The bodily-self encompasses two related capacities: body ownership and sense of agency (SoA), which are typically seamlessly interwoven into our experience to such a degree that we are typically not explicitly aware of them, rather they are pre-reflective [5,6]. Body ownership, the identification with one's body, relies on the integration of multisensory signals constructing a coherent representation of the self in the present moment. For example, synchronous visual–tactile stimulation can create an illusory sense of body ownership over a rubber hand or a virtual body [7–9]. SoA, the feeling of being in control of one's actions, also relies on multisensory integration but incorporates internal neural efferent signals originating in the agent's volition [10–12].

SoA primarily relies on the comparison of the predicted consequences of our actions (i.e., forwards models) with the actual afferent sensory outcomes via a comparator mechanism (but see other approaches such as Cue Integration, e.g., [13–15] and Postdictive accounts of SoA, e.g., [16,17]). If the predicted and actual outcome of the action match, then SoA arises, whereas if they are incongruent, the outcome will likely be attributed to an external cause [18–20]. For example, while reading this article on a computer screen, when you scroll the mouse with your finger to continue reading, and the screen scrolls, an SoA arises for these actions and outcomes. Importantly, two forms of SoA can be discerned in this example [21,22]. The first, embodied SoA, focuses on the immediate, often pre-reflective, connection between the intention to perform the action and the action itself (i.e., moving your finger) [23]. This form of SoA is inherently tied to the body of the agent that performs the action. The second, non-embodied SoA, focuses on the link between the action performed by the agent (i.e., moving your finger) and the intended outcome (i.e., screen scrolling). This SoA is related to a more general sense of causation, linking an action to its predicted outcome that is often detached spatially and temporally from the agent's body and action. Historically, there has been no clear distinction between these two forms of agency, which are often conflated in the literature [11,24–29]. However, we argue that embodied SoA, with its close affinity to the bodily-self, introduces unique characteristics. The importance of this distinction is intuitively demonstrated by the hypothetical reaction to the failure of each form of agency. Imagine the profound shock and fear you would experience if you intended to move your finger, and it did not move (i.e., embodied SoA). Whereas, if you scrolled your mouse and the screen failed to scroll (i.e., non-embodied SoA), you would likely dismiss it as a problem with your laptop. In line with this distinction, the exclusive focus of the current paper is embodied SoA.

In the literature, various experimental paradigms have been used to examine SoA, yet these diverging paradigms probe different aspects of agency that are often conflated (see [22] for an extensive discussion). Thus, some paradigms (e.g., [30,31]) use an additional actor within the experimental setting, and probe agentic authorship by asking participants whether they or the other actor performed the presented action. While other paradigms have examined the role of active as opposed to passive actions on SoA (e.g., [26,28,32–34]), examining how the agent's volition and the availability of neural efferent signals shape agency. In line with the theoretical suggestion that agency arises primarily from the congruence of predicted and actual sensory outcomes of action ([35–37]), and in line with a well-established line of research examining the effects of sensorimotor congruence on agency (e.g., [28,34,38–41]), the focus of the current paper is on examining how embodied agency is affected by the introduction of conflicts between actions and their visual consequences

1.2. Embodied SoA and Its Metacognition: Exteroceptive and Interoceptive Contributions

In line with our theoretical definition of embodied SoA that focuses on intention and motor actions, experimental operationalizations of embodied SoA use naturalistic representations of the body and focus on the motor action itself. Despite its theoretical and philosophical importance, experimentally examining embodied SoA has been somewhat limited, requiring creativity and ingenuity, such as using mirror set-ups and video systems [31,34], to create realistic distortions of self-generated movements. Recent advances in virtual reality (VR) technology allow for easier, more complex, and better-controlled manipulations of the bodily-self [9,42,43] and embodied SoA [28,44–48]. Such research has enabled significant advances in understanding the cognitive and neural processes by which sensory and motor signals shape the self [1,49,50]. In addition to the integration of exteroceptive signals, research has highlighted the importance of cardiac signals in the formation of the bodily-self. The neural processing of cardiac signals is modified by experimental changes in body ownership [51,52]. Moreover, cardiac signals can be used to induce body ownership over virtual hands [53] and bodies [54]. Within the realm of SoA, cardiac signals have been related to the subjective awareness of motor actions and errors [55,56]. Given the role of cardiac signals in body ownership and actions, we posited that awareness of one's cardiac activity might be linked to awareness of one's actions and embodied SoA.

Within judgments of SoA, we can distinguish between first-order and second-order processes [46,57,58]. First-order processes are related to the initial judgment of agency and include sensitivity—the ability to detect sensorimotor conflicts, and criteria—the decision threshold for asserting agency. Whereas, second-order processes concern the assessment of one's initial judgment and include measures of confidence and metacognition. Importantly, metacognition is a bridge between immediate judgments of agency and reflective awareness and self-knowledge of one's agency [5,57]. Both processes are central in delineating the self and are impaired in psychiatric populations such as psychosis [20,57,58]. Recently, we found that sensitivity and criteria of embodied SoA were both highly correlated across distortions in both the temporal and spatial domains introduced on a virtual hand presentation of self-generated movements [46]. These findings suggest an integrated mechanism of first-order processes that extends beyond specific domains and supports the processing of self-generated actions [4,10].

To briefly summarize, embodied SoA is a fundamental process contributing to our experience of the bodily-self. Accordingly, we hypothesize that SoA will be closely related to other facets of the bodily-self, such as body ownership and interoceptive processing. Furthermore, we expect that SoA and its metacognition will be correlated across domains, pointing to central processing and awareness of embodied actions.

1.3. Open Questions: The Effect of Stress

It is well documented that adverse situations such as stress and anxiety are a contributing factor to a wide range of psychopathological conditions entailing breakdowns of the self. Following trauma, people often experience dissociative states such as depersonalization that entail a deep sense of detachment from themselves, their body, and experiences [59–62]. Likewise, it is widely acknowledged that stress has a prominent role in the inception of psychosis [63–65]. Large-scale epidemiological studies have found that adverse life-events and extreme stress during childhood increase the odds of later psychotic experiences by 2–8 times [66,67]. Psychosis is characterized by disturbance of the minimal self, affecting the basic, pre-reflexive manner in which we experience ourselves, our body, and surroundings [3]. Accordingly, psychosis and disturbance of the bodily-self are closely linked to impaired SoA [68,69]. Across the psychosis continuum, impairments related to SoA are prominent both in the early prodromal phase [70,71] and in chronic schizophrenia patients [20,47]. Despite compelling evidence linking stress to psychosis and impairments of SoA, there is a paucity of experimental research examining how stress affects SoA. Experimentally understanding the effects of stress on SoA may allow us to uncover the underlying mechanisms and better understand the etiological factors affecting impaired SoA.

1.4. The Present Study: Goals and Predictions

The goal of the current study was to investigate two central questions using a VR paradigm of embodied SoA [46]. First, what is the relationship between embodied SoA and other facets of the bodily-self? Second, how is embodied SoA impacted by stress? These two questions were examined in a series of four experiments. Specifically, the following predictions were derived: (1) We hypothesized that increased sensorimotor conflict would significantly decrease subjective ratings of SoA and body ownership (Exp. 1). (2) We hypothesized that SoA processing (sensitivity, criterion and metacognition) would be correlated across different domains of sensorimotor conflict, suggesting a generalized mechanism for embodied SoA (Exp. 2). (3) In line with the role of cardiac signals in the formation of the bodily-self and motor awareness, we expected that interoceptive accuracy and embodied SoA would be positively correlated (Exp. 3). Concerning our second question, given the role of stress in the etiology of disturbances of the self, we expected that stress would be related to impaired SoA. Specifically, (4) we predicted that self-reported trait anxiety, in line with its close relation to stress [72], would be correlated with impaired SoA (Exp. 3). (5) Furthermore, we expected that experimentally manipulated psychosocial stress would affect SoA (Exp. 4). (6) Finally, in line with impairments of SoA in clinical populations with psychosis, we expected to find a correlation between a high presence of self-reported Attenuated Psychotic Symptoms (APS) in healthy individuals and impaired SoA (Exp. 2–4).

2. Participants

Participants in the study were 70 undergraduate students at Bar-Ilan University (37 women) aged 20–48 years (mean 25.4) All participants were right-handed, with normal or corrected-to-normal vision, and self-reported no history of neurological or psychiatric disease. They gave their informed consent to participate in the experiment and in return, were paid or given course credit. The study was approved by the Internal Review Board of Bar-Ilan University and was carried out in accordance with the relevant guidelines and regulations. Participants were excluded from the analysis if they did not have a sufficient number of trials (less than 80%), or failed to comply with instructions (see Supplemental Material Section A for details of participants excluded from each experiment).

3. Procedure

3.1. Experiment 1

In experiment 1 we examined whether increased magnitude of the sensorimotor conflict decreases subjective ratings of SoA and body ownership in order to validate that our experimental paradigm indeed assesses embodied SoA. Fourteen participants performed a VR-based paradigm of recognition of self-generated movements [46]. The technical set-up of the paradigm is described in detail in Krugwasser et al. (2019). In brief, participants' right hand was placed 18 cm below a Leap Motion controller (Leap Motion Inc., San Francisco, CA, USA) and their hand was hidden from them via a barrier. A realistic Virtual Hand (VH) that mimicked the real hand's position and movement was presented on a screen placed in front of the participant, positioned approximately 30 cm from the participant and at the same angle that the real hand was placed behind the barrier (see Figure 1A for set-up). In each trial, participants were presented with a fixation cross (1.5 s) followed by a presentation of the VH (2 s), during which they were instructed to fold only their index finger, while the rest of their hand remained static. A sensorimotor conflict was introduced in some trials by presenting the VH's finger's movement with one of four magnitudes of temporal delay (i.e., 0/100/200/300 ms) between the actual movement and the presentation of the VH's movement. After the presentation of the VH, participants rated their subjective SoA (i.e., "I felt as if the movement presented was my own?"; questions were presented in Hebrew) and body ownership (i.e., "I felt as if the hand presented was my own") on a Likert scale ranging from −3 (i.e., "completely disagree") to 3 (i.e., "completely agree") that were adapted from similar studies [26,28,73,74]. The order of the questions was counterbalanced across participants to avoid confusion. Thirty trials of each magnitude were presented, resulting in a total of 120 trials. A practice block consisting of 15 trials was performed with the experimenter present in order to ensure compliance with task demands at the start of the experiment and was not included in analyses. Trials were not analyzed if a camera malfunction occurred, as reported in the camera logs, if the participant did not respond to one of the questions, or if the reaction time exceeded four seconds.

A

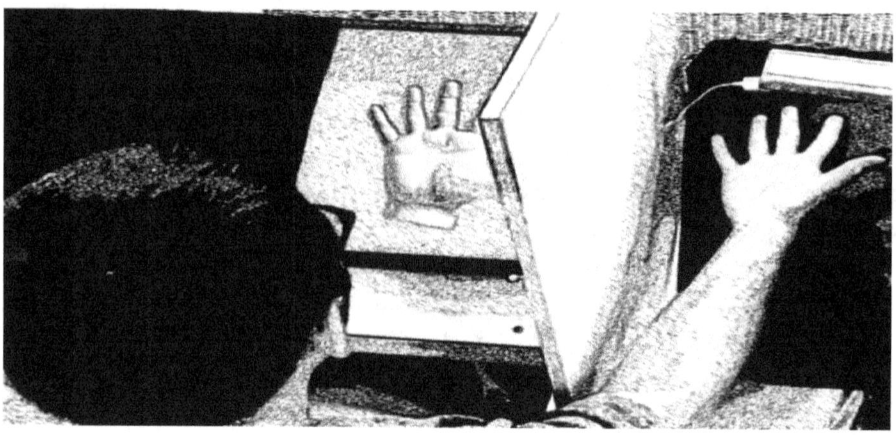

Figure 1. *Cont.*

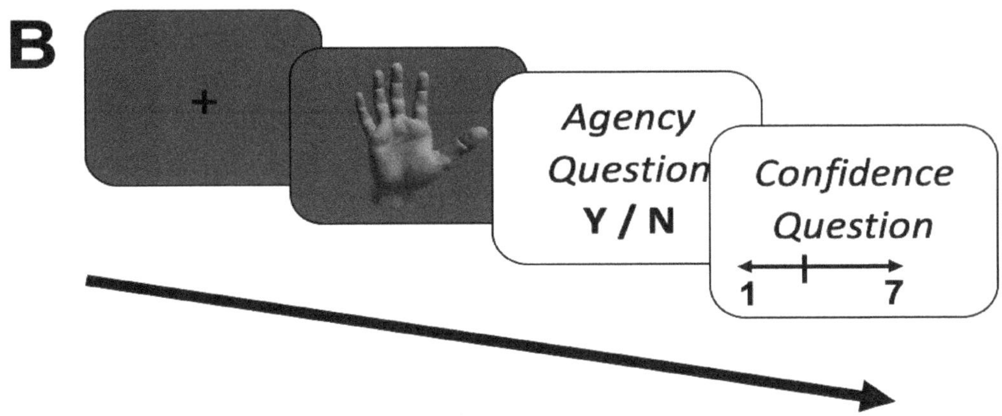

Figure 1. Experimental set-up and trial flow for the experiment. (**A**) Experimental set-up. The participant's hand is hidden from his view by the barrier, and the camera mounted above his hand records movement and presents it on the screen in front of him as a VH. (**B**) Trial flow. In each trial, a fixation cross was followed by a VH that moved with/without an alteration. Following the VH's presentation, in experiments 2–4, participants judged "same"/"not same" in response to the question "Was the movement of the VH identical to my movement?" (i.e., agency question) and rated their confidence in their response to the question, "How confident are you?" (i.e., confidence question) on a scale ranging from 1 (i.e., "not at all") to 7 (i.e., "completely"). In experiment 1, participants rated their subjective experience of SoA (i.e., "I felt as if the movement presented was my own?") and body ownership (i.e., "I felt as if the hand presented was my own?") on a Likert scale ranging from −3 (i.e., "completely disagree") to 3 (i.e., "completely agree"). Please note that across all experiments, the agency question included no explicit mention of the word 'agency'.

3.2. Experiment 2

In experiment 2 we examined whether SoA performance across different sensorimotor domains is correlated, supporting a domain-general mechanism for embodied SoA. Nineteen participants performed the VH paradigm, with three key differences from experiment 1. First, in some trials, the VH was presented with an alteration either in the temporal or spatial domain and in other trials without an alteration. Importantly, alteration in both domains was not presented together in any of the trials. In the temporal domain, as in experiment 1, one of four magnitudes of delay (i.e., 0/100/200/300 ms) between the actual movement and the VH's was inserted. In the spatial domain, an angular deviation of the VH's movement was introduced, with four magnitudes of angular deviation (0°, 6°, 10°, 14°) inserted in the presentation of the bending movement of the index finger. Thus, during a 6° deviation trial the movement of the VH's index finger would diverge in a lateral trajectory (i.e., towards the thumb) from the real index finger's movement by 6°. The finger's motion kinematics were modeled to ensure a natural-looking motion (see [46] for full details). Second, after the presentation of the VH, participants judged whether the VH's movement was identical to their actual movement using a two-alternative forced-choice question (2 AFC), "Was the movement of the VH identical to my movement?" (i.e., agency question), and rated their confidence in their response (i.e., confidence question; see Figure 1B for trial flow). We used this phrasing for the agency question as it probes the psychophysical aspect of SoA (i.e., the sensorimotor correspondence), and is in line with previous studies that have involved altered feedback of self-generated movements [46,75–77], although other approaches using 3 AFC have also been employed (e.g., [24]). Third, participants performed in each domain, 40 trials of the zero (i.e., no alteration) and first magnitude, and 20 trials of the final two magnitudes. Thus, a total of 240 trials in random order were presented.

From this task, we calculated four measures pertaining to SoA and its metacognition. First, we calculated SoA as the proportion of trials in each magnitude of alteration in each domain that participants responded that the VH's movement was identical to their movement. Second, we assessed confidence in SoA by averaging the confidence ratings of the trials with correct SoA (i.e., participants responded that the movement was identical when no alteration was present, or that it was different when an alteration was present). This was extracted for each magnitude of the alteration in each domain. Third, to allow for comparison of performance between domains, a signal detection framework was used to calculate sensitivity and criteria for each domain across the different magnitudes of alteration. Sensitivity reflects the capacity to accurately recognize trials in which the VH's movement was identical to the real hand and trials that it was altered. Criterion reflects the individual's decision boundary in order to judge that the VH movement was identical [78]. Finally, we calculated metacognitive confidence. In contrast to the measure of confidence described above, metacognitive confidence examines whether trials that were correct were rated with higher confidence than trials that were incorrect. This was calculated as the within-participant Goodman–Kruskal gamma correlation [79] between ratings of confidence and correctness of answers, capturing the degree to which confidence was linked to performance [80]. To ensure a sufficient number of observations, metacognitive confidence was calculated across the different magnitudes in each domain, yielding a single value per domain.

Following the completion of the task, participants completed the Prodromal Questionnaire Brief version (PQ-B) [81], as a self-report measure of APS that constitutes mild psychotic symptoms that have been experienced in the past month. We examined the number of items endorsed.

3.3. Experiment 3

In experiment 3 we examined the relation between SoA, interoception and self-reported anxiety. 23 participants performed the VH task identical to the task performed in experiment 2, except for two differences. First, in this experiment, only a temporal delay was administered. Second, 80 trials of each magnitude were administered in random order, resulting in a total of 320 trials. Following the VH task, participants performed a heartbeat tracking task. During the task, they were presented with a fixation cross for three time periods (25, 35, 45 s), in random order. They were instructed to press a button each time they perceived a heartbeat. During this period, the heart rate was recorded. Interoceptive accuracy was calculated as: $\frac{1}{3} \times \sum 1 - \frac{|recorded\ heartbeats - counted\ heartbeats|}{recorded\ heartbeats}$ [82–85]. Accordingly, interoceptive accuracy values range from one, signifying perfect accuracy, to zero. Following the completion of the VH and heartbeat tracking task, they completed both the PQ-B, as in experiment 2, and the State-Trait Anxiety Inventory (STAI) [86]. The ratings of the STAI items were averaged, resulting in a score ranging from 0, reflecting low anxiety, to 4, reflecting high anxiety.

3.4. Experiment 4

In experiment 4 we examined the effects of experimentally induced stress on SoA. Fourteen participants performed a VH task similar to that in experiment 2 except for two differences. First, the VH task was split into two blocks, a 'neutral' block succeeded by a 'stress' block. Second, only the temporal domain was administered. For each magnitude of delay in each of the two blocks, 30 trials were presented, resulting in a total of 240 trials displayed in random order.

To experimentally induce stress, we used an adaptation of well-accepted stress manipulations such as the Trier Social Stress Test [87] and the Montreal Imaging Stress Task [88] that use peer-evaluation and assessment of performance as stressors. Specifically, at the start of the neutral block following the actual practice session with the experimenter, participants were informed that they would now perform a 'practice' block alone that is aimed at acclimating them to the task and that their performance will not be monitored. Following the 'practice' (i.e., neutral) block, the experimenter re-entered the room and briefed the participants that they will now perform the task as a test, and their performance will be monitored. To increase psychosocial stress associated with performing the task as a test, participants were briefed about a fictitious concept of 'physical intelligence', described in such a manner that it is a positive concept related to their self-esteem, and informed that the VH task is a measure of 'physical intelligence'. They were informed that their performance in the current block will be compared to other participants', and that high performers would be recruited for future studies that include high monetary reimbursement (see Supplemental Material Section B for description provided to participants). To further exacerbate social stress, a camera was set up opposite their face and they were informed that their facial expressions would be analyzed during this block, (in effect the camera did not record). Finally, participants were informed that their heart rate would be recorded during this block.

To assess the physiological reaction to the stress induction, during both blocks, heart rate was recorded from three electrodes placed on participants' torso and connected to a G-Nautilus EEG system (250 Hz sampling rate) [89], and heart rate variability (HRV) was calculated. Briefly stated, HRV is a measure of the variability in the duration of succeeding R-peaks and is a robust biomarker of the body's response to stressors [90–92]. Under stress, HRV is typically decreased, whereas during relaxation HRV is relatively high. Physiological stress reactivity was calculated by subtracting the HRV of the neutral block from the stress block. Importantly, negative values of this difference indicated increased stress during the stress block.

Following the completion of both blocks, participants completed a post-experiment interview with the experimenter in which they rated their subjective feeling of stress in the neutral and stress blocks on a Likert scale ranging from 1 (i.e., "not at all") to 5 (i.e., "completely"). Subjective experience of stress was calculated by subtracting the neutral block's score from the stress block's score. In addition, the credibility of the stress induction was assessed in the interview. Finally, participants completed the PQ-B questionnaire.

Importantly, because this task will also be administered to clinical populations such as individuals at 'clinical high-risk' to develop psychosis in the future, we chose a stress manipulation that did not include negative feedback and could be successfully applied to them. Previous findings highlight that this population perceives even mildly stressful situations (i.e., solving simple mathematical problems with feedback introduced as a 'neutral' block) as extremely stressful [93], essentially equating them with the 'stress' block. Furthermore, based on our previous experience with clinical high-risk individuals in experimental settings in which participants were given negative feedback, we sought a mild stress manipulation that would ensure that they would complete the experiment and not leave due to the feedback.

4. Data Analysis

Data were processed using in-house Matlab scripts [94]. Statistical analyses were performed using JASP 0.9 [95]. To assess the effects of different magnitudes of alteration, domains, and blocks on subjective ratings of SoA and body ownership (Exp. 1), as well as SoA accuracy and confidence (Exp. 2–4), a within-subject repeated-measures ANOVA was used. In cases where the assumption of sphericity was violated, we performed Greenhouse–Geisser corrections. Post-hoc comparisons were Bonferroni corrected. To examine the correlations between variables, Pearson correlations were calculated. Finally, Bayesian statistics were used to assess evidence of null results [96,97].

5. Results

5.1. Experiment 1

To examine the effects of magnitude of alteration on subjective ratings of SoA and body ownership, two one-way repeated-measures ANOVAs with the factor magnitude (0/1/2/3) were performed. For SoA we found a significant main effect of magnitude ($F_{3,39} = 6.72$, $p = 0.01$, $\eta^2_p = 0.34$; see Figure 2A), such that as magnitude of alteration increased ratings of SoA decreased. For body ownership we also found a significant main effect ($F_{3,39} = 7.71$, $p = 0.006$, $\eta^2_p = 0.37$; see Figure 2B) similar to that of SoA. Thus, increased alteration of the VH's movement decreased the subjective experience of both SoA and body ownership. To assess if SoA and body ownership were indeed experienced by the participants in the no alteration condition (i.e., M0), we performed a one-sample t-test examining whether M0 ratings significantly differed from the baseline rating of zero. Both SoA ($t_{13} = 4.13$, $p = 0.001$ Cohen's $d = 1.1$) and body ownership ($t_{13} = 4.13$, $p = 0.001$, Cohen's $d = 1.1$) were significantly greater than baseline, further strengthening the ecological validity of the VH paradigm. Finally, to compare the effect of alteration magnitude on SoA as opposed to body ownership, a 2 × 4 repeated-measures ANOVA with the factors magnitude (0/1/2/3) and embodiment aspect (SoA/body ownership) was performed. As expected, the effect of magnitude was significant ($F_{3,39} = 8.03$, $p = 0.006$, $\eta^2_p = 0.38$); however, neither embodiment aspect ($F_{1,13} = 1.29$, $p = 0.28$), nor its interaction with magnitude ($F_{3,13} = 1.36$, $p = 0.27$) were significant. To assess this null finding, we examined the contribution of the embodiment aspect and its interaction with magnitude via the Bayes factor of inclusion ($BF_{Inclusion}$). Briefly stated, $BF_{Inclusion}$ is a measure of the evidence supporting the inclusion of a given factor, by comparing the effect of including or stripping a given factor from a group of models with an equivalent number of parameters [98]. This analysis yielded inconclusive evidence for the inclusion of the embodiment aspect ($BF_{Inclusion} = 2.7$), and moderately supported not including the interaction ($BF_{Inclusion} = 0.11$). To further elucidate the relation between SoA and body ownership, for each participant we examined the correlation between the two ratings on each question. For all participants, the correlation was positive and significant (all p's < 0.005) and the mean correlation across participants was 0.65 (SD = 0.25), with a range of 0.26 to 0.98. Thus, these two facets of the bodily-self are strongly entwined, and both were strongly affected by magnitude of alteration.

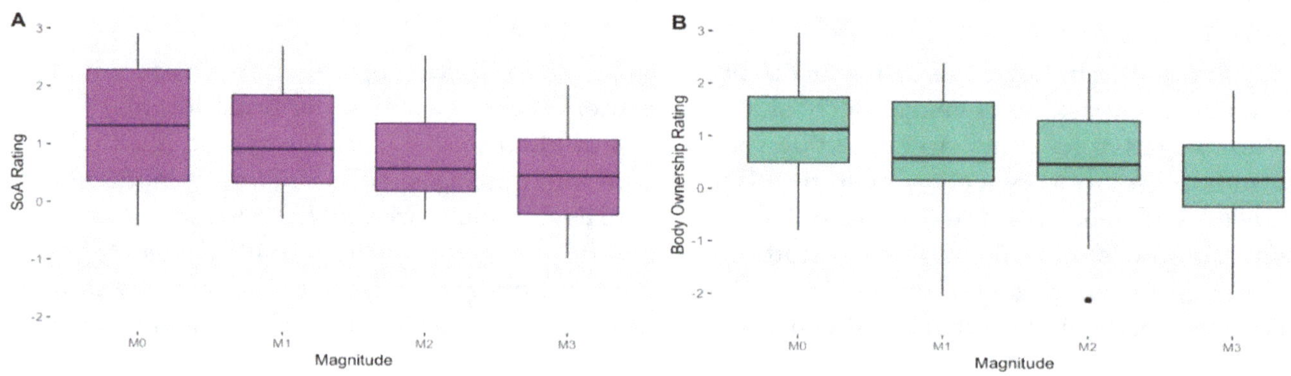

Figure 2. Subjective ratings of SoA (i.e., "I felt as if the movement presented was my own?"; Panel (**A**)) and body ownership (i.e., "I felt as if the hand presented was my own?"; Panel (**B**)) in experiment 1. *X*-axis is the magnitude of temporal alteration; *Y*-axis is the subjective rating that ranged from −3 (i.e., "completely disagree") to 3 (i.e., "completely agree").

5.2. Experiment 2

To examine the effects of domain and magnitude of alteration on SoA, a 2 × 4 repeated-measures ANOVA with the factor domain (temporal/spatial) and magnitude (0/1/2/3) was used. A significant main effect of domain was found ($F_{1,54} = 8.87$, $p = 0.008$, $\eta^2_p = 0.33$; see Figure 3A), such that in the temporal domain participants tended to judge VH movements to be identical to their own more than in the spatial domain. Importantly due to the distribution of trials across the magnitude of alteration, this main effect reflects participants' increased tendency to mistake altered trials in the temporal domain. In light of this main effect of domain, in order to examine the effect of magnitude on SoA, we performed a one-way repeated-measures ANOVA with the factor magnitude (0/1/2/3) for each domain separately. In the temporal domain we found a significant main effect of magnitude ($F_{3,54} = 57.44$, $p < 0.001$, $\eta^2_p = 0.76$; see Table S1 in the Supplemental Material for summary statistics and pairwise comparisons), as well as in the spatial domain ($F_{3,54} = 78.35$, $p < 0.001$, $\eta^2_p = 0.81$). As expected, in both domains, as the magnitude of alteration increased, VH movements were correctly judged as not identical to the participants' actual movements. Finally, there was a significant interaction between magnitude and domain ($F_{3,54} = 6.41$, $p < 0.001$, $\eta^2_p = 0.26$). As can be seen in Figure 3A, the differences between domains were most prominent in magnitude one and two, with participants showing a greater tendency to misattribute movements in the temporal domain in these magnitudes.

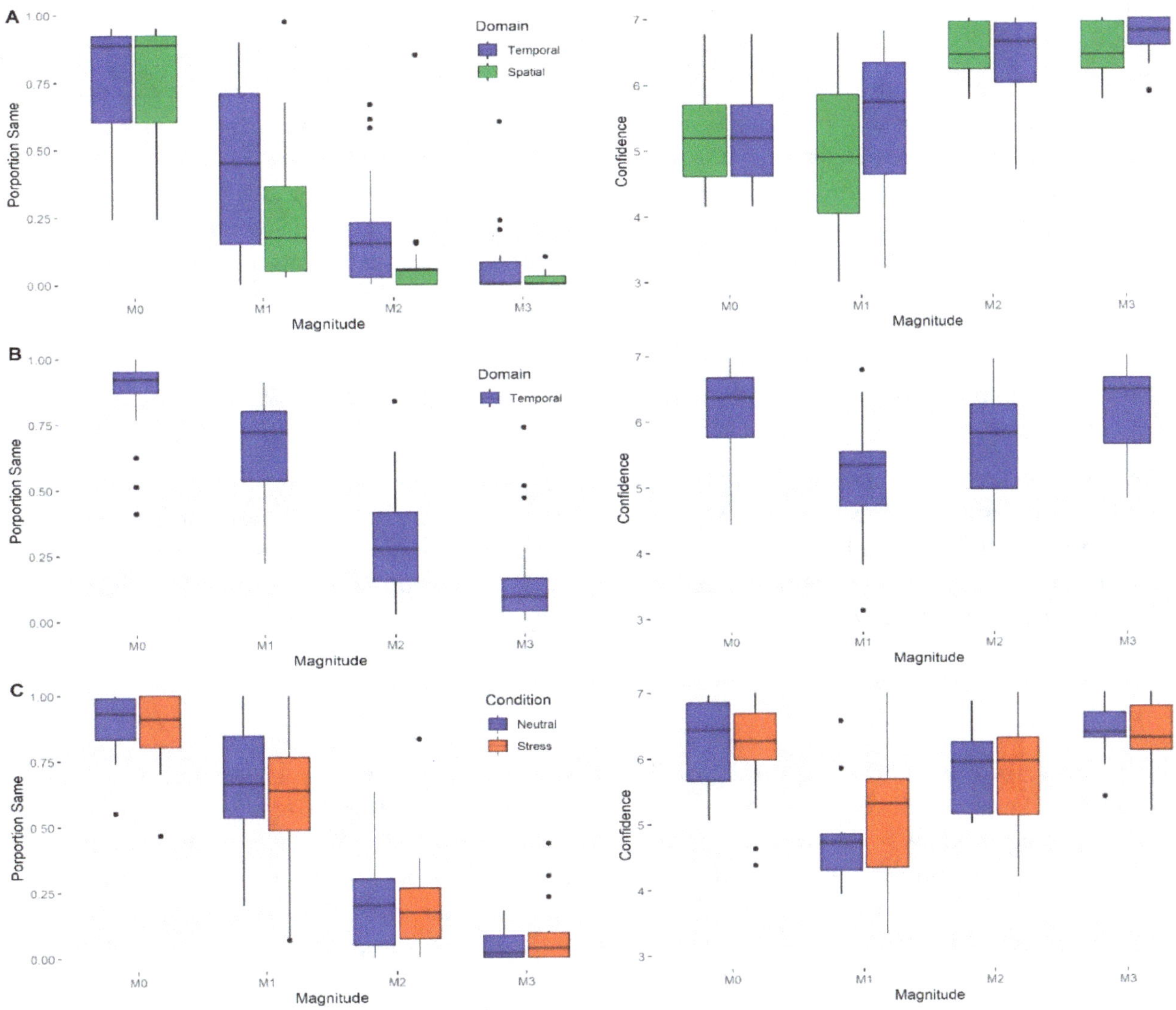

Figure 3. Judgments of SoA (left panels) and confidence (right panels) across three experiments (2–4; **A**–**C**). In the left panels, the *Y*-axis is the proportion of trials in which participants responded that VH's movement was the same as the actual movement, across the different magnitudes of alteration. Importantly, only in M0 (i.e., no alteration) was it correct to respond 'same'. In the right panels, the *Y*-axis is the participants' mean confidence rating (rated on a scale of 1–7) of their response to the agency question in which their response was correct. Lines within colored boxes are medians. (**A**) Experiment 2. Alterations were introduced in both the spatial (green) and temporal (blue) domain. (**B**) Experiment 3. Alterations were only introduced in the temporal domain. (**C**) Experiment 4. Alterations were introduced only in the temporal domain, and assessed in a neutral (blue) and stress (red) block.

An equivalent repeated-measures ANOVA was used to examine the effects of domain and magnitude of alteration on the confidence of correct trials. A significant main effect of domain was revealed ($F_{1,51} = 6.64$, $p = 0.02$, $\eta^2_p = 0.27$; see Figure 3A), such that participants were more confident in the spatial domain. This finding complements our previous findings that participants were more accurate in the spatial domain. In light of this main effect of domain, in order to examine the effect of magnitude on confidence, we performed a one-way repeated-measures ANOVA with the factor alteration magnitude (0/1/2/3) for each domain separately. In the temporal domain we found a significant main effect of magnitude ($F_{3,51} = 13.89$, $p < 0.001$, $\eta^2_p = 0.45$; see Table S2 in Supplemental Material for summary statistics and pairwise comparisons), as well as in the spatial domain ($F_{3,54} = 25.77$, $p < 0.001$, $\eta^2_p = 0.60$). Contrary to our expectations and findings in subsequent experiments, in the no alteration magnitude, confidence ratings were relatively low. This may be due to the high number of trials with alterations of magnitude zero (i.e., no alteration) and one, that caused participants to be uncertain whether a slight alteration or no alteration occurred.

To further elucidate the relation between SoA in the different domains, we examined the between-subject correlation of sensitivity, criterion and metacognitive confidence between the temporal and spatial domains. For sensitivity, we found a strong correlation between domains ($r = 0.71$, $p < 0.001$). Likewise, for criterion, there was a strong correlation between domains ($r = 0.89$, $p < 0.001$), reflecting that the threshold for evidence used for judgments of agency were related across domains. Finally, for metacognitive confidence we also found a strong correlation between domains ($r = 0.83$, $p < 0.001$). These findings demonstrate that the mechanism underlying embodied SoA and its metacognition are not domain-specific rather rely on a domain-general mechanism perhaps related to the bodily-self. Importantly, these findings are a strong replication of our previous findings concerning across domain correlations for sensitivity and bias [46], and also extend them to the capacity of metacognitive confidence.

Finally, we examined the relation between SoA and APS, assessed via the PQ-B questionnaire. We found a significant negative correlation between APS and sensitivity in the spatial domain ($r = -0.68$, $p = 0.001$) and in the temporal domain ($r = -0.49$, $p = 0.03$). Thus, participants that reported more APS symptoms showed lower sensitivity in both domains. Furthermore, the relation to metacognitive confidence, in both the spatial ($r = -0.65$, $p = 0.003$) and the temporal ($r = -0.57$, $p = 0.01$) domains was significant. Thus, participants that reported higher APS had lower metacognitive confidence.

5.3. Experiment 3

To examine the effect of the magnitude of alteration on SoA a one-way repeated-measures ANOVA with the factor of magnitude (0/1/2/3) was applied. Replicating our finding in experiment 2, a significant main effect of magnitude was found ($F_{3,66} = 121.3$, $p < 0.001$, $\eta^2_p = 0.85$). As the magnitude of alteration increased the proportion of trials judged to be identical decreased (see Figure 3B). Examining the effects of magnitude on the confidence of correct trials, using an equivalent ANOVA, also revealed a significant effect of magnitude ($F_{3,66} = 15.33$, $p < 0.001$, $\eta^2_p = 0.41$). As can be seen in Figure 3B, a U-shaped curve of confidence was observed, with the lowest confidence exhibited in magnitude one of alteration. Presumably, this magnitude of alteration is the most difficult, in line with its high proportions of incorrect responses. As expected, and in contrast to experiment 2, the no alteration condition (i.e., magnitude 0) also exhibited high levels of confidence. Presumably, this reflects the relative ease of correctly identifying movements that are identical.

Examining the correlation between interoceptive accuracy, assessed via the heartbeat counting task, and sensitivity of SoA, assessed via the VH task, we found a significant positive correlation ($r = 0.52$, $p = 0.02$). Similarly, the correlation to metacognitive confidence was also significantly correlated ($r = 0.47$, $p = 0.04$). Thus, individual differences in interoceptive accuracy and both sensitivity and metacognition of embodied SoA were closely linked, as would be expected due to these capacities' close affinity to the bodily-self.

Concerning the relation between the self-reported measures of APS and trait anxiety, and the performance measures of SoA and interoceptive accuracy. Contrary to our hypothesis and the results of experiment 2, the correlation between sensitivity of SoA and APS was not significant ($r = -0.05$, $p = 0.81$), with Bayesian statistics providing anecdotal evidence for lack of a correlation ($BF_{01} = 2.97$). Neither was the correlation between metacognitive confidence and APS significant ($r = -0.17$, $p = 0.45$), with Bayesian statistics providing anecdotal evidence for a lack of correlation ($BF_{01} = 2.94$). Concerning trait anxiety, the sensitivity of SoA was not significantly correlated ($r = -0.15$, $p = 0.52$), with Bayesian statistics providing moderate evidence in favor of a lack of correlation ($BF_{01} = 3.1$). Meanwhile, interoceptive accuracy and anxiety showed a non-significant negative correlation ($r = -0.36$, $p = 0.13$), such that participants with higher levels of anxiety had lower interoceptive accuracy.

5.4. Experiment 4

In this experiment, we examined the effects of experimentally manipulated stress on SoA. First, we assessed the validity of the stress induction both via the subjective experience of stress as reported in the post-experiment interview in which participants rated on a Likert scale ranging from 1–5 how stressful they experienced each block to be, and via the physiological change in HRV between blocks. As expected, the mean rating of stress experienced in the stress block (M = 2.68, SEM = 0.24) was higher than in the neutral block (M = 2.00, SEM = 0.22), and this difference was significant ($t_{18} = 3.24$, $p = 0.005$, Cohen's $d = 0.74$). In contrast, the difference between HRV in the stress block (M = 0.049, SEM = 0.005) and the neutral block (M = 0.052, SEM = 0.005) was not significant ($t_{13} = 0.49$, $p = 0.63$). Importantly, the subjective experience of stress was correlated with the change in HRV ($r = -0.64$, $p = 0.014$). Thus, changes in HRV reflect individual differences in the subjective experience of stress following its induction. Accordingly, in the analyses concerning the effects of stress, we included HRV as a covariate to capture these individual differences.

We examined the effect of stress on SoA via a repeated-measures ANOVA with the factors block (neutral/stress) and magnitude of alteration (0/1/2/3), and change in HRV as a covariate. There was a significant main effect of magnitude ($F_{3,36} = 86.71$, $p < 0.001$, $\eta^2 = 0.87$; see Figure 3C), replicating our previous findings concerning the decrease in SoA as magnitude increases. The main effect of block was not significant ($F_{1,12} < 1$, $p = 0.40$). Meanwhile, the interaction between block and delay was significant ($F_{3,24} = 3.56$, $p = 0.024$, $\eta^2 = 0.20$), with participants under stress more likely to misattribute their movement in the largest magnitude of alteration. Yet none of the post-hoc comparisons between blocks across the different magnitudes of alteration were significant ($p > 0.12$). Comparing sensitivity of SoA between blocks, contrary to our expectation the difference between sensitivity in the stress block (M = 1.78, SEM = 0.22) and the neutral block (M = 1.75, SEM = 0.19), was not significant ($F_{1,12} < 1$, $p = 0.37$). The equivalent Bayesian analysis yielded anecdotal evidence in favor of the null effect of the block ($BF_{01} = 2.67$). Thus, it seems that the stress induction did not affect overall SoA.

Examining the effect of stress on confidence with the equivalent ANOVA used for SoA, we found a significant main effect of magnitude ($F_{3,24} = 9.74$, $p < 0.001$, $\eta^2 = 0.54$; see Figure 3C). Replicating experiment 3, confidence across magnitudes displayed a U-shaped curve with the lowest confidence in the first magnitude of alteration. The main effect of block was not significant ($F_{1,8} = 2.63$, $p = 0.14$), nor was the interaction of block and magnitude ($F_{3,24} = 1.1$, $p = 0.37$). Comparing metacognitive confidence between blocks, under stress metacognitive confidence was higher (M = 0.43, SEM = 0.08) in comparison to the neutral block (M = 0.41, SEM = 0.07), and this difference was significant ($F_{1,12} = 10.6$, $p = 0.007$, ${\eta^2}_p = 0.47$). Thus, contrary to our hypothesis, stress significantly improved metacognitive confidence.

Finally, examining the correlation between sensitivity of SoA and APS, contrary to our expectation, we did not find a significant correlation ($r = -0.07$, $p = 0.79$), with Bayesian analysis providing anecdotal to moderate evidence for lack of a correlation ($BF_{01} = 2.98$).

5.5. The Relation between APS and SoA across Experiments

To further examine the relation between APS and SoA with increased statistical power, we pooled the participants from the three experiments (i.e., Exp. 2–4) in which the binary judgment of SoA was used and sensitivity could be extracted, and examined only SoA in the temporal domain, because it was measured in all three studies (in experiment 4 we included only the neutral block). APS showed a negative correlation to sensitivity ($r = -0.17$, $p = 0.19$; see Figure 4A) and metacognition of SoA ($r = -0.20$, $p = 0.12$; see Figure 4B), yet contrary to our expectation these correlations were not significant. Noting that one participant in experiment 4 endorsed an extremely high number of APS symptoms (18 out of 21 items), we reexamined the correlation, excluding this participant as an outlier. There are two justifications for this decision. First, clinical cutoffs of the PQB are typically set at between 3 to 8 items [81,99]; thus the participant's high number of items endorsed likely points to his misunderstanding of the questionnaire or extreme clinical distress that was not evident in his functioning. Second, the number of items endorsed by this participant is more than three standard deviations from the participants' mean number of items endorsed. Excluding this participant, there was a significant correlation between APS and sensitivity ($r = -0.27$, $p = 0.04$) and metacognitive confidence ($r = -0.32$, $p = 0.01$) of SoA. Yet, it should be noted that these correlations were not corrected for multiple comparisons.

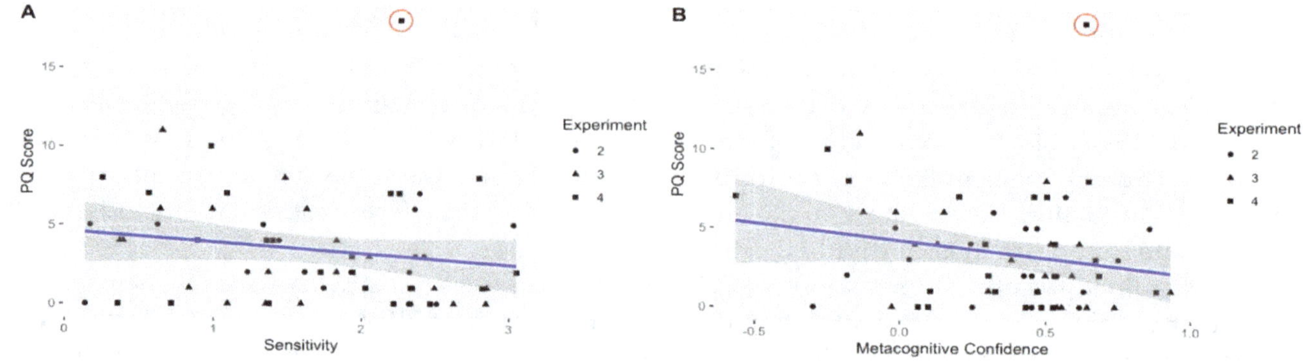

Figure 4. Correlation between APS and sensitivity (**A**) and metacognitive confidence (**B**) across the three experiments (experiment 2–4). The blue line denotes the linear regression fit and the shaded area is 95% confidence interval of fit. A red circle surrounds the participant identified as an outlier.

6. Discussion

Across four experiments, using a virtual reality paradigm, we examined two questions pertaining to embodied SoA. The first question focused on the relationship between embodied SoA and other facets of the bodily-self, such as body ownership and interoception. All of our predictions derived from this question were corroborated. First, we found that increased magnitude of alteration significantly decreased graded subjective ratings of both SoA and body ownership, validating the ecological validity of our experimental paradigm of embodied SoA (prediction1; experiment1). These two measures exhibited strong within-trial correlations, further supporting a unified construct of the bodily-self. This finding is in contrast to theoretical and empirical accounts [26,100] that argue for a dissociation between these two processes and is in line with previous studies that have found the two to be correlated [28,73]. Second, our prediction that sensitivity and criteria would be correlated across temporal and spatial domain (prediction 2; experiment 2) was strongly supported and replicates the findings of our previous study [46]. These correlations support an account of a domain-general processing of embodied SoA, differing between individuals but stable across different sensorimotor prediction domains. The current study also expanded this correlation across domains to the capacity of metacognitive confidence of SoA. Metacognitive confidence, reflecting the degree to which the participant is aware of his performance, bridges between immediate judgments of agency and more reflexive knowledge pertaining to the certainty of these judgments [57]. Correlated metacognition together with correlated criterion point to similar subjective processes inherently related to embodied SoA, lending further support to the existence of a central, domain-general representation of the bodily-self. Future neuroimaging studies may attempt to examine whether embodied SoA across domains involves similar or distinct neural mechanisms and regions. In line with our third prediction and further supporting embodied SoA's connection to the bodily-self [2,52,101–103], we found that interoceptive accuracy was significantly correlated with SoA (prediction 3; experiment 3). Previous studies have found that interoceptive accuracy is linked to body ownership [84] and peripersonal space [85]. The current finding demonstrates the importance of awareness to cardiac signals in influencing enactment, that alongside embodiment, shape our representation of the bodily-self.

A limitation pertaining to our finding that SoA was closely related to the bodily-self is that in the current study (Exp. 2–4) we only examined one aspect of SoA, namely the effect of sensorimotor alterations on SoA. Importantly, it should be noted that SoA entails additional aspects [22], such as agentic authorship (i.e., did I or someone else perform the action [24,31]) as well as the effect of passive as opposed to active actions and the effect of volition on SoA [29,104,105]. Furthermore, the wording of experiment 1's question (i.e., "I felt as if the movement presented was my own") is ambiguous in the sense that it may be interpreted as probing either the sensorimotor congruency or the agentic authorship aspect of SoA. Hence, additional studies are needed in order to disentangle the relationship of these additional aspects of SoA to the bodily-self. Additionally, Exp. 1 only probed the effect of alterations in the temporal domain on SoA. In light of previous findings that have found significant differences between domains and their effect on different aspects of SoA [24], future studies should also examine the effects of spatial alterations on the subjective experience of SoA.

Examining the relation between impaired SoA and APS yielded precarious results (prediction 6). Only in experiment 2 was the correlation to SoA in both domains significant, whereas in both experiments 3 and 4, we did not find significant correlations and Bayesian analyses provided anecdotal to moderate evidence for lack of a correlation. Pooling participants from all three experiments, the correlation was only significant when excluding an outlier. From these mixed findings, we derive two preliminary conclusions that although consistent with existing research, nonetheless need to be replicated in future studies. First, the significant correlations found between self-reported APS and embodied SoA are in line with the 'psychosis continuum' that posits the existence of psychotic-like experiences also in normative functioning populations [106]. Importantly, the current study expands previous studies [70] by showing that APS is related to both impaired sensitivity of embodied SoA and its metacognition. Interestingly, a recent study using VR to manipulate other aspects of the embodied Self (i.e., making the participant bigger or smaller) also showed a correlation between sensitivity to this alteration and APS [107]. Our correlation between self-reported psychotic symptoms and metacognition points to the potential role metacognition may play in attenuating and translating experimentally measured impairments into real-world functioning [108–110]. Second, the precariousness of the correlations highlights the wide range of symptoms endorsed in the general population, which especially affects small sample sizes. To clarify, we fully acknowledge the seminal importance of self-report questionnaires in the early stages of screening for risk of psychosis [81,99,111]. Yet, due to the low specificity of the questionnaires, some individuals endorse a high number of items that may not be indicative of actual APS and introduces additional noise to correlational analyses. Accordingly, we interpret these mixed findings with cautious enthusiasm and believe that they require further replication.

Our second question based on the pivotal role of stress in breakdowns of the self and psychosis examined the effects of stress on SoA. It yielded complex findings that did not corroborate our two predictions. The first prediction (prediction 4; experiment 3) concerning the correlation between trait anxiety and SoA was not corroborated. Although stress and anxiety are closely related concepts [72], a single self-report questionnaire of anxiety may not capture the 'stress-sensitivity' that has been found to be elevated during the early stages of psychosis. It is typically assessed at numerous time points over an extended period, via the experience sampling method that allows us to assess participants' reaction to daily stressors [112–114]. Future studies will use this method, which captures minute fluctuations in both anxiety and subjective stress, as well as obtaining a more stable measure of stress reactivity over an extended period. We also note the small sample size and low statistical power may have impaired the detection of a potential relationship. Furthermore, contrary to our prediction, we found that experimentally manipulating mild psychosocial stress in healthy individuals improved metacognitive confidence and did not affect the sensitivity of SoA (prediction 5; experiment 4). In line with the well-established inverted U-shape effect of stress on performance [115], we hypothesize that the mild stress placed healthy participants in the upward part of the inverted U, as evidenced by their enhanced metacognition. This finding highlights the importance of using a graded manipulation of stress that will allow us to calibrate the effects of the stress manipulation on the participant's subjective experience, allowing us to compare participants' performance at an equated level of subjective stress.

Although stress did not impair SoA in the current experiments, we nonetheless believe that paradigms integrating virtual reality and stress inductions are a promising avenue. It is well recognized that preceding full-blown psychosis and schizophrenia, most individuals undergo a period of heightened APS, in a risk period often coined 'clinical high-risk' [116–118]. Improving our ability to accurately predict which at-risk individuals will eventually convert to full-blown schizophrenia is a pressing goal that holds a potential to improve the harsh prognosis of schizophrenia. This has led to an ongoing search for neurocognitive characteristics and biomarkers specific to the clinical high-risk population in general and convertors in particular [71,119,120]. Yet the correlation between various impairments and the actual prognosis is typically weak at best. In line with the prominent role of stress in the etiology of psychosis and at-risk individual's heightened reactivity to mild daily stressors [112,113], we have recently hypothesized that neurocognitive performance under stress may be of greater predictive value than neurocognitive performance per se [108]. Analogous to cardiac patients that during rest exhibit an electrocardiogram similar to healthy controls and only under cardiac stress (i.e., walking on a treadmill) is their signal differentiable. Neurocognitive deficits during the at-risk phase may only be identifiable in a stressful environment that mimics the environment in which psychosis typically occurs [108,121]. Importantly, experiment 4 served as a pilot study to examine the effect of stress on neurocognitive capacities associated with the bodily-self in at-risk populations. In the hope that performance under stress will yield insight into the etiology of psychosis and improve our ability to predict conversion.

7. Conclusions

The current study examined embodied SoA using a virtual reality paradigm. We found a strong connection between embodied SoA and other facets of the bodily-self, both replicating our previous finding [46] that SoA is highly correlated across different domains of alteration, and finding that it is correlated with interoceptive accuracy and body ownership. In addition, embodied SoA was correlated with self-reported psychotic symptoms, further supporting the disturbance of the bodily-self in the psychosis continuum. Finally, examining how embodied SoA is impacted by stress in a normative population, we found that it was not impaired. Despite this finding, which was contrary to our hypothesis, we believe that examining the effects of stress on embodied SoA in clinical populations holds promise for better understanding the role of stress in the etiology of psychosis.

Supplementary Materials:
Supplemental Material Section A: Exclusion Criteria and Number of Participants Excluded from Experiments, Supplemental Material Section B: Description of Brief included in the Stress Induction of Experiment 4, Supplemental Material Section C: Tables of Summary Statistics for VH task, Table S1. Summary statistics of the VH task across the four experiments, Mean (S.E.M), Table S2. Summary statistics of the confidence rating of correct responses in the VH task across the experiments 2–4, Mean (S.E.M).

Author Contributions: Conceptualization and methodology, Y.S., D.K., and R.S.; software, Y.S. and R.S.; data curation, Y.S., R.M. and G.P.; investigation, Y.S., R.M. and G.P.; formal analysis, Y.S. and R.S.; resources and funding acquisition, R.S.; project administration, Y.S.; writing—original draft preparation, Y.S. and R.S.; writing—review and editing, Y.S., D.K. and R.S. All authors have read and agreed to the published version of the manuscript.

Acknowledgments: We wish to thank Amit Regev Krugwasser and Yair Zvilichovsky for their assistance with the technical set-up of the experimental paradigm.

References

1. Blanke, O.; Metzinger, T. Full-body illusions and minimal phenomenal selfhood. *Trends Cogn. Sci.* **2009**, *13*, 7–13. [CrossRef] [PubMed]
2. Blanke, O.; Slater, M.; Serino, A. Behavioral, Neural, and Computational Principles of Bodily Self-Consciousness. *Neuron* **2015**, *88*, 145–166. [CrossRef] [PubMed]
3. Sass, L.A.; Parnas, J. Schizophrenia, consciousness, and the self. *Schizophr. Bull.* **2003**, *29*, 427–444. [CrossRef] [PubMed]

4. Salomon, R. The Assembly of the Self from Sensory and Motor Foundations. *Soc. Cogn.* **2017**, *35*, 87–106. [CrossRef]
5. Gallagher, S. The Natural Philosophy of Agency. *Philos. Compass* **2007**, *2*, 347–357. [CrossRef]
6. Metzinger, T. Self models. *Scholarpedia* **2007**, *2*, 4174. [CrossRef]
7. Botvinick, M.; Cohen, J. Rubber hands 'feel' touch that eyes see. *Nature* **1998**, *391*, 756. [CrossRef]
8. Ehrsson, H.H.; Wiech, K.; Weiskopf, N.; Dolan, R.J.; Passingham, R.E. Threatening a rubber hand that you feel is yours elicits a cortical anxiety response. *Proc. Natl. Acad. Sci. USA* **2007**, *104*, 9828–9833. [CrossRef]
9. Lenggenhager, B.; Tadi, T.; Metzinger, T.; Blanke, O. Video ergo sum: Manipulating bodily self-consciousness. *Science* **2007**, *317*, 1096–1099. [CrossRef]
10. De Vignemont, F.; Fourneret, P. The sense of agency: A philosophical and empirical review of the "Who" system. *Conscious. Cogn.* **2004**, *13*, 1–19. [CrossRef]
11. Haggard, P. Sense of agency in the human brain. *Nat. Rev. Neurosci.* **2017**, *18*, 196. [CrossRef] [PubMed]
12. Kalckert, A.; Ehrsson, H.H. The moving rubber hand illusion revisited: Comparing movements and visuotactile stimulation to induce illusory ownership. *Conscious. Cogn.* **2014**, *26*, 117–132. [CrossRef] [PubMed]
13. Aarts, H.; Custers, R.; Wegner, D.M. On the inference of personal authorship: Enhancing experienced agency by priming effect information. *Conscious. Cogn.* **2005**, *14*, 439–458. [CrossRef]
14. Moore, J.W.; Fletcher, P.C. Sense of agency in health and disease: A review of cue integration approaches. *Conscious. Cogn.* **2012**, *21*, 59–68. [CrossRef]
15. Synofzik, M.; Vosgerau, G.; Lindner, A. Me or not me–An optimal integration of agency cues? *Conscious. Cogn.* **2009**, *18*, 1065–1068. [CrossRef] [PubMed]
16. Wegner, D.M.; Sparrow, B.; Winerman, L. Vicarious agency: Experiencing control over the movements of others. *J. Personal. Soc. Psychol.* **2004**, *86*, 838. [CrossRef] [PubMed]
17. Wegner, D.M. The mind's best trick: How we experience conscious will. *Trends Cogn. Sci.* **2003**, *7*, 65–69. [CrossRef]
18. Frith, C.; Blakemore, S.-J.; Wolpert, D. Abnormalities in the awareness and control of action. *Philos. Trans. R. Soc. Lond. Ser. B Biol. Sci.* **2000**, *355*, 1771–1788. [CrossRef]
19. Wolpert, D.M. Computational approaches to motor control. *Trends Cogn. Sci.* **1997**, *1*, 209–216. [CrossRef]
20. Jeannerod, M. The sense of agency and its disturbances in schizophrenia: A reappraisal. *Exp. Brain Res.* **2009**, *192*, 527. [CrossRef]
21. Christensen, M.S.; Grünbaum, T. Sense of agency for movements. *Conscious. Cogn.* **2018**, *65*, 27–47. [CrossRef] [PubMed]
22. Christensen, M.S.; Grünbaum, T. Sense of moving: Moving closer to the movement. *Sensat. Mov.* **2017**, 64–84. [CrossRef]
23. Anscombe, G.E.M. *Intention*; Harvard University Press: Cambridge, MA, USA, 2000.
24. Farrer, C.; Bouchereau, M.; Jeannerod, M.; Franck, N. Effect of distorted visual feedback on the sense of agency. *Behav. Neurol.* **2008**, *19*, 53–57. [CrossRef] [PubMed]
25. Gentsch, A.; Kathmann, N.; Schütz-Bosbach, S. Reliability of sensory predictions determines the experience of self-agency. *Behav. Brain Res.* **2012**, *228*, 415–422. [CrossRef] [PubMed]
26. Kalckert, A.; Ehrsson, H.H. Moving a rubber hand that feels like your own: A dissociation of ownership and agency. *Front. Hum. Neurosci.* **2012**, *6*, 40. [CrossRef]
27. Ma, K.; Hommel, B. The role of agency for perceived ownership in the virtual hand illusion. *Conscious. Cogn.* **2015**, *36*, 277–288. [CrossRef]
28. Salomon, R.; Fernandez, N.B.; Van Elk, M.; Vachicouras, N.; Sabatier, F.; Tychinskaya, A.; Llobera, J.; Blanke, O. Changing motor perception by sensorimotor conflicts and body ownership. *Sci. Rep.* **2016**, *6*, 1–13. [CrossRef]
29. Salomon, R.; Lim, M.; Kannape, O.; Llobera, J.; Blanke, O. "Self pop-out": Agency enhances self-recognition in visual search. *Exp. Brain Res.* **2013**, *228*, 173–181. [CrossRef]
30. Jeannerod, M. Visual and action cues contribute to the self-other distinction. *Nat. Neurosci.* **2004**, *7*, 422–423. [CrossRef]
31. Sirigu, A.; Daprati, E.; Pradat-Diehl, P.; Franck, N.; Jeannerod, M. Perception of self-generated movement following left parietal lesion. *Brain* **1999**, *122*, 1867–1874. [CrossRef]
32. Caspar, E.A.; Cleeremans, A.; Haggard, P. The relationship between human agency and embodiment. *Conscious. Cogn.* **2015**, *33*, 226–236. [CrossRef]

33. Engbert, K.; Wohlschläger, A.; Haggard, P. Who is causing what? The sense of agency is relational and efferent-triggered. *Cognition* **2008**, *107*, 693–704. [CrossRef] [PubMed]
34. Salomon, R.; Malach, R.; Lamy, D. Involvement of the intrinsic/default system in movement-related self recognition. *PLoS ONE* **2009**, *4*, e7527. [CrossRef] [PubMed]
35. Frith, C.; Done, D. Experiences of alien control in schizophrenia reflect a disorder in the central monitoring of action. *Psychol. Med.* **2009**, *19*, 359–363. [CrossRef] [PubMed]
36. Wolpert, D.M.; Kawato, M. Multiple paired forward and inverse models for motor control. *Neural Netw.* **1998**, *11*, 1317–1329. [CrossRef]
37. Wolpert, D.M.; Ghahramani, Z.; Jordan, M.I. An internal model for sensorimotor integration. *Science* **1995**, *269*, 1880. [CrossRef]
38. Blakemore, S.-J.; Wolpert, D.M.; Frith, C.D. Central cancellation of self-produced tickle sensation. *Nat. Neurosci.* **1998**, *1*, 635–640. [CrossRef]
39. Nielsen, T. Volition: A new experimental approach. *Scand. J. Psychol.* **1963**, *4*, 225–230. [CrossRef]
40. Sato, A.; Yasuda, A. Illusion of sense of self-agency: Discrepancy between the predicted and actual sensory consequences of actions modulates the sense of self-agency, but not the sense of self-ownership. *Cognition* **2005**, *94*, 241–255. [CrossRef]
41. Synofzik, M.; Thier, P.; Lindner, A. Internalizing agency of self-action: Perception of one's own hand movements depends on an adaptable prediction about the sensory action outcome. *J. Neurophysiol.* **2006**, *96*, 1592. [CrossRef]
42. Bergouignan, L.; Nyberg, L.; Ehrsson, H.H. Out-of-body-induced hippocampal amnesia. *Proc. Natl. Acad. Sci. USA* **2014**, *111*, 4421–4426. [CrossRef] [PubMed]
43. Bohil, C.J.; Alicea, B.; Biocca, F.A. Virtual reality in neuroscience research and therapy. *Nat. Rev. Neurosci.* **2011**, *12*, 752. [CrossRef]
44. Debarba, H.G.; Bovet, S.; Salomon, R.; Blanke, O.; Herbelin, B.; Boulic, R. Characterizing first and third person viewpoints and their alternation for embodied interaction in virtual reality. *PLoS ONE* **2017**, *12*, e0190109. [CrossRef] [PubMed]
45. Kannape, O.A.; Schwabe, L.; Tadi, T.; Blanke, O. The limits of agency in walking humans. *Neuropsychologia* **2010**, *48*, 1628–1636. [CrossRef]
46. Krugwasser, A.R.; Harel, E.V.; Salomon, R. The boundaries of the self: The sense of agency across different sensorimotor aspects. *J. Vis.* **2019**, *19*, 14. [CrossRef] [PubMed]
47. Synofzik, M.; Thier, P.; Leube, D.T.; Schlotterbeck, P.; Lindner, A. Misattributions of agency in schizophrenia are based on imprecise predictions about the sensory consequences of one's actions. *Brain* **2010**, *133*, 262–271. [CrossRef]
48. Limanowski, J.; Kirilina, E.; Blankenburg, F. Neuronal correlates of continuous manual tracking under varying visual movement feedback in a virtual reality environment. *NeuroImage* **2017**, *146*, 81–89. [CrossRef]
49. Herbelin, B.; Salomon, R.; Serino, A.; Blanke, O. 5. Neural Mechanisms of Bodily Self-Consciousness and the Experience of Presence in Virtual Reality. *Hum. Comput. Conflu. Transform. Hum. Exp. Symbiotic Technol.* **2015**. [CrossRef]
50. Sanchez-Vives, M.V.; Slater, M. From presence to consciousness through virtual reality. *Nat. Rev. Neurosci.* **2005**, *6*, 332–339. [CrossRef]
51. Park, H.-D.; Bernasconi, F.; Bello-Ruiz, J.; Pfeiffer, C.; Salomon, R.; Blanke, O. Transient Modulations of Neural Responses to Heartbeats Covary with Bodily Self-Consciousness. *J. Neurosci.* **2016**, *36*, 8453–8460. [CrossRef]
52. Park, H.-D.; Blanke, O. Coupling Inner and Outer Body for Self-Consciousness. *Trends Cogn. Sci.* **2019**, *23*, 377–388. [CrossRef] [PubMed]
53. Suzuki, K.; Garfinkel, S.N.; Critchley, H.D.; Seth, A.K. Multisensory integration across exteroceptive and interoceptive domains modulates self-experience in the rubber-hand illusion. *Neuropsychologia* **2013**, *51*, 2909–2917. [CrossRef] [PubMed]
54. Aspell, J.E.; Heydrich, L.; Marillier, G.; Lavanchy, T.; Herbelin, B.; Blanke, O. Turning Body and Self Inside Out: Visualized Heartbeats Alter Bodily Self-Consciousness and Tactile Perception. *Psychol. Sci.* **2013**, *24*, 2445–2453.
55. Bury, G.; García-Huéscar, M.; Bhattacharya, J.; Ruiz, M.H. Cardiac afferent activity modulates early neural signature of error detection during skilled performance. *NeuroImage* **2019**, *199*, 704–717. [CrossRef]

56. Wessel, J.R.; Danielmeier, C.; Ullsperger, M. Error awareness revisited: Accumulation of multimodal evidence from central and autonomic nervous systems. *J. Cogn. Neurosci.* **2011**, *23*, 3021–3036. [CrossRef]
57. Chambon, V.; Filevich, E.; Haggard, P. What is the human sense of agency, and is it Metacognitive? In *The Cognitive Neuroscience of Metacognition*; Springer: Berlin/Heidelberg, Germany, 2014; pp. 321–342.
58. Metcalfe, J.; Van Snellenberg, J.X.; DeRosse, P.; Balsam, P.; Malhotra, A.K. Judgements of agency in schizophrenia: An impairment in autonoetic metacognition. *Philos. Trans. R. Soc. Lond. B Biol. Sci.* **2012**, *367*, 1391–1400. [CrossRef] [PubMed]
59. Carlson, E.B.; Dalenberg, C.; McDade-Montez, E. Dissociation in posttraumatic stress disorder part I: Definitions and review of research. *Psychol. Trauma Theory Res. Pract. Policy* **2012**, *4*, 479–489. [CrossRef]
60. Sass, L.; Pienkos, E.; Nelson, B.; Medford, N. Anomalous self-experience in depersonalization and schizophrenia: A comparative investigation. *Conscious. Cogn.* **2013**, *22*, 430–441. [CrossRef]
61. Schauer, M.; Elbert, T. Dissociation following traumatic stress etiology and treatment. *J. Psychol.* **2010**, *218*, 109–127. [CrossRef]
62. Stein, D.J.; Koenen, K.C.; Friedman, M.J.; Hill, E.; McLaughlin, K.A.; Petukhova, M.; Ruscio, A.M.; Shahly, V.; Spiegel, D.; Borges, G.; et al. Dissociation in posttraumatic stress disorder: Evidence from the world mental health surveys. *Biol. Psychiatry* **2013**, *73*, 302–312. [CrossRef]
63. Fowles, D.C. Schizophrenia: Diathesis-stress revisited. *Annu. Rev. Psychol.* **1992**, *43*, 303–336. [CrossRef] [PubMed]
64. Walker, E.F.; Diforio, D. Schizophrenia: A neural diathesis-stress model. *Psychol. Rev.* **1997**, *104*, 667–685. [CrossRef] [PubMed]
65. Pruessner, M.; Cullen, A.E.; Aas, M.; Walker, E.F. The neural diathesis-stress model of schizophrenia revisited: An update on recent findings considering illness stage and neurobiological and methodological complexities. *Neurosci. Biobehav. Rev.* **2017**, *73*, 191–218. [CrossRef]
66. Croft, J.; Heron, J.; Teufel, C.; Cannon, M.; Wolke, D.; Thompson, A.; Houtepen, L.; Zammit, S. Association of Trauma Type, Age of Exposure, and Frequency in Childhood and Adolescence with Psychotic Experiences in Early Adulthood. *JAMA Psychiatry* **2019**, *76*, 79–86. [CrossRef] [PubMed]
67. McGrath, J.J.; McLaughlin, K.A.; Saha, S.; Aguilar-Gaxiola, S.; Al-Hamzawi, A.; Alonso, J.; Bruffaerts, R.; De Girolamo, G.; De Jonge, P.; Esan, O.; et al. The association between childhood adversities and subsequent first onset of psychotic experiences: A cross-national analysis of 23 998 respondents from 17 countries. *Psychol. Med.* **2017**, *47*, 1230–1245. [CrossRef]
68. Frith, C. *The Cognitive Neuropsychology of Schizophrenia*; Psychology Press: London, UK, 2014.
69. Nelson, B.; Whitford, T.J.; Lavoie, S.; Sass, L.A. What are the neurocognitive correlates of basic self-disturbance in schizophrenia?: Integrating phenomenology and neurocognition. Part 2 (Aberrant salience). *Schizophr. Res.* **2014**, *152*, 20–27. [CrossRef]
70. Asai, T.; Tanno, Y. Highly schizotypal students have a weaker sense of self-agency. *Psychiatry Clin. Neurosci.* **2008**, *62*, 115–119. [CrossRef]
71. Nelson, B.; Lavoie, S.; Li, E.; Sass, L.A.; Koren, D.; McGorry, P.D.; Jack, B.N.; Parnas, J.; Polari, A.; Allott, K.; et al. The neurophenomenology of early psychosis: An integrative empirical study. *Conscious. Cogn.* **2020**, *77*, 102845. [CrossRef]
72. Eysenck, M.W.; Derakshan, N.; Santos, R.; Calvo, M.G. Anxiety and cognitive performance: Attentional control theory. *Emotion* **2007**, *7*, 336–353. [CrossRef]
73. Kalckert, A.; Ehrsson, H.H. The spatial distance rule in the moving and classical rubber hand illusions. *Conscious. Cogn.* **2014**, *30*, 118–132. [CrossRef]
74. Salomon, R.; Lim, M.; Pfeiffer, C.; Gassert, R.; Blanke, O. Full body illusion is associated with widespread skin temperature reduction. *Front. Behav. Neurosci.* **2013**, *7*, 65. [CrossRef] [PubMed]
75. Hara, M.; Pozeg, P.; Rognini, G.; Higuchi, T.; Fukuhara, K.; Yamamoto, A.; Higuchi, T.; Blanke, O.; Salomon, R. Voluntary self-touch increases body ownership. *Front. Psychol.* **2015**, *6*, 1509. [CrossRef] [PubMed]
76. Leube, D.T.; Knoblich, G.; Erb, M.; Grodd, W.; Bartels, M.; Kircher, T.T. The neural correlates of perceiving one's own movements. *Neuroimage* **2003**, *20*, 2084–2090. [CrossRef] [PubMed]
77. Sato, A. Both motor prediction and conceptual congruency between preview and action-effect contribute to explicit judgment of agency. *Cognition* **2009**, *110*, 74–83. [CrossRef] [PubMed]
78. Stanislaw, H.; Todorov, N. Calculation of signal detection theory measures. *Behav. Res. Methods Instrum. Comput.* **1999**, *31*, 137–149. [CrossRef] [PubMed]

79. Goodman, L.A.; Kruskal, W.H. Measures of Association for Cross Classifications. *J. Am. Stat. Assoc.* **1954**, *49*, 732–764.
80. Nelson, T.O. A comparison of current measures of the accuracy of feeling-of-knowing predictions. *Psychol. Bull.* **1984**, *95*, 109. [CrossRef]
81. Loewy, R.L.; Pearson, R.; Vinogradov, S.; Bearden, C.E.; Cannon, T.D. Psychosis risk screening with the Prodromal Questionnaire—Brief Version (PQ-B). *Schizophr. Res.* **2011**, *129*, 42–46. [CrossRef]
82. Schandry, R. Heart beat perception and emotional experience. *Psychophysiology* **1981**, *18*, 483–488. [CrossRef]
83. Garfinkel, S.N.; Seth, A.K.; Barrett, A.B.; Suzuki, K.; Critchley, H.D. Knowing your own heart: Distinguishing interoceptive accuracy from interoceptive awareness. *Biol. Psychol.* **2015**, *104*, 65–74. [CrossRef]
84. Tsakiris, M.; Tajadura-Jiménez, A.; Costantini, M. Just a heartbeat away from one's body:Interoceptive sensitivity predicts malleability of body-representations. *Proc. R. Soc. B Biol. Sci.* **2011**, *278*, 2470–2476. [CrossRef]
85. Ardizzi, M.; Ferri, F. Interoceptive influences on peripersonal space boundary. *Cognition* **2018**, *177*, 79–86. [CrossRef]
86. Spielberger, C.D.; Gorsuch, R.L.; Lushene, R.E. Manual for the State-Trait Anxiety Inventory (Self Evaluation Questionnaire). *Palo Alto Calif. Consult. Psychol.* **1970**, *22*, 1–24.
87. Kirschbaum, C.; Pirke, K.-M.; Hellhammer, D.H. The 'Trier Social Stress Test—A tool for investigating psychobiological stress responses in a laboratory setting. *Neuropsychobiology* **1993**, *28*, 76–81. [CrossRef] [PubMed]
88. Dedovic, K.; Renwick, R.; Mahani, N.K.; Engert, V. The Montreal Imaging Stress Task: Using functional imaging to investigate the effects of perceiving and processing psychosocial stress in the human brain. *J. Psychiatry Neurosci.* **2005**, *30*, 319–325.
89. *G.Nautilus Wireless 64-Channel EEG Acquisition System*; g.tec Medical Engineering GmbH: Schiedlberg, Austria. Available online: https://www.gtec.at/product/gnautilus-pro/ (accessed on 1 August 2019).
90. Thayer, J.F.; Lane, R.D. A model of neurovisceral integration in emotion regulation and dysregulation. *J. Affect. Disord.* **2000**, *61*, 201–216. [CrossRef]
91. Kim, H.G.; Cheon, E.J.; Bai, D.S.; Lee, Y.H.; Koo, B.H. Stress and heart rate variability: A meta-analysis and review of the literature. *Psychiatry Investig.* **2018**, *15*, 235–245. [CrossRef] [PubMed]
92. Quintana, D.S.; Alvares, G.A.; Heathers, J.A.J. Guidelines for Reporting Articles on Psychiatry and Heart rate variability (GRAPH): Recommendations to advance research communication. *Transl. Psychiatry* **2016**, *6*, e803. [CrossRef]
93. Castro, M.N.; Villarreal, M.F.; Bolotinsky, N.; Papávero, E.; Goldschmidt, M.G.; Costanzo, E.Y.; Drucaroff, L.; Wainsztein, A.; de Achával, D.; Pahissa, J.; et al. Brain activation induced by psychological stress in patients with schizophrenia. *Schizophr. Res.* **2015**, *168*, 313–321. [CrossRef] [PubMed]
94. MathWorks, T. *Matlab Version 9.6.0 (R2019a)*; The MathWorks: Natick, MA, USA, 2019.
95. *JASP*, Version 0.9; Computer software; JASP Team: Amsterdam, The Netherlands, 2018.
96. Wagenmakers, E.J.; Marsman, M.; Jamil, T.; Ly, A.; Verhagen, J.; Love, J.; Selker, R.; Gronau, Q.F.; Šmíra, M.; Epskamp, S.; et al. Bayesian inference for psychology. Part I: Theoretical advantages and practical ramifications. *Psychon. Bull. Rev.* **2018**, *25*, 35–57. [CrossRef]
97. Kruschke, J.K.; Liddell, T.M. Bayesian data analysis for newcomers. *Psychon. Bull. Rev.* **2018**, *25*, 155–177. [CrossRef]
98. Keysers, C.; Gazzola, V.; Wagenmakers, E.-J. Using Bayes factor hypothesis testing in neuroscience to establish evidence of absence. *Nat. Neurosci.* **2020**, *23*, 788–799. [CrossRef] [PubMed]
99. Savill, M.; Ambrosio, J.D.; Cannon, T.D.; Loewy, R.L. Psychosis risk screening in different populations using the Prodromal Questionnaire: A systematic review. *Early Interv. Psychiatry* **2017**, *12*, 1–12. [CrossRef] [PubMed]
100. Gallagher, S. Philosophical conceptions of the self: Implications for cognitive science. *Trends Cogn. Sci.* **2000**, *4*, 14–21. [CrossRef]
101. Marshall, A.C.; Gentsch, A.; Schütz-Bosbach, S. The interaction between interoceptive and action states within a framework of predictive coding. *Front. Psychol.* **2018**, *9*, 1–14. [CrossRef] [PubMed]
102. Salomon, R.; Ronchi, R.; Dönz, J.; Bello-Ruiz, J.; Herbelin, B.; Martet, R.; Faivre, N.; Schaller, K.; Blanke, O. The insula mediates access to awareness of visual stimuli presented synchronously to the heartbeat. *J. Neurosci.* **2016**, *36*, 5115–5127. [CrossRef]

103. Seth, A.K. Interoceptive inference, emotion, and the embodied self. *Trends Cogn. Sci.* **2013**, *17*, 565–573. [CrossRef] [PubMed]
104. Haggard, P.; Clark, S.; Kalogeras, J. Voluntary action and conscious awareness. *Nat. Neurosci.* **2002**, *5*, 382–385. [CrossRef]
105. Tsakiris, M.; Prabhu, G.; Haggard, P. Having a body versus moving your body: How agency structures body-ownership. *Conscious. Cogn.* **2006**, *15*, 423–432. [CrossRef]
106. Van Os, J.; Linscott, R.J.; Myin-Germeys, I.; Delespaul, P.; Krabbendam, L. A systematic review and meta-analysis of the psychosis continuum: Evidence for a psychosis proneness–persistence–impairment model of psychotic disorder. *Psychol. Med.* **2009**, *39*, 179–195. [CrossRef]
107. Drori, G.; Bar-Tal, P.; Stern, Y.; Zvilichovsky, Y.; Salomon, R. UnReal? Investigating the Sense of Reality and Psychotic Symptoms with Virtual Reality. *J. Clin. Med.* **2020**, *9*, 1627. [CrossRef] [PubMed]
108. Koren, D.; Scheyer, R.; Reznik, N.; Adres, M.; Apter, A.; Parnas, J.; Seidman, L.J. Basic self-disturbance, neurocognition and metacognition: A pilot study among help-seeking adolescents with and without attenuated psychosis syndrome. *Early Interv. Psychiatry* **2017**. [CrossRef]
109. Koren, D.; Scheyer, R.; Stern, Y.; Adres, M.; Reznik, N.; Apter, A.; Seidman, L.J. Metacognition strengthens the association between neurocognition and attenuated psychosis syndrome: Preliminary evidence from a pilot study among treatment-seeking versus healthy adolescents. *Schizophr. Res.* **2019**, *210*, 207–214. [CrossRef]
110. Koren, D.; Seidman, L.J.; Goldsmith, M.; Harvey, P.D. Real-world cognitive—And metacognitive—Dysfunction in schizophrenia: A new approach for measuring (and remediating) more "right stuff". *Schizophr. Bull.* **2006**, *32*, 310–326. [CrossRef]
111. McDonald, M.; Christoforidou, E.; Van Rijsbergen, N.; Gajwani, R.; Gross, J.; Gumley, A.I.; Lawrie, S.M.; Schwannauer, M.; Schultze-Lutter, F.; Uhlhaas, P.J. Using online screening in the general population to detect participants at clinical high-risk for psychosis. *Schizophr. Bull.* **2018**, *45*, 600–609. [CrossRef] [PubMed]
112. Myin-Germeys, I.; van Os, J. Stress-reactivity in psychosis: Evidence for an affective pathway to psychosis. *Clin. Psychol. Rev.* **2007**, *27*, 409–424. [CrossRef] [PubMed]
113. Klippel, A.; Viechtbauer, W.; Reininghaus, U.; Wigman, J.; van Borkulo, C.; Myin-Germeys, I.; Wichers, M. The Cascade of Stress: A Network Approach to Explore Differential Dynamics in Populations Varying in Risk for Psychosis. *Schizophr. Bull.* **2017**, *44*, 328–337. [CrossRef] [PubMed]
114. Reininghaus, U.; Kempton, M.J.; Valmaggia, L.; Craig, T.K.J.; Garety, P.; Onyejiaka, A.; Gayer-Anderson, C.; So, S.H.; Hubbard, K.; Beards, S.; et al. Stress sensitivity, aberrant salience, and threat anticipation in early psychosis: An experience sampling study. *Schizophr. Bull.* **2016**, *42*, 712–722. [CrossRef] [PubMed]
115. Yerkes, R.M.; Dodson, J.D. The relation of strength of stimulus to rapidity of habit-formation. *J. Comp. Neurol. Psychol.* **1908**, *18*, 459–482. [CrossRef]
116. Fusar-Poli, P.; Borgwardt, S.; Bechdolf, A.; Addington, J.; Riecher-Rössler, A.; Schultze-Lutter, F.; Keshavan, M.; Wood, S.; Ruhrmann, S.; Seidman, L.J.; et al. The psychosis high-risk state: A comprehensive state-of-the-art review. *Arch. Gen. Psychiatry* **2013**, *70*, 107–120. [CrossRef] [PubMed]
117. van der Gaag, M.; Smit, F.; Bechdolf, A.; French, P.; Linszen, D.H.; Yung, A.R.; McGorry, P.; Cuijpers, P. Preventing a first episode of psychosis: Meta-analysis of randomized controlled prevention trials of 12 month and longer-term follow-ups. *Schizophr. Res.* **2013**, *149*, 56–62. [CrossRef] [PubMed]
118. Tsuang, M.T.; Van Os, J.; Tandon, R.; Barch, D.M.; Bustillo, J.; Gaebel, W.; Gur, R.E.; Heckers, S.; Malaspina, D.; Owen, M.J.; et al. Attenuated psychosis syndrome in DSM-5. *Schizophr. Res.* **2013**, *150*, 31–35. [CrossRef] [PubMed]
119. Light, G.A.; Swerdlow, N.R. Bending the curve on psychosis outcomes. *Lancet Psychiatry* **2015**, *2*, 365–367. [CrossRef]
120. Tsuang, M.T.; Shapiro, D.I.; Ronzio, A.; Bearden, C.E.; Cadenhead, K.S.; Addington, J.; McGlashan, T.H.; Walker, E.F.; Stone, W.S.; Perkins, D.O.; et al. Association of Neurocognition with Transition to Psychosis. *JAMA Psychiatry* **2016**, *73*, 1239. [CrossRef]
121. Gupta, S.; Ranganathan, M.; Dsouza, D.C. The early identification of psychosis: Can lessons be learnt from cardiac stress testing? *Psychopharmacology* **2016**, *233*, 19–37. [CrossRef]

5

Neurorehabilitation of Spatial Memory Using Virtual Environments

Jessica Isbely Montana [1,*], Cosimo Tuena [2], Silvia Serino [3], Pietro Cipresso [2,4] and Giuseppe Riva [2,4]

1 Department of Human Sciences for Education, University of Milano-Bicocca, Piazza dell'Ateneo Nuovo 1, 20126 Milano, Italy
2 ATN-P Lab, Department of Psychology, IRCSS Auxologico Italiano, Via Magnasco 2, 20149 Milano, Italy; cosimotuena@gmail.com (C.T.); p.cipresso@auxologico.it (P.C.); giuseppe.riva@unicatt.it (G.R.)
3 MySpace Lab, Department of Clinical Neurosciences, University Hospital Lausanne-CHUV, CH-1011 Lausanne, Switzerland; silvia.serino@chuv.ch
4 Department of Psychology, Catholic University of the Sacred Heart, Largo Gemelli,1, 20100 Milan, Italy
* Correspondence: jessica.montana@unimib.it

Abstract: In recent years, virtual reality (VR) technologies have become widely used in clinical settings because they offer impressive opportunities for neurorehabilitation of different cognitive deficits. Specifically, virtual environments (VEs) have ideal characteristics for navigational training aimed at rehabilitating spatial memory. A systematic search, following PRISMA guidelines, was carried out to explore the current scenario in neurorehabilitation of spatial memory using virtual reality. The literature on this topic was queried, 5048 papers were screened, and 16 studies were included, covering patients presenting different neuropsychological diseases. Our findings highlight the potential of the navigational task in virtual environments (VEs) for enhancing navigation and orientation abilities in patients with spatial memory disorders. The results are promising and suggest that VR training can facilitate neurorehabilitation, promoting brain plasticity processes. An overview of how VR-based training has been implemented is crucial for using these tools in clinical settings. Hence, in the current manuscript, we have critically debated the structure and the length of training protocols, as well as a different type of exploration through VR devices with different degrees of immersion. Furthermore, we analyzed and highlighted the crucial role played by the selection of the assessment tools.

Keywords: navigation; neurorehabilitation; spatial memory; systematic review; virtual environment; virtual reality

1. Introduction

Virtual reality (VR) is a computer application by which humans interact with computer-generated environments in a way that simulates real life and involves various senses [1] and gives the user an experience of being "immersed" in the VR [2,3]. The experience created in VR depends on output tools (visual, aural, and haptic) that immerse the user in the virtual environments (VEs), input tools (trackers, gloves, or mice) that continually track the position and movements of the users, and the human interaction [4,5]. The degree of physical stimulation impacting on the sensory systems and the sensitivity of the system to motor inputs characterize the immersion experience. The product of immersion is *presence*, defined as the psychological sensation of "being there" in the VE instead of the physical and real environment [1,2,6] or as the "feeling of being in a world that exists outside the self" [4,7–10]. The most commonly used forms of sensory stimulation in VR systems are visual displays. A virtual camera controls the viewpoint from which the subject experiences the computer-generated image. The user's perspective changes according to where he is looking; therefore, it is indispensable to track their location by an incorporated, highly sensitive head and body tracking systems. Sensors monitor the subject's position to provide an egocentric reference frame for the simulation. The images can be delivered either by a head-mounted display (HMD) or by a computer monitor or projection screen. HMDs may be more immersive but can induce cybersickness in vulnerable subjects, whose symptoms are a headache, eye strain, nausea, or, in extreme cases, vomiting [11,12]. In this sense, display screens, semi-immersive systems, are generally more comfortable to use. Auditory and haptic stimulations are often combined with a visual display and are increasingly able to provide a strong sense of physical contact with the VE [13]. In less immersive systems, the input is retrieved from standard joystick controllers, mouse, and keyboard. These control devices are easy to use and naturalistic interfaces that simulate real-world interactions are largely used [1]. The use of VR in neurorehabilitation has grown in a meaningful way, and experimental evidence suggests that this technology could have a positive impact on functional recovery in neuropsychological disorders [8,14]. It is a fascinating tool in neurorehabilitation for its peculiarities. First, the possibility of creating tailor-made training that has the value of highlighting how each rehabilitation process must be individualized, addressing the recovery of the patient's specific disorder and adaptation request [1]. The active involvement that this tool can generate in the subjects is due to the possibility of creating new and appealing environments without forgetting the valuable immediate and concrete feedback that comes to the person. The movement accomplished can be reproduced by the avatar within the VR and this is crucial feedback for the patient [15–18]. VR also offers the opportunity for controlled, ecological, and secure testing environments with different degrees of immersion and interaction [1,19]. Thus, an increasing number of cognitive rehabilitation programs have started using VE to simulate daily activities, such as shopping, traveling [20], or exploring a city [21].

The literature shows that virtual reality is an acceptable and promising therapeutic tool for several pathological fields [13], such as mental health disorders in patients with post-traumatic stress disorder, anxiety and depression [22,23], or eating disorders [14,24,25] and in neuropsychological deficits, for instance, in patients with traumatic brain injury (TBI) [26]. Interesting are the results in which VR has been shown to have potential for improving the assessment and treatment of TBI and dementia [27–29], even in cases where the probabilities of recovery appear low [30]. It has been demonstrated as a successful tool in spatial memory and navigational abilities, particularly in Alzheimer's disease (AD) and in mild cognitive impairment (MCI) [13,31,32].

Spatial memory is reflected in a person's navigation and orientation abilities, fundamental requirements for moving in the surrounding environment. The ability to reach landmarks efficiently depends upon the ability to form, retain, and utilize a cognitive representation of the environment [33]. Human navigation involves several cognitive functions and processes. It can be based on self-motion cues and static environmental cues. The tracking of a person's position and orientation is based on self-motion cues, motor efferences, and vestibular and proprioceptive feedback [34]. Environmental cues are based on landmarks and extended boundaries that can provide one's position and orientation relative to the environment. Self-motion and static environmental cues can inform allocentric and egocentric reference frames [35,36]. Allocentric representation is independent of the position of the navigator and does not change with the navigator through space. An egocentric frame, however, involves the representation of locations based on the subject's viewpoint [37]. The self-reference system uses self-motion cues to update body location and face direction relative to an allocentric, orientation-free, immediately available, object-to-object map [38].

Spatial memory problems, such as forgetting the orientation and the position of objects or getting lost, are often a result of hippocampal damage in humans [32,37,39,40]. The consequence of these representations can be dissociated in terms of behavioral and developmental elements, and, finally, of their neural bases. Thus, the hippocampus and medial temporal lobe offer allocentric environmental representations, whereas the parietal lobe egocentric representations and the retrosplenial cortex and parieto-occipital sulcus allow both types of representation to interact with each other [37,39,41,42].

In human navigation, the role of the hippocampus and associated mesial temporal lobe structures has been widely demonstrated [37]. Meanwhile, differential activity in the hippocampus and caudate correspond to the acquisition and expression of information about locations derived from environmental boundaries or landmarks, respectively [43]. Changes in the navigation network may be a result of cognitive decline and can manifest in impaired spatial navigation [35].

In conclusion, the environments recreated using VR technology represent a context through which the user has the opportunity to experience real-life scenarios and increase their abilities and experience new adaptation strategies [13]. In [44], it is suggested that patients are able to transfer information about the environment acquired from VE to real life. They suggest that mental representations of space in VE are rather like those implicated in the navigation of the real world. Concerning the growing interest in VR and high potential applications in neurorehabilitation, it is necessary to examine the treatment procedures and the results obtained so far. According to these premises, we aimed at providing a systematic review of the experiments in the field of spatial memory neurorehabilitation to comprehend if VR navigational training, compared to treatment as usual, is effective in improving navigational abilities. The specific objectives of the present work are two-fold. First, to provide an overview of which apparatus are available for neurorehabilitation and understanding how these VR training regimes have been implemented in clinical settings. We analyzed different types of software and procedures for implementing the training. Finally, in light of the cognitive and neural theories of spatial processing, we attempted to compare different VR navigational training used and analyzed which is more useful.

2. Method

2.1. Search Methodology

Preferred Reporting Items for Systematic Reviews and Meta-Analysis (PRISMA) guidelines were followed [45]. Two high-profile databases (PubMed and Web of Science) were used to perform the computer-based research on the 6 July 2019. According to PICO format, we defined the question (following the identification of problem, intervention, comparison group, and outcome) as "In spatial memory disorder, is VR navigational training, compared to treatment as usual, effective in improving navigation abilities?". We then proceeded with the definition of keywords for the search strategy. The string used to carry out the search strategy was virtual-realit* OR virtual-environment* AND neurorehabilitation OR rehabilitation OR training OR stimulation OR navigation OR learning OR abilit* OR memor* AND spatial OR space.

From the search of both databases, we obtained 5048 articles, excluding duplicates. Title and abstract screening was carried out, and 24 articles passed to the full-text screening phase. Eight studies were excluded with reasons as follow: Not Controlled trial (= 1); Results of neuropsychological outcome for spatial memory not reported (= 3); Qualitative/descriptive study (= 2); Not neuropsychological rehabilitation for spatial memory (= 2).

2.2. Inclusion Criteria

The review considered randomized control trials, nonrandomized control trials, intervention studies, and case-control studies in clinical patient populations with an overt spatial memory disorder. Studies on rehabilitation's programs of navigation abilities with virtual reality (VR) devices in different population of patients (such as mild cognitive impairment (MCI), Alzheimer's disease (AD), traumatic brain injury (TBI), multiple sclerosis (MS), stroke, cerebral palsy, epilepsy, incomplete cervical vertebro-spinal trauma, topographical disorientation disorders and neglect) were included. We only included studies in the English language and which satisfied strict criteria for eligibility for the review (research studies, clinical patient population, VR training, spatial memory disorders, rehabilitation programs). The qualitative component also considered the type of VR navigational training and methodological design. We excluded articles which lacked necessary information for review in the full-text or the abstract. Reviews, meeting abstracts, proceedings, notes, case reports, letters to the editor, assessment protocols, editorials, and other editorial materials were also excluded. Retrospective studies were not included because the area of interest requires performing experiments.

2.3. *Risk of Bias Assessment*

To assess the risk of bias, the reviewers followed the methods recommended by The Cochrane Collaboration Risk of Bias Tool [46] and the STROBE Statement [47]. Two reviewers (J.M. and C.T.) independently assessed the risk of bias of each included study against key criteria: random sequence generation, allocation concealment, blinding of participants, personnel, and outcomes, incomplete outcome data, selective outcome reporting, and other sources of bias. The following judgments were used: low risk, high risk, or unclear (either lack of information or uncertainty over the potential for bias). Disagreements were resolved through consensus, and a third author was consulted to resolve disagreements if necessary. In particular, the selected studies followed strict criteria in the methods, including presenting critical elements of study design, clearly defining all outcomes, describing the setting and relevant dates, including periods of recruitment and exposure, giving sources of data and details of methods of assessment (measurement).

2.4. *PRISMA Flow Diagram*

PRISMA guidelines were strictly followed; all titles and abstracts were screened according to the abovementioned inclusion criteria after removing the duplicates. Full texts of eligible articles were retrieved and assessed by two reviewers (J.M. and C.T.) for individual selection of papers to reduce the risk of bias and resolving disagreements through consensus as explained in Section 2.1. See Figure 1 for the paper selection procedure.

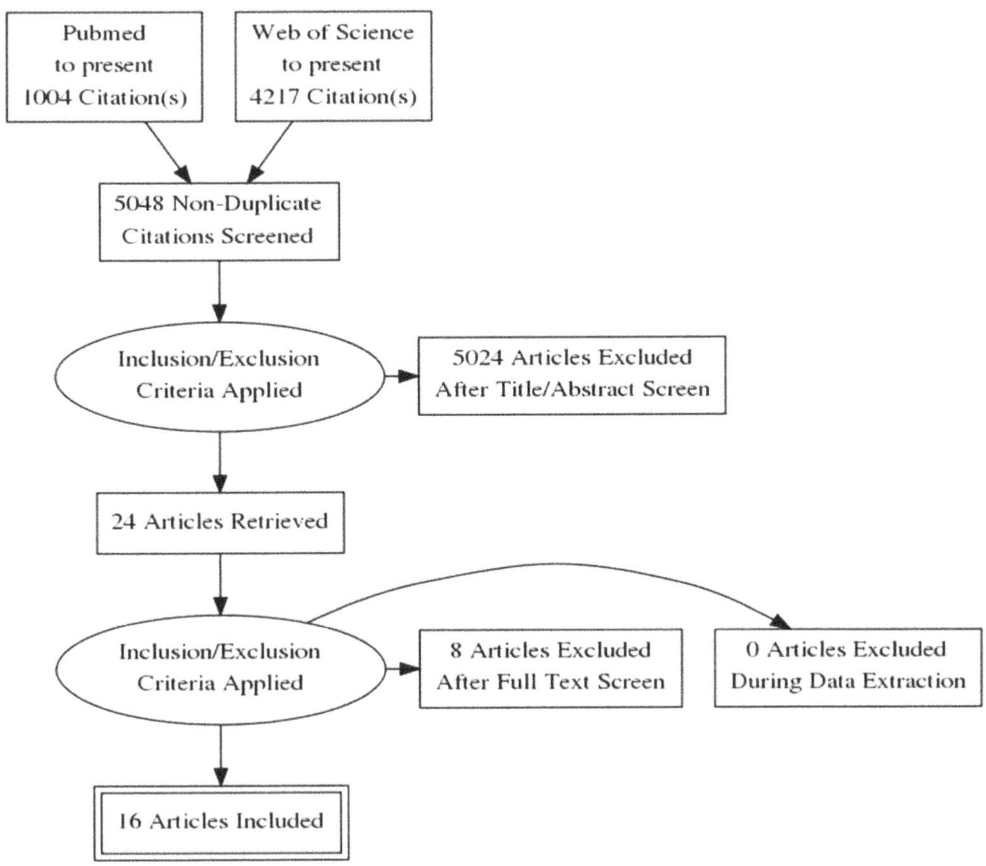

Figure 1. PRISMA flow diagram.

3. Results

Sixteen studies were analyzed to test the usefulness of rehabilitative interventions using virtual reality (VR) systems. However, growing interest in VR has led researchers to question how the characteristics of VR equipment and different aspects of the training tasks could influence the treatment outcomes, with particular regard to the results that reflect on the patient's daily life in an ecological way. In our review, we aim at giving more awareness to the researchers and at guiding them in the selection of the most appropriate VR device to use. Considering the studies mentioned in this analysis, it could be possible to understand which is the most suitable program for the treatment of spatial memory disorders, in terms of the type of apparatus used and the training method. Furthermore, it is essential to understand which kind of patient will benefit from the intervention. To satisfy our aims and to facilitate the understanding, we considered the following clusters: (1) Authors; (2) Year; (3) Sample (N); (4) Sample characteristics; (5) Mean age; (6) VR Task; (7) Virtual Apparatus; (8) Neuropsychological assessment; (9) Primary Outcomes. Results are reported in Table 1.

Table 1. Papers included in the PRISMA systematic review. MMSE—Mini-Mental State Assessment; MoCA—Montreal Cognitive Assessment; ACE—Addenbrooke's Cognitive Examination; ADAS—Alzheimer's Disease Assessment Scale; WAIS-III—Weschler Adult Intelligent Scale; RAVLT—Rey Auditory verbal Learning Test; RBMT—Rivermead Behavioural Memory Test; CBTT—Corsi Block-Tapping Test; DART—Dutch Version of Reading Test; BIT—Behavioural Inattention Test; FIM—Functional Independence Measure; FAB—Frontal Assessment Battery; AM—attentive Matrices; TMT A- B- A/B—Trial Making Test; BIT—Behavioural Inattention Test; WMS IV—Wechsler memory scale; WTAR—Wechsler Scale of adult Reading; VOSP—Visual Object and Space Perception Battery; CFMT—Cambridge Face Memory Test; CFPT—Cambridge Face Perception Test; BRLD—Bergen Left-Right Discrimination Test; ROCF—Rey–Osterrieth Complex Figure Test; RWT—Regensburg Verbal Fluency Test; VLMT—German adaptation of the Rey Verbal Learning Test; LPS 50+—The Achievement Measure System 50+; LVT—Visual Pursuit Test.

	Authors	Year	Sample (N)	Sample Characteristics	Mean Age (SD or Range)	VR Task	VR Apparatus	Pre- and Post- Assessment	Primary Outcomes
1	Pugnetti et al. [48]	1998	30	**Experimental Group (EG)** 15 MS patients. **Control Group (CG)** 15 healthy controls.	**EG** active condition mean age = 39.1; Standard Deviation (SD) =11.1/passive condition mean age = 37.7; SD = 8.1. **CG** active condition mean age = 35.8; SD = 9.41/passive condition mean age = 35.4; SD = 12.2	The aim was to explore the VE of a house, composed of four rooms and corridors, in search of an object.	Nonimmersive Virtual Reality (Superscape Software, version 4).	ROF, CBTT, Raven's matrices IQ.	Spatial memory improved in the active subject (MS and healthy) suggesting that direct interaction with the environment can enhance navigation ability.
2	Akhutina et al. [49]	2003	EXP 1. 21 EXP 2. 45	EXP 1. **EG/CG** 21 patients with a diagnosis of cerebral palsy. EXP 2. **EG/CG** 45 patients with a diagnosis of cerebral palsy.	EXP 1. **EG** 12 (range 7–14) **CG** 9 (range 7–14) EXP 2. **EG** 23 (range 7–14) **CG** 22 (range 7–14)	The aim in each version of the task (drawn, real or virtual) was to move through a maze to reach a tree.	Non immersive environments IBM-PC and a mouse (Super Scape VRT 3-D Software) displayed on a 40,630 cm monitor.	EXP1. computer versions of the Koos Block Design Test, and a Clown Assembly Test. Decentration of Viewpoint Test, and Directional Pointing to a Hidden Object Test. EXP 2. Additional measures: Raven Progressive Matrices; The Benton Judgment of Line Orientation Test; The arrows subtest of the Nepsy; The Roads Test.	The studies have demonstrated that the general spatial abilities of a group of children with motor disabilities can be enhanced using a battery of training tasks that demand the use of various spatial skills. The battery included VEs that provided the children with navigational spatial experience, of a kind that most would rarely (if ever) experience in the course of their daily lives.

Table 1. *Cont.*

	Authors	Year	Sample (N)	Sample Characteristics	Mean Age (SD or Range)	VR Task	VR Apparatus	Pre- and Post- Assessment	Primary Outcomes
3	Caglio et al. [50]	2012	1	TBI patient with hemorrhagic contusions in the bilateral frontal, temporal and parietal lobes.	24 (male)	The aim was to explore part of a virtual town (London) from a ground-level perspective.	Nonimmersive Virtual Reality (Midtown Madness 2 videogame).	Corsi Block-Tapping Test, Corsi Supra-Span Test, Backward digit span, RAVLT, TMT A-B, Phonemic fluency, ADAS, RBMT.	Improvement in immediate verbal learning, immediate and delayed spatial learning and everyday-spatial memory persisted at follow-ups.
4	Grewe et al. [20]	2013	24	**EG** 5 patients with focal epilepsy (2 right temporo-parietal; 1 right hippocampal; 1 bilateral temporal; 1 bilateral occipital periventricular). **CG** 19 healthy participants	**EG** mean age = 35.04; SD = 8.08; **CG** mean age = 23; SD = 3.45	The aim was to navigate into a virtual medium-sized supermarket, modeled according to a real standard supermarket, in search of a specific list of objects.	OctaVis, semi-immersive Virtual Reality device.	ROF	The supermarket training provided preliminary evidence of effectiveness, but significant improvement was not found. A strong limitation was due to the small sample size.

Table 1. *Cont.*

	Authors	Year	Sample (N)	Sample Characteristics	Mean Age (SD or Range)	VR Task	VR Apparatus	Pre- and Post- Assessment	Primary Outcomes
5	Kober et al. [51]	2013	23	**EG** 23 patients: 3 right and 1 arteria cerebri media stroke, 1 basal ganglia and thalamus stroke, 1 right arteria cerebri media, 1 basal ganglia stroke, 1 right fronto-parietal stroke, 2 right aneurysm and subsequent infarct (arteria cerebri posterior and arteria communicans with parietal infarct), 1 arteria cerebri media hemorrhage, 1 TBI (left hippocampus and pons). **CG** 11 healthy participants	**EG** mean age = 66.09; SD = 3.30 CG mean age = 66.18; SD = 2.97	The aim was a route-finding in a district of the real-world town of Graz, Austria.	Nonimmersive Virtual Reality.	Four spatial tests before and after the five VR training sessions: the Benton Test, the LPS 50+, the LVT, and the CBTT.	Route finding ability in the VR task increased over the five training sessions. Moreover, both groups improved different aspects of spatial abilities after VR training in comparison to the spatial performance before VR training.

Table 1. *Cont.*

	Authors	Year	Sample (N)	Sample Characteristics	Mean Age (SD or Range)	VR Task	VR Apparatus	Pre- and Post- Assessment	Primary Outcomes
6	Grewe et al. [52]	2014	33	**EG** 14 patients with focal epilepsy (frontal = 3, temporal = 8, central = 2, parietal = 1). **CG** 19 healthy participants	**EG** mean age = 31.29; SD = 9.44; 8 males. **CG** mean age = 31.21; SD = 14.26; 4 males	The aim was to navigate into a virtual medium-sized supermarket, modeled according to a real standard supermarket, in search of a specific list of objects.	OctaVis, semi-immersive Virtual Reality device.	BRLD-A, BRLD-B; ROCF copy, ROCF immediate and delayed recall; RWT Total Score; Digit Span Forward and Backward; VLMT immediate recallB, VLMT total learningB Trials, VLMT loss after InterferenceB, VLMT loss after delayB.	Spatial navigation and memory performance (n° of correct products, movements trajectories, time) significantly increased in the course of the 8-day training. Due to the small sample sizes in the subgroups, it could not be established the effects of different sites of epileptic foci.
7	Claessen et al. [53]	2015	6	6 stroke patients with left (N = 3), right (N = 2) and bilateral (N = 1) supratentorial stroke. No control group.	mean age = 57; SD = 8.9; 2 males	The aim was a route-finding in the Virtual Tubingen town.	Nonimmersive Virtual Reality with a joystick (Virtual Tübingen).	CBTT, TMT A-B, WAIS-III, DART, Virtual Tübingen Test (Scene recognition, Route continuation/sequence/ order/progression/ distance, Pointing to start/to end, Map drawing/recognition).	Navigation abilities clearly improved in one patient, partially in four cases. For other cases, were successful in adopting an alternative navigation strategy and improved on most of the trained abilities. VR was judged as highly feasible by the patients.
8	Faria et al. [54]	2016	18	**EG** 9 stroke patients. **CG** 9 stroke patients	**EG** mean age = 58 – 71; male = 44%. **CG** mean age = 53; male = 44%	The aim was to navigate in order to accomplish some common ADL's (in a supermarket, a post office, a bank, and a pharmacy) in a virtual city with streets, sidewalks, commercial buildings, parks and moving cars.	Nonimmersive Virtual Reality with a joystick (Reh@City).	ACE, TMT A-B, Picture Arrangement Test, SIS 3.0.	VR group improved in attention, visuospatial abilities, memory, executive functions, emotion, global cognition, and overall recovery. Between comparisons showed training effect on global cognition, executive functions and attention for VR group.

Table 1. *Cont.*

	Authors	Year	Sample (N)	Sample Characteristics	Mean Age (SD or Range)	VR Task	VR Apparatus	Pre- and Post- Assessment	Primary Outcomes
9	White & Moussavi [55]	2016	1	MCI patient with probable development of AD	74 (male)	The aim was to navigate into a virtual building in search of specific targets.	Immersive Virtual Reality system with Head-mounted Display and joypad.	MoCA, VRN task (Byagowi & Moussavi, 2012), navigation diary.	The patient improved navigation during the sessions assessed with the VRN task and as reported with the wife's diary.
10	Bate et al. [56]	2017	1	Patient with developmental prosopagnosia with concurrent topographical disorientation	58 (female)	The aim was to navigate in a virtual city, (containing six landmarks such as cinema, restaurant, pub, hotel, pharmacy, and florist) and recall the position of each landmark on a top-view map of the city.	Nonimmersive Virtual Reality with the keypad.	WAIS-III, WMS-IV, Wisconsin Card Sorting Test, CBTT, Rey's complex figures, Picture Naming, WTAR, VOSP. Face processing tasks: CFMT, famous faces, CFPT, Ekman 60, navigational assessment: Benton, Santa Barbara Sense of direction Scale, Memory of building, 'O clock task, route map.	Following the last session of treatment, the patient was able to form a cognitive map faster than the first one and the performance in the retrieval task was improved. A similar performance was observed at the one-week follow-up session.

Table 1. *Cont.*

	Authors	Year	Sample (N)	Sample Characteristics	Mean Age (SD or Range)	VR Task	VR Apparatus	Pre- and Post- Assessment	Primary Outcomes
11	De La Torre - Luque et al. [57]	2017	20	20 patients with a neurological diagnosis included cerebral palsy (20%), intellectual development disorder (20%) and both disorders (55%); TBI (5%).	mean age= 34.35, SD= 10.2; 13 males and 7 females.	The aim was to move through the virtual environment, and then through the equivalent real-life one and to find the same two rooms for both environments.	Semi-immersive Virtual Reality with a joystick and a mouse. A Mitsubishi® projector (model XL8U), projecting onto a × 1.5-m screen.	For the assessment of cognitive visuospatial planning and orientation, 2 tests: Porteus Maze Test; Mindscape's Brain Trainer® 2 Maze Stair Test.	Both groups improved in a similar way, though we can say that the best. results in the virtual and the real building and generalization goals were due to virtual training. Firstly, a reduction in errors and time needed to locate the objectives in the virtual building was found after the training, so as to point out that the active navigational training showed changes. In addition, the participants had better scores in the posttest and generalization tasks in the real environment and when using maps of the building, and these tasks were not directly trained.
12	De Luca et al. [58]	2017	1	Neglect patient (subarachnoid hemorrhage, right fronto-temporal- parietal region).	57	The aim was to move in the virtual environment and manipulate specific objects, in order to realize specific associations.	Semi-immersive VR (BTs Nirvana PC System connected to a projector or a big screen).	MMSE, BIT; line crossing and bisection, letter and star cancellation, map navigation, card, and coin sorting, drawing and copying tests, phone dialing, menu and article reading, telling and setting the time.	The training enhanced spatial cognition, visual search, and attention. In addition, with standard cognitive treatment was observed a nearly complete recovery of Unilateral Spatial Neglect.

Table 1. *Cont.*

	Authors	Year	Sample (N)	Sample Characteristics	Mean Age (SD or Range)	VR Task	VR Apparatus	Pre- and Post- Assessment	Primary Outcomes
13	Serino et al. [21]	2017	28	**EG** 10 patients with AD. 8 healthy participants. **CG** 10 patients with AD	**EG** patients mean age = 86.60; SD = 6.13; 1male. healthy mean age = 86.62; SD = 6.19; 4 males. **CG** patients mean age = 88.7; SD = 3.59; 2 males	The aim was to navigate inside the virtual environment, to discover one, two or three hidden objects (i.e., a bottle of milk, a plant in a vase and a trunk) to retrieve their positions in the last phase.	Nonimmersive VR (NeuroVR software).	MMSE, Phonemic fluency, Categorical fluency, FAB, Attentional Matrices Test, Digit span test, Corsi Block-Tapping Test, Corsi Supra-Span Test.	The training enhanced spatial learning in the VR group-AD compared to control group-AD and VR healthy group improved executive functions compared to VR group-AD.
14	De Luca et al. [59]	2018	12	**EG** 6 post-stroke patients. **CG** 6 post-stroke patients	**EG/CG** mean age = 40; SD = 14	The aim was to move in the virtual environment and manipulate specific objects, in order to realize specific associations.	Semi-immersive VR (BTs Nirvana PC System connected to a projector or a big screen).	MoCA, FIM, FAB, AM, TMT A, TMT B, TMT A/B.	VR can be useful in potentiating the cognitive recovery in post-stroke chronic phase. It improved visuospatial and attention in the experimental group.

Table 1. *Cont.*

	Authors	Year	Sample (N)	Sample Characteristics	Mean Age (SD or Range)	VR Task	VR Apparatus	Pre- and Post- Assessment	Primary Outcomes
15	Maresca et al. [60]	2018	1	A right-handed patient affected by incomplete cervical vertebro-spinal trauma, presented with a moderate tetraparesis, mainly involving the left side.	60 (male)	The aim was to move in the virtual environment and manipulate specific objects, and to realize specific associations.	A nonimmersive virtual reality rehabilitation system (VRRS) by Khymeia, interacting with a touch screen or a magnetic tracking sensor.	MoCA, AM, TMT, digit span, RAVLI, RAVLR, Wigl's sorting test, Raven's colored matrices, VFT, SFT, HRS-D, HRS-A.	The combined approach using VRRS demonstrated a significant improvement in different cognitive domains as spatial abilities, executive functions, selective attention, and memory abilities.
16	Mrakic-Sposta et al. [61]	2018	10	**EG** 5 MCI patients with compromise visuospatial abilities. **CG** 5 MCI patients with compromise visuospatial abilities	**EG/CG** aged > 65 years; 4 males and 6 females	The aim was to navigate and to orientate inside three virtual environments (ride a bike in a park, crossroads in a city and shopping in a supermarket).	Semi-immersive scenarios with a finger touch projector and a PlayStation controller and cycle-ergometer, a Wearable smart garment (heart rate)	MMSE; RAVLT-I and RAVLT-D; ROCFT; AM; TMT-A and TMT-B; FAB; VFT.	The presented results suggest that the adopted training protocol was able to affect MMSE tasks and to increase the global cognition levels of MCI patients.

Analysis of results in spatial navigation rehabilitation programs was carried out starting from the outcomes of 16 studies, taking into consideration the patient population, the VR apparatus (immersive/semi- or nonimmersive) and the type of training used. We analyzed clinical, methodological, and technical outcomes to cast research and clinical applications of VR in the context of VR navigational training. The results were argued in response to the following three questions.

3.1. Which Virtual Apparatus Is Recommended for Spatial Memory Rehabilitation?

3.1.1. Type of Device and Controllers During Navigation

Among all the studies reviewed, the only one that used an immersive virtual reality (VR) system with a head-mounted display HMD Oculus Rift DK2, using the Unity 5 game engine, and a joypad is described in [39] (see Table 1 for an overview of VR equipment). Several studies [20,52,57–59,61], used semi-immersive systems: the previous one used OctaVis, a circle of eight screens in which the participant can freely rotate on a fixed chair and interact with a joystick; while [58,59] used a BTs Nirvana PC System connected to a projector or a big screen and to an infrared sensor for movements; in [61], a finger touch projector was used and the scenarios were developed using Unity 3D. In order to increase the user's presence in the VE, attention was paid to elements such as the visual flow synchronized with the cycling velocity in real-time, realistic 3D sound, perception of the wind through the movement of trees; [57] used a projector on a big screen (2 × 1.5 m) and a viewing height of 1.8 m. Virtual Scene Designer was used to create the scenarios. The advantage conferred by the semi-immersive system is that it allows sensorial isolation, but it presents fewer signs of cybersickness. Even this system demonstrates the generalizability of VR measures by correlations with subjective estimations of cognitive abilities and real-life shopping performance [52]. Immersive and semi-immersive systems have proved to be useful tools in navigational training for improving spatial cognition and attention processes [55,58].

Nine further studies reviewed used nonimmersive systems. In [50] the rehabilitation training was based on a navigational task, exploring part of a virtual town (London) from a ground-level perspective, using a computer videogame driving simulator (Midtown Madness 2, Microsoft Game Studios). Other studies have used nonimmersive VR training on a computer with joystick or keypad to navigate the city, using Unity 3D software—Reh@city [54,56]—on a standard IBM-PC computer and in an environment developed with the Super Scape VRT-3D construction package [49]; or a specific software developed by authors—Virtual Tübingen [53]. Other studies used Superscape software version 4 and NeuroVR. NeuroVR is a free VR-platform for customizing a large number of predeveloped virtual environments [9,21,48,62]. One study [51] created a simulation of the real-world town of Graz (Austria) using Instantreality software, a high-performance Mixed-Reality framework that provides a comprehensive set of features to support classic virtual reality [63]. Another study [60] used a certified medical device with high customization capacity, the virtual reality rehabilitation system (VRSS), which comprises a central hub connected to specialized peripheral devices, such as magnetic sensors for movements, which is fully synchronized and integrated with the system. Also, the rehabilitation programs that used a nonimmersive system showed promising enhancement of different cognitive abilities through spatial and navigational training [21,48,50–53,58].

3.1.2. VR Spatial Navigation

The usefulness of VR navigational tasks in rehabilitation programs for spatial memory has been highlighted. Promising results have been demonstrated with the use of navigation tasks on simple display screens of a computer (nonimmersive devices). However, better performance can be achieved through immersive rather than semi-immersive systems by using head-mounted displays. This is explained by the greater sense of presence [4,8], with integrated systems that record the user's movement and take advantage of up to six degrees of freedom, and providing feedback to the user about their performance [15]. Since navigation in virtual environments can trigger the same brain mechanisms as navigation in the real world, spatial "presence" can be generated [64].

3.2. *Which Virtual Training Method Is Suitable for Spatial Memory Rehabilitation?*

The studies included in the current review are all focused on the rehabilitation of spatial memory and navigation abilities in different neurologic patients, including mild cognitive impairment (MCI), Alzheimer's disease (AD), traumatic brain injury (TBI), multiple sclerosis (MS), stroke, cerebral palsy, epilepsy, incomplete cervical vertebro-spinal trauma, prosopagnosia with topographical disorientation disorders, and neglect. all patients have used virtual reality (VR) devices in different rehabilitation programs, and nobody had any difficulty in following the training. Overall, the emerging outcomes are positive, and they present improvements to different degrees. All of the mentioned studies had a control group [20,21,48,49,51,52,54,57,59,61] except one [53]. Five of them reported results of single case studies [50,55,56,58,60]. Virtual rehabilitation enables clinicians to control the specific features of the virtual environment, enabling tailoring of the challenge to suit individual patient needs [65]. The characteristics of virtual training (detailed in the following paragraphs) that are crucially important are the overall duration of the training, the frequency, the intensity of each session, and, last but not least, the time elapsed since the damage [57]. Additionally, some studies have already demonstrated that the use of a map as a navigational aid improved the performance of users performing complex navigational tasks [66]. Furthermore, the presence of a small-scale interactive aerial view facilitated the retrieval of stored spatial layout and an arrow or salient landmarks, giving more comprehensive information about the egocentric heading in environment, were effective in supporting the navigation [67,68]. Also, findings in the studies examined underline the importance of using active navigation protocols to promote the neurorehabilitation of spatial memory [62,67], and that the degree of the visual similarities between the virtual world and the real one boosts the transfer of learning between contexts [57].

3.2.1. VR Training Duration

The protocol duration turned out to be an important variable for rehabilitation training outcomes (details are visible in Table 2). The training proposed by [50,60] was the most intensive. The first regime consisted of 15 sessions of 90 min each, amounting to 22.5 h. The second regime consisted of three weekly sessions of 60 min for a total of 36 treatments. The improvements are visible after a certain period of time, as evidenced by two-month and one-year follow-ups [50]. One study [55] proposed 21 sessions of 45 min each, amounting to 15.75 h, and [61] proposed 18 sessions lasting 40–45 min each for a total of 13.5 h. In these studies, the patients showed substantial improvement in navigation ability. Another study [59] conducted 20 sessions for stroke patients in which an intensive and long training program was essential for obtaining substantial improvements. Other rehabilitation programs, which lasted between eight to 15 sessions, showed an improvement in long-term spatial memory after VR-based training [21,52,57]. Transference of improvements from the VR-based training to more general aspects of spatial cognition was observed [21]. Interesting results are also connected with high frequency and intensity of sessions [21,50,52,55,58,59] rather than low-intensity training regimes [49]. A protocol lasting less than four hours returns vulnerable outcomes [20,51,53,54,56,62]. For example, one study [53] based on four sessions of 1 h each was only able to significantly improve one patient's performance.

Table 2. Training characteristics.

	Authors	Type of Training	Single Session Duration (min)	Repetitions	Frequency/Period	Total Hours
1	Pugnetti et al. (1998)	Navigational training with active and passive conditions + recall landmarks	30	1		30 min
2	Akhutina et al. (2003)	Navigational task	30–60	6–8	within a month	3–8 h
3	Caglio et al. (2012)	Navigational training	90	15	3 times a week for 5 weeks	22.5 h
4	Grewe et al. (2013)	Navigational training + free recall of objects list and positions (at last session)	20	8	daily	2.6 h
5	Kober et al. (2013)	Navigational training + recall up to maximal three different routes	20	6	-	2 h
6	Grewe et al.	Navigational training + free recall of objects list and positions (at last session) + real-life performance	30	8	Every 1–3 days within 2 weeks	4 h
7	Claessen et al. (2015)	Navigational training	60	4	-	4 h
8	Faria et al. (2016)	Navigational training	20	12	4–6 weeks	4 h
9	White & Moussavi (2016)	Navigational training	45	21	3 times a week for 7 weeks	15.75 h
10	Bate et al. (2017)	Navigational training + recall landmarks	60-70	7	Every 3–4 days	7–8 h
11	De La Torre Luque et al. (2017)	Navigational training	20	15	daily	5 h
12	De Luca et al. (2017)	Navigational training + association of object position	45	20	5 times a week for 1 month	15 h
13	Serino et al. (2017)	Navigational training + recall object positions	30	10	3 times a week for 3–4 weeks	5 h
14	De Luca et al. (2018)	Navigational training + association of object position	45	24	3 times a week for 8 weeks	18 h
15	Maresca et al. (2018)	Navigational training	60	36	3 times a week for 12 weeks	36 h
16	Mrakic et al (2018)	Navigational training	45	18	3 times a week for 6 weeks	13.5 h

3.2.2. Time Elapsed Since Damage

Another important variable is the time elapsed from the brain injury to the starting point of cognitive rehabilitation. One study [54] found an overall recovery and showed a positive training effect on global cognitive functions in post-stroke patients which started the treatment within 7 months from the stroke. A long-distance from the traumatic event, instead, does not promise good results, as happened in patients who started an average of 43 months after stroke [53]. A short interval was also important in other disorders. One study [50] have gained promising results with a single traumatic brain injury (TBI) patient that began the training within 1 year. The shorter the period between the traumatic event and the beginning of treatment, the higher the probability of achieving a better outcome [50,52,54].

3.2.3. Training Procedure

A detailed description of the different procedures is outlined below. In one study [50], the patient was given the instruction "You must cut down poles and trees that you find all along the way", with the aim of inducing the participant to explore the virtual town, avoiding passing the same roads twice. The spatial memory task was implicit, while the explicit task was a simple game, which entertained the participant. The participant did not have access to a city map during the task.

One study [53] used training divided into implicit (free exploration) and explicit tasks (following specific routes). During the sessions, the patients were encouraged to practice the instructed navigational strategy learned in a previous psycho-educational phase. The participants had access to a city map during the task. Two studies [54,56] used implicit tasks. In the first study, the participant was guided by instructions such as "Go to the supermarket". Visual feedback elements (time and point counters) were used to reward successful actions. The participant had access to a mini-map in the lower half of the screen and/or a guidance arrow. In the second study, the participant was asked to follow three routes, differing in length, as quickly and as accurately as possible. In the next learning phase, the patient was required to create a mental representation of the city, incorporating the spatial location of six landmarks. In the retrieval phase, he was required to navigate via the city in order to reach a location as quickly as possible and using the shortest route possible.

In [55], the participant was instructed to enter a building and find the correct window, which had been previously shown from an external view of the building. Two studies [21,51] used specific tasks with encoding and retrieval phases. In the first study, the neuropsychologist asked participants to find and memorize the position of hidden objects within the virtual city. Then, they were asked to retrieve the position of the objects identified before, starting from another point of the city. Participants had access to a city map during the task. In the second study, the participant had to learn a route by following verbal instructions and subsequently had to recall the correct directions. In two studies [48,57], the participants received explicit instructions to explore and memorize a route in the virtual environment (VE) during the research of an object. Subsequently, in the first study, they were asked to draw the layout of the VE, and in the second study they had to move through the equivalent real-life environment. Also, in [49], the participants were asked to move through a maze to reach a tree. In the first and second versions, the plan of the maze was visible, and the target always remained visible. In the third version, the target tree could be seen only from a short distance when not hidden by the maze walls. In [20,52], the participants had to memorize an auditory shopping list of 20 items as an implicit spatial memory task and subsequently buy all the items remembered in a VR supermarket. In the second study, the same authors presented a new interfering list with 20 distractor items during the training.

Three studies [58–60] included a series of exercises involving different cognitive functions. The participants were asked to remember the positions and the name of elements observed or to program movements to manipulate specific objects and to realize specific associations with dynamic interaction in VE. In [61], three scenarios were used, in which patients had to navigate freely to accomplish the task explicitly requested, for example, purchasing five items form a supermarket. The spatial memory task was explicit, and only in the last version was no aid was given for completing the task. In conclusion, independently from the simulation, the outcomes showed that VR training enhanced spatial memory abilities in the clinical population.

3.2.4. Visual Cues

In terms of guide elements which facilitate the patient during the training, different cues have been included in some of the tasks, such as maps [21,53,54], guidance arrows [54], and lists of objects. In particular, [54] employed a method of fading cues, decreasing assistance (DA), in which the training continues with all the cues until correct performance is achieved on three consecutive sessions and then they are gradually removed. Furthermore, in [21], the number of objects to be memorized depended on the level reached by each participant; if the patient was not able to locate the first object, the other ones were not presented. The task presented to the participant was guided in some cases by explicit navigational instructions [21,53,56] that needed to be followed to memorize the route.

3.3. Which Assessment Method Is Best for Spatial Memory?

3.3.1. Spatial Memory Outcomes

In clinical practice, the most common neuropsychological test for the evaluation of short and long-term spatial memory, given its psychometric characteristics, is the Supraspan Corsi Test. In these studies, the Supraspan Corsi Test has proved to be adequately sensitive and has indicated a significant improvement in spatial memory [50], with a medium effect size $r = 0.474$ and $p = 0.03$ [21]. Another ecological spatial memory assessment tests, Route delayed recall (RBMT), has generated desirable changes (0/5 to 4/5) that persisted at 2-month and 1-year follow-ups (respectively 4/5 and 5/5) [50]. One study [53] has shown that the virtual reality (VR) system is a sensitive assessment tool for the same cognitive function (Virtual Tübingen Test). They found that one patient improved in nine out of the 10 virtual navigation subtasks. To assess spatial navigation and memory performance in the VR supermarket, [52] analyzed the enhancements in "number of correctly bought products", "number of the correct products relative to distance", and "number of the correct products relative to time". Other authors asked the participant to form a cognitive map of the VE, and active participants showed significantly better performance [48] and were quicker [56] than the control group. A similar performance pattern was observed at the one-week follow-up session. VR neurorehabilitation programs for spatial memory can also provide a positive effect on other cognitive domains. By using specific-domain assessments, it is possible to observe if a transference of improvements occurs from VR-based training to more general aspects of spatial cognition. Following the treatment, however, general enhancement of cognitive functions occurs and is reflected in several assessment tests. The Rey Auditory Verbal Learning Test (RAVLT) has shown significant improvement in the immediate recall that persists at 1-year follow-up [50]. A considerable improvement can be observed in screening tests, such as in Addenbrooke's Cognitive Examination (ACE) ($r = 0.85, p = 0.011$), particularly in visuospatial ($r = 0.80, p = 0.017$), attention ($r = 0.79, p = 0.018$), and memory ($r = 0.79, p = 0.017$) domains and in the Mini-Mental State Examination (MMSE) ($r = 0.75, p = 0.025$) [54]. Montreal Cognitive Assessment (MoCA) results significantly improved in the experimental group after treatment in visuospatial and attention domains [59]. However, [55] did not observe consistent changes in MoCA. However, after the training, the participant was able to complete the VRN Building navigational task correctly, and the effects persisted at 5- and 28-week follow-ups. Improvements in navigational abilities have also been confirmed in daily life as recorded in wives' diaries. In [51], the patient group showed significantly higher scores in the Achievement Measure System LSP 50+, a German standardized intelligence test developed for older people between 50 and 90 years, and in the Benton Visual Retention Test, which assesses visual perception and visual memory. Also, in the Visual Pursuit Test (LVT) for visual orientation assessment, the authors observed a significant result [51]. De La-Torre [57] showed the existence of a main effect between the targets and the average errors committed to locate them within the virtual building (F adjusted (1.37, 28.01) = 8.55, $p < 0.01$; η^2 partial = 0.32, observed potency = 0.87).

One study [52] to analyze changes following treatment made correlations between VR measures and cognitive performances in the patient group. They observed that the mean number of correct products per time across all learning trials was correlated with higher performance on the Bergen Right-Left Discrimination Test (BRLD-B) to assess mental rotation. The percentile of the Digit Span Forward for short-term verbal memory was significantly correlated with the number of correctly bought products in the last learning trial on day 6 and number of correct products on the free recall trial after interference on day 7. The mean number of correct products per time and per distance across all learning trials were correlated with better performance on, respectively, the delayed free recall and immediate and delayed free recall of the Rey-Osterrieth Complex Figure (ROCF) for the assessment of visuo-construction, planning, and long term visual memory. A significant improvement was also observed in ROF [48]. In [56], the patients' face recognition performance significantly improved as measure by the Cambridge Face Memory Test (CFMT) following training. The effects persisted at one-week and 6-month follow-ups.

3.3.2. Traditional and Virtual Assessment

Results of the current review support the idea that virtual reality-based training improves orientation and navigation abilities in different neuropsychological disorders. Although the efficacy of treatment needs to be critically analyzed using a scientifically validated method, for this reason, the use of validated measures with adequate psychometric properties is fundamental. Over the past decade, evidence-based clinical guidelines have become a significant feature of healthcare services to improve the quality of care [69]. Indeed, among the studies analyzed, those that used specific-domain assessments (Corsi Supraspan, Virtual Tübingen, Route delayed recall RBMT, cognitive maps, or variables extracted from the supermarket task) were more able to demonstrate clear and significant results after the spatial memory rehabilitation training [21,48,50,53,56], highlighting the crucial role played by the selection of the assessment tools. In addition to the traditional paper-and-pencil tests used, new virtual assessment measures also emerged in the analyzed studies. These last have shown that the virtual reality (VR) system could be a sensitive assessment tool for detecting spatial memory improvements. Therefore, it is urgent to find more scientific evidence regarding the psychometric validity of these new measuring instruments, particularly concerning navigation abilities.

4. Discussion

In the current review, we provided initial, positive results concerning the effect of virtual reality (VR) training on spatial memory rehabilitation, highlighting the potential of navigational tasks in virtual environments (VEs) to enhance navigation and orientation abilities in patients with spatial memory disorders. The rapid development and diffusion of VR technologies are amending the accessibility landscape of VR technology for the average consumer. Lower-cost VR systems such as the Oculus Rift, Go, Quest, and the HTC Vive are already issued on the market and have significantly reduced the cost barrier of VR hardware. Even lower-cost options are currently available using a smartphone, for example, Gear VR is compatible with specific Samsung phones, and both Google Cardboard and Google Daydream can be used with several smartphones. Although the review underlined encouraging results, current research in this topic has some limitations that researchers need to overcome. The current work is meant to provide methodological solutions for future studies.

As the first result of the review, we have found clear improvements in spatial memory through the application of navigational tasks in VR. Both immersive and nonimmersive VR systems have shown appropriate enhancements for navigation and orientation abilities, underling the power of the navigational tasks proposed. Furthermore, the results have shown a transference of improvements from VR-based training to more general aspects of spatial cognition. However, the mode of exploration influences the spatial learning of a new environment. The active exploration has an essential role in the acquisition of spatial knowledge and it is characterized by five components: motor orders that determine the path of locomotion, proprioceptive and vestibular information for self-motion, allocation of attention to navigation-related features of the environment, and cognitive decisions about the direction during navigation and mental manipulation of spatial information [70]. If immersive systems are able to target all these components, nonimmersive systems do not allow the activation of the idiothetic and motor systems, even if input devices require motor planning and execution. In this review, only one study [55] used an immersive virtual reality system with the Oculus Rift DK2 head-mounted display and a joypad. Instead, other studies [20,52,58,59] used semi-immersive systems: the first one used OctaVis, a circle of eight screens in which the participants can freely rotate on a fixed chair and interact with a joystick; the latter used the BTs Nirvana PC system connected to a projector or a big screen and an infrared sensor for movements. The recent availability of lower-cost options for immersive VR may change the situation soon, allowing more protocols that fully support active exploration.

Another important element for the rehabilitation program is the structure and length of the training protocol. Some studies have already demonstrated that the use of visual cueing, such as a map as a navigational aid, improved the performance of users performing complex navigational tasks [66] and in patients with Alzheimer's disease or mild cognitive impairment [70]. The presence of an interactive aerial view facilitated the retrieval of stored spatial layout and arrows or salient landmarks, giving more comprehensive information about the egocentric heading in the environment, were effective in supporting the navigation [67,68]. Also, the current review underlined the importance of cues in the tasks, such as maps, guidance arrows, methods of fading cues, and instructions (explicit or implicit), to support the patient during the training [21,53,54]. It has been demonstrated that a large visual arrow supports the neurorehabilitation of spatial memory due to the cognitive synchronization between the allocentric viewpoint-independent representation (including object-to-object information) and the allocentric viewpoint-dependent representation (i.e., comprising information about the current egocentric heading in the environment), as suggested by the "mental frame syncing hypothesis" [32,71]. Furthermore, the duration of the protocol [50,60] and time elapsed since damage onset are also key factors [50,52,54]. The analysis of these studies showed that a short duration—less than four hours—is insufficient to provide consistent changes. Concerning the distance from onset, the shorter the period between the traumatic event and the beginning of treatment, the higher the probability of better outcomes.

The rehabilitation programs analyzed all focused on spatial memory and navigation abilities in different neurologic patients, including mild cognitive impairment (MCI), Alzheimer's disease (AD), traumatic brain injury (TBI), stroke, epilepsy, prosopagnosia with topographical disorientation disorders, and neglect. An important aspect to keep in mind is the clear characterization of the sample of patients to whom the therapeutic procedure is provided. The severity and the qualitative characteristics of the mnestic deficit are extremely variable from subject to subject. Furthermore, memory disorders rarely occur in an isolated form, and are often accompanied by an impairment of other cognitive functions, such as attention, language, reasoning. In this view, the most effective protocols are the ones that target a specific pathology.

The difficulty in finding homogeneous groups of patients is the reason why most of the experimental studies reported in the literature are based on the treatment of a single patient or a tiny group of patients. However, to monitor the improvements due to the treatment, the presence of an adequate control group is necessary to ensure that the observed improvement is not due to spontaneous recovery nor is the result of generic cognitive stimulation. In this view, the most reliable control condition is the repeated evaluation of the same patients receiving the experimental treatment, for example, through cross-over trials [72]. Another possible approach is the involvement of patients who, in the immediately preceding period, were followed in the absence of therapy or using another type of cognitive treatment. Moreover, the studies that used domain-specific assessments (Corsi Supraspan, Virtual Tübingen, Route delayed recall RBMT, cognitive maps, or variables extracted from the supermarket) were more able to demonstrate clear and significant results after the spatial memory rehabilitation training [21,48,50,53,56], highlighting the crucial role played by the selection of the assessment tools. Among the tests used (Corsi Supraspan, Virtual Tübingen, Route delayed recall RBMT), only the Virtual Tübingen can investigate the several aspects (scene recognition, route continuation/sequence/order/progression/distance, pointing to start/to end, map drawing recognition) involved in navigation. Thus, the scarcity of tools for spatial memory assessment is evident, particularly concerning navigation abilities.

This review was subject to certain limitations. Extensive literature research was performed to deliver these findings; however, only two databased were queried. A second limitation of this review may be the selection of the keywords in the search strategy. In order to provide a considerable quantity of studies in the field, the authors decided to use wider keywords. However, the inclusion criteria reduced the focus to only studies according to the objectives of the review. A final limitation may be the fact that the discussion on duration and intensity of VR navigational training cannot draw firm conclusions due to the heterogeneity of interventions. Moreover, the difficulty of finding a homogeneous group of patients is the reason why most of the experimental studies reported in the literature are based on the treatment of a single patient or a tiny group of patients. Because our findings are positive, we hope that the literature could soon be enriched with clinical trials investigating VR's effectiveness in more specific and larger clinical populations.

5. Conclusions

In conclusion, the results of this systematic review demonstrate that all studies, although to varying degrees, suggest that patients improved their spatial memory following treatment. This result highlights the potential of navigational tasks performed in virtual environments (VEs) for enhancing navigation and orientation abilities in patients with spatial memory disorders. In neuroscience, researchers have long faced the challenge of conducting ecologically valid measurements of experimental variables while maintaining strict experimental control over visual displays. Virtual reality (VR) systems enable the researchers to design and consequently control dynamic, realistic, and immersive environments, while closely monitoring behavioral and physiological responses during experimentation [1,73]. In this view, VR systems offer impressive opportunities as an ecological tool which is currently available for neuropsychologists to assess and enhance spatial memory, particularly navigation and orientation abilities using the "affordances" [74] offered to the patients in the virtual environment. One of the significant advantages of VR is the high degree of experimental control that is afforded to investigate the cognitive and behavioral components that are involved in spatial navigation [75]. VR training can facilitate neurorehabilitation, promoting brain plasticity processes through complex mechanisms related to the reactivation of brain neurotransmitter capacities, maximizing the results compared to those obtained by conventional treatment [66,76]. Monitoring EEG activities of the patients could be a suitable practice to assess the biomarkers of neuroplasticity and to measure rehabilitation progress [67,77]. The results are promising; hence, we encourage researchers to develop new spatial memory VR-based protocols for neurorehabilitation. However, more research is required to validate and support this result.

References

1. Bohil, C.J.; Alicea, B.; Biocca, F.A. Virtual reality in neuroscience research and therapy. *Nat. Rev. Neurosci.* **2011**, *12*, 752–762. [CrossRef] [PubMed]
2. Steuer, J. Defining Virtual Reality: Characteristics Determining Telepresence. *J. Commun.* **1992**, *42*, 73–94. [CrossRef]
3. Sanchez-Vives, M.V.; Slater, M. Opinion: From presence to consciousness through virtual reality. *Nat. Rev. Neurosci.* **2005**, *6*, 332–339. [CrossRef] [PubMed]
4. Riva, G. From Virtual to Real Body. *J. Cyberther. Rehabil.* **2008**, *1*, 7–22.
5. Riva, G.; Baños, R.M.; Botella, C.; Mantovani, F.; Gaggioli, A. Transforming Experience: The Potential of Augmented Reality and Virtual Reality for Enhancing Personal and Clinical Change. *Front. Psychol.* **2016**, *7*, 164. [CrossRef] [PubMed]

6. Slater, M. Place illusion and plausibility can lead to realistic behaviour in immersive virtual environments. *Philos. Trans. R. Soc. B Boil. Sci.* **2009**, *364*, 3549–3557. [CrossRef] [PubMed]
7. Riva, G.; Waterworth, J.A.; Waterworth, E.L. The Layers of Presence: A Bio-cultural Approach to Understanding Presence in Natural and Mediated Environments. *CyberPsychol. Behav.* **2004**, *7*, 402–416. [CrossRef] [PubMed]
8. Riva, G.; Castelnuovo, G.; Mantovani, F. Transformation of flow in rehabilitation: The role of advanced communication technologies. *Behav. Res. Methods* **2006**, *38*, 237–244. [CrossRef] [PubMed]
9. Riva, G.; Gaggioli, A.; Villani, D.; Preziosa, A.; Morganti, F.; Corsi, R.; Faletti, G.; Vezzadini, L. NeuroVR: An open source virtual reality platform for clinical psychology and behavioral neurosciences. *Stud. Health Technol. Inform.* **2007**, *125*, 394–399.
10. Witmer, B.G.; Singer, M.J. Measuring Presence in Virtual Environments: A Presence. *Presence* **1998**, *7*, 225–241. [CrossRef]
11. Laviola, J.J. A discussion of cybersickness in virtual environments. *ACM SIGCHI Bull.* **2000**, *32*, 47–56. [CrossRef]
12. Pot-kolder, R.; Veling, W.; Counotte, J.; van der Gaag, M. Anxiety Partially Mediates Cybersickness Symptoms in Immersive Virtual Reality Environments. *Cyberpsychol. Behav. Soc. Netw.* **2017**, *21*, 187–193. [CrossRef] [PubMed]
13. Gatica-Rojas, V.; Méndez-Rebolledo, G. Virtual reality interface devices in the reorganization of neural networks in the brain of patients with neurological diseases. *Neural Regen. Res.* **2014**, *9*, 888–896. [CrossRef] [PubMed]
14. Riva, G.; Dakanalis, A.; Gaggioli, A. From body dissatisfaction to obesity: How virtual reality may improve obesity prevention and treatment in adolescents. *Stud. Health Technol. Inform.* **2011**, *184*, 356–362.
15. Slater, M.; Sanchez-Vives, M.V. Enhancing Our Lives with Immersive Virtual Reality. *Front. Robot. AI* **2016**, *3*, 1–47. [CrossRef]
16. Slater, M. Grand Challenges in Virtual Environments. *Front. Robot. AI* **2014**, *1*, 1–4. [CrossRef]
17. Slater, M.; Spanlang, B.; Corominas, D. Simulating virtual environments within virtual environments as the basis for a psychophysics of presence. *ACM Trans. Grapghics* **2010**, *29*, 1–9. [CrossRef]
18. Slater, M.; Marcos, D.P.; Ehrsson, H.H.; Sanchez-Vives, M.V. Inducing Illusory Ownership of a Virtual Body. *Front. Mol. Neurosci.* **2009**, *3*, 214–220. [CrossRef] [PubMed]
19. Serino, S.; Baglio, F.; Rossetto, F.; Realdon, O.; Cipresso, P.; Parsons, T.D.; Cappellini, G.; Mantovani, F.; De Leo, G.; Nemni, R.; et al. Picture Interpretation Test (PIT) 360°: An Innovative Measure of Executive Functions. *Sci. Rep.* **2017**, *7*, 16000. [CrossRef]
20. Grewe, P.; Kohsik, A.; Flentge, D.; Dyck, E.; Botsch, M.; Winter, Y.; Markowitsch, H.J.; Bien, C.G.; Piefke, M. Learning real-life cognitive abilities in a novel 360 degrees -virtual reality supermarket: A neuropsychological study of healthy participants and patients with epilepsy. *J. Neuroeng. Rehabil.* **2013**, *10*, 42. [CrossRef]
21. Serino, S.; Pedroli, E.; Tuena, C.; De Leo, G.; Stramba-Badiale, M.; Goulene, K.; Mariotti, N.G.; Riva, G. A novel virtual reality-based training protocol for the enhancement of the 'mental frame syncing' in individuals with Alzheimer's disease: A development-of-concept trial. *Front. Aging Neurosci.* **2017**, *9*, 1–12. [CrossRef] [PubMed]
22. Mishkind, M.C.; Norr, A.M.; Katz, A.C.; Reger, G.M. Review of Virtual Reality Treatment in Psychiatry: Evidence Versus Current Diffusion and Use. *Curr. Psychiatry Rep.* **2017**, *19*, 80. [CrossRef] [PubMed]
23. Zeng, N.; Pope, Z.; Lee, J.E.; Gao, Z. Virtual Reality Exercise for Anxiety and Depression: A Preliminary Review of Current Research in an Emerging Field. *J. Clin. Med.* **2018**, *7*, 42. [CrossRef] [PubMed]
24. Ferrer-García, M.; Gutiérrez-Maldonado, J.; Pla-Sanjuanelo, J.; Vilalta-Abella, F.; Riva, G.; Clerici, M.; Ribas-Sabaté, J.; Andreu-Gracia, A.; Fernandez-Aranda, F.; Forcano, L.; et al. A Randomised Controlled Comparison of Second-Level Treatment Approaches for Treatment-Resistant Adults with Bulimia Nervosa and Binge Eating Disorder: Assessing the Benefits of Virtual Reality Cue Exposure Therapy. *Eur. Eat. Disord. Rev.* **2017**, *25*, 479–490. [CrossRef] [PubMed]
25. Clus, D.; Larsen, M.E.; Lemey, C.; Berrouiguet, S. The Use of Virtual Reality in Patients with Eating Disorders: Systematic Review. *J. Med. Internet Res.* **2018**, *20*, 1–9. [CrossRef] [PubMed]
26. Spreij, L.A.; Visser-Meily, J.M.A.; Van Heugten, C.M.; Nijboer, T.C.W. Novel insights into the rehabilitation of memory post acquired brain injury: A systematic review. *Front. Hum. Neurosci.* **2014**, *8*, 1–19. [CrossRef] [PubMed]

27. Valladares-Rodriguez, S.; Perez-Rodriguez, R.; Facal, D.; Fernandez-Iglesias, M.J.; Anido-Rifon, L.; Mouriño-Garcia, M. Design process and preliminary psychometric study of a video game to detect cognitive impairment in senior adults. *PeerJ* **2017**, *5*, 1–35. [CrossRef] [PubMed]
28. Schedlbauer, A.M.; Copara, M.S.; Watrous, A.J.; Ekstrom, A.D. Multiple interacting brain areas underlie successful spatiotemporal memory retrieval in humans. *Sci. Rep.* **2014**, *4*, 6431. [CrossRef]
29. Carrieri, M.; Petracca, A.; Lancia, S.; Moro, S.B.; Brigadoi, S.; Spezialetti, M.; Ferrari, M.; Placidi, G.; Quaresima, V. Prefrontal Cortex Activation Upon a Demanding Virtual Hand-Controlled Task: A New Frontier for Neuroergonomics. *Front. Hum. Neurosci.* **2016**, *10*, 1–13. [CrossRef]
30. Zanier, E.R.; Zoerle, T.; Di Lernia, D.; Riva, G. Virtual Reality for Traumatic Brain Injury. *Front. Neurol.* **2018**, *9*, 1–4. [CrossRef]
31. Colombo, D.; Serino, S.; Tuena, C.; Pedroli, E.; Dakanalis, A.; Cipresso, P.; Riva, G. Egocentric and allocentric spatial reference frames in aging: A systematic review. *Neurosci. Biobehav. Rev.* **2017**, *80*, 605–621. [CrossRef] [PubMed]
32. Serino, S.; Riva, G. Getting lost in Alzheimer's disease: A break in the mental frame syncing. *Med. Hypotheses* **2013**, *80*, 416–421. [CrossRef] [PubMed]
33. Allison, S.L.; Fagan, A.M.; Morris, J.C.; Head, D. Spatial Navigation in Preclinical Alzheimer's Disease. *J. Alzheimers Dis.* **2016**, *52*, 77–90. [CrossRef] [PubMed]
34. Kuehn, E.; Perez-Lopez, M.B.; Diersch, N.; Döhler, J.; Wolbers, T.; Riemer, M. Embodiment in the aging mind. *Neurosci. Biobehav. Rev.* **2018**, *86*, 207–225. [CrossRef] [PubMed]
35. Lester, A.W.; Moffat, S.D.; Wiener, J.M.; Barnes, C.A.; Wolbers, T. The Aging Navigational System. *Neuron* **2017**, *95*, 1019–1035. [CrossRef] [PubMed]
36. E Cullen, K.; Taube, J.S. Our sense of direction: Progress, controversies and challenges. *Nat. Neurosci.* **2017**, *20*, 1465–1473. [CrossRef]
37. Bird, C.M.; Burgess, N. The hippocampus and memory: Insights from spatial processing. *Nat. Rev. Neurosci.* **2008**, *9*, 182–194. [CrossRef] [PubMed]
38. Holmes, M.C.; Sholl, M.J. Allocentric Coding of Object-to-Object Relations in Overlearned and Novel Environments. *J. Exp. Psychol. Learn. Mem. Cogn.* **2005**, *31*, 1069–1087. [CrossRef]
39. Hartley, T.; Lever, C.; Burgess, N.; O'Keefe, J. Space in the brain: How the hippocampal formation supports spatial cognition. *Philos. Trans. R. Soc. B Biol. Sci.* **2013**, *369*, 20120510. [CrossRef]
40. Burgess, N. Spatial cognition and the brain. *Ann. N. Y. Acad. Sci.* **2008**, *1124*, 77–97. [CrossRef]
41. D'Esposito, M.; Aguirre, G.K. Topographical disorientation: A synthesis and taxonomy. *Brain* **1999**, *122*, 1613–1628.
42. Vann, S.D.; Aggleton, J.P.; Maguire, E.A. What does the retrosplenial cortex do? *Nat. Rev. Neurosci.* **2009**, *10*, 792–802. [CrossRef] [PubMed]
43. Doeller, C.F.; King, J.A.; Burgess, N. Parallel striatal and hippocampal systems for landmarks and boundaries in spatial memory. *Proc. Natl. Acad. Sci. USA* **2008**, *105*, 5915–5920. [CrossRef] [PubMed]
44. Borrego, A.; Latorre, J.; Llorens, R.; Alcañiz, M.; Noé, E. Feasibility of a walking virtual reality system for rehabilitation: Objective and subjective parameters. *J. Neuroeng. Rehabil.* **2016**, *13*, 68. [CrossRef] [PubMed]
45. Moher, D.; Liberati, A.; Tetzlaff, J.; Altman, D.G.; Grp, P. Preferred Reporting Items for Systematic Reviews and Meta-Analyses: The PRISMA Statement (Reprinted from Annals of Internal Medicine). *Phys. Ther.* **2009**, *89*, 873–880. [PubMed]
46. Higgins, J.; Green, S. *Cochrane Handbook for Systematic Reviews of Interventions*; Version 5; The Cochrane Collaboration: London, UK, 2011.
47. Von Elm, E.; Altman, D.G.; Egger, M.; Pocock, S.J.; Gøtzsche, P.C.; Vandenbroucke, J.P. The Strengthening the Reporting of Observational Studies in Epidemiology (STROBE) Statement: Guidelines for reporting observational studies. *Lancet* **2007**, *370*, 1453–1457. [CrossRef]
48. Pugnetti, L.; Mendozzi, L.; Brooks, B.; Attree, E.; Barbieri, E.; Alpini, D.; Motta, A.; Rose, D. Active versus passive exploration of virtual environments modulates spatial memory in MS patients: A yoked control study. *Ital. J. Neurol. Sci.* **1998**, *19*, S424–S430. [CrossRef]
49. Akhutina, T.; Foreman, N.; Krichevets, A.; Matikka, L.; Närhi, V.; Pylaeva, N.; Vahakuopus, J. Improving spatial functioning in children with cerebral palsy using computerized and traditional game tasks. *Disabil. Rehabil.* **2003**, *25*, 1361–1371. [CrossRef]
50. Caglio, M.; Latini-Corazzini, L.; D'Agata, F.; Cauda, F.; Sacco, K.; Monteverdi, S.; Zettin, M.; Duca, S.;

Geminiani, G. Virtual navigation for memory rehabilitation in a traumatic brain injured patient. *Neurocase (Psychology Press)* **2012**, *18*, 123–131. [CrossRef]
51. Kober, S.E.; Wood, G.; Hofer, D.; Kreuzig, W.; Kiefer, M.; Neuper, C. Virtual reality in neurologic rehabilitation of spatial disorientation. *J. Neuroeng. Rehabil.* **2013**, *10*, 1–13. [CrossRef]
52. Grewe, P.; Lahr, D.; Kohsik, A.; Dyck, E.; Markowitsch, H.; Bien, C.; Botsch, M.; Piefke, M. Real-life memory and spatial navigation in patients with focal epilepsy: Ecological validity of a virtual reality supermarket task. *Epilepsy Behav.* **2014**, *31*, 57–66. [CrossRef] [PubMed]
53. Claessen, M.H.G.; van der Ham, I.J.M.; Jagersma, E.; Visser-Meily, J.M.A. Navigation strategy training using virtual reality in six chronic stroke patients: A novel and explorative approach to the rehabilitation of navigation impairment. *Neuropsychol. Rehabil.* **2016**, *26*, 822–846. [CrossRef] [PubMed]
54. Faria, A.L.; Andrade, A.; Soares, L.; I Badia, S.B. Benefits of virtual reality based cognitive rehabilitation through simulated activities of daily living: A randomized controlled trial with stroke patients. *J. Neuroeng. Rehabil.* **2016**, *13*, 1–12. [CrossRef] [PubMed]
55. White, P.J.; Moussavi, Z. Neuro-Cognitive Treatment for an Alzheimer's Patient using a Virtual Reality Navigational Environment. *J. Exp. Neurosci.* **2016**, *10*, 129–135. [CrossRef] [PubMed]
56. Bate, S.; Adams, A.; Bennetts, R.; Line, H. Developmental prosopagnosia with concurrent topographical difficulties: A case report and virtual reality training programme. *Neuropsychol. Rehabil.* **2017**, *29*, 1–23.
57. De La Torre-Luque, A.; Valero-Aguayo, L.; De La Rubia-Cuestas, E.J. Visuospatial Orientation Learning through Virtual Reality for People with Severe Disability. *Int. J. Disabil. Dev. Educ.* **2017**, *64*, 420–435. [CrossRef]
58. De Luca, R.; Buono, V.L.; Leo, A.; Russo, M.; Aragona, B.; Leonardi, S.; Buda, A.; Naro, A.; Calabrò, R.S. Use of virtual reality in improving poststroke neglect: Promising neuropsychological and neurophysiological findings from a case study. *Appl. Neuropsychol.* **2017**, *26*, 1–5. [CrossRef]
59. De Luca, R.; Russo, M.; Naro, A.; Tomasello, P.; Leonardi, S.; Santamaria, F.; Desireè, L.; Bramanti, A.; Silvestri, G.; Bramanti, P.; et al. Effects of virtual reality-based training with BTs-Nirvana on functional recovery in stroke patients: Preliminary considerations. *Int. J. Neurosci.* **2018**, *7454*, 1–6. [CrossRef]
60. Maresca, G.; Maggio, M.G.; Buda, A.; la Rosa, G. A novel use of virtual reality in the treatment of cognitive and motor de fi cit in spinal cord injury. *Medicine (Baltimore)* **2018**, *97*, e13559. [CrossRef]
61. Mrakic-Sposta, S.; Di Santo, S.G.; Franchini, F.; Arlati, S.; Zangiacomi, A.; Greci, L.; Moretti, S.; Jesuthasan, N.; Marzorati, M.; Rizzo, G.; et al. Effects of Combined Physical and Cognitive Virtual Reality-Based Training on Cognitive Impairment and Oxidative Stress in MCI Patients: A Pilot Study. *Front. Aging Neurosci.* **2018**, *10*, 1–11. [CrossRef]
62. Cipresso, P.; Serino, S.; Riva, G. Psychometric assessment and behavioral experiments using a free virtual reality platform and computational science. *BMC Med. Inform. Decis. Mak.* **2016**, *16*, 1–11. [CrossRef] [PubMed]
63. Behr, J.; Bockholt, U.; Fellner, D. Instantreality—A Framework for Industrial Augmented and Virtual Reality Applications. In *Virtual Reality & Augmented Reality in Industry*; Ma, D., Fan, X., Gausemeier, J., Grafe, M., Eds.; Springer: Berlin/Heidelberg, Germany, 2011.
64. Brotons-Mas, J.R.; O'Mara, S.; Sanchez-Vives, M.V. Neural processing of spatial information: What we know about place cells and what know about place cells and what they can tell us about presence. *Presence Teleoperators Virtual Environ.* **2006**, *15*, 485–499. [CrossRef]
65. De Luca, R.; Portaro, S.; Le Cause, M.; De Domenico, C.; Maggio, M.G.; Ferrera, M.C.; Giuffrè, G.; Bramanti, A.; Calabrò, R.S. Cognitive rehabilitation using immersive virtual reality at young age: A case report on traumatic brain injury. *Appl. Neuropsychol. Child* **2019**, 1–6. [CrossRef] [PubMed]
66. Darken, R.P.; Sibert, J.L. Navigating Large Virtual Spaces. *Int. J. Hum-Comput. Interact.* **1996**, *8*, 49–72. [CrossRef]
67. Serino, S.; Mestre, D.; Mallet, P.; Pergandi, J.; Cipresso, P.; Riva, G. *Don't Get Lost in Translation: The Role of Egocentric Heading in Spatial Orientation*; Elsevier: Amsterdam, The Netherlands, 2015.
68. Cogné, M.; Auriacombe, S.; Vasa, L.; Tison, F.; Klinger, É.; Sauzeon, H.; Joseph, P.-A.; N'kaoua, B. Are visual cues helpful for virtual spatial navigation and spatial memory in patients with mild cognitive impairment or Alzheimer's disease? *Neuropsychology* **2018**, *32*, 385–400.

69. Flores-Mateo, G.; Argimon, J.M. Evidence based practice in postgraduate healthcare education: A systematic review. *BMC Health Serv. Res.* **2007**, *7*, 1–8. [CrossRef] [PubMed]
70. Chrastil, E.R.; Warren, W.H. Active and passive contributions to spatial learning. *Psychon. Bull. Rev.* **2012**, *19*, 1–23. [CrossRef]
71. Serino, S.; Riva, G. What is the role of spatial processing in the decline of episodic memory in Alzheimer's disease? The 'mental frame syncing' hypothesis. *Front. Aging Neurosci.* **2014**, *6*, 1–7. [CrossRef]
72. Senn, S. *Cross-over Trials in Clinical Research*; John Wiley & Sons, Ltd: Hoboken, NJ, USA, 2002.
73. Loomis, J.M.; Blascovich, J.J.; Beall, A.C. Immersive virtual environment technology as a basic research tool in psychology. *Behav. Res. Methods Instrum. Comput.* **1999**, *31*, 557–564. [CrossRef]
74. Gibson, J.J. The Theory of Affordances. In *The Ecological Approach to Visual Perception*; Routledge: Abingdon, UK, 1979.
75. Meade, M.E.; Meade, J.G.; Fernandes, M.A. Active Navigation in Virtual Environments Benefits Spatial Memory in Older Adults. *Brain Sci.* **2019**, *9*, 47. [CrossRef]
76. Maggio, M.G.; Maresca, G.; De Luca, R.; Stagnitti, M.C.; Porcari, B.; Ferrera, M.C.; Galletti, F.; Casella, C.; Manuli, A.; Calabrò, R.S. The Growing Use of Virtual Reality in Cognitive Rehabilitation: Fact, Fake or Vision? A Scoping Review. *J. Natl. Med. Assoc.* **2019**. [CrossRef] [PubMed]
77. Wen, D.; Lan, X.; Zhou, Y.; Li, G.; Hsu, S.-H.; Jung, T.-P. The Study of Evaluation and Rehabilitation of Patients with Different Cognitive Impairment Phases Based on Virtual Reality and EEG. *Front. Aging Neurosci.* **2018**, *10*, 1–6. [CrossRef] [PubMed]

6

Be a Mom's Efficacy in Enhancing Positive Mental Health among Postpartum Women Presenting Low Risk for Postpartum Depression: Results from a Pilot Randomized Trial

Fabiana Monteiro *, Marco Pereira, Maria Cristina Canavarro and Ana Fonseca

Center for Research in Neuropsychology and Cognitive Behavioral Intervention (CINEICC), Faculty of Psychology and Educational Sciences, the University of Coimbra Rua do Colégio Novo, 3000-315 Coimbra, Portugal; marcopereira@fpce.uc.pt (M.P.); mccanavarro@fpce.uc.pt (M.C.C.); ana.fonseca77@gmail.com (A.F.)

* Correspondence: fgmonteiro.91@gmail.com

Abstract: In this study, we conducted a preliminary investigation of the efficacy of *Be a Mom*, a web-based self-guided intervention, in enhancing positive mental health among postpartum women at low risk for postpartum depression. Additionally, we examined *Be a Mom*'s efficacy regarding secondary outcomes as well as its acceptability and adherence. A total of 367 participants were randomly assigned to the *Be a Mom* group (n = 191) or to the waiting-list control group (n = 176) and completed baseline (T1) and postintervention (T2) assessments. The intervention group reported significant increases in positive mental health between T1 and T2 compared to the control group. Additionally, group effects were found for depressive and anxiety symptoms. A significantly higher proportion of participants in the *Be a Mom* group had an improvement trajectory (from not flourishing at T1 to flourishing at T2). A total of 62 (32.5%) women completed *Be a Mom*, and most would use it again if needed (n = 82/113; 72.6%). This study provides preliminary evidence of *Be a Mom*'s efficacy in increasing positive mental health among low-risk postpartum women. Our findings support mental health promotion strategies in the postpartum period and highlight the important role of web-based CBT interventions.

Keywords: web-based intervention; be a mom; randomized controlled trial; positive mental health; flourishing; postpartum period

---

1. Introduction

The transition to motherhood is often depicted as a joyful period filled with excitement, but it also involves demanding adjustments to a new role and new responsibilities [1]. Research in this area has suggested that this is a period of increased mental health vulnerability due to the considerable number of stressors that are often experienced, such as increased physical health needs, adjusting to infant care tasks, changes in marital and social relationships, financial strains or transitioning back to work [2–7]. Even under optimal circumstances, the early postpartum period is full of challenging tasks. Although some women may present risk factors that make them more vulnerable to mental illness, such as postpartum depression (PPD; e.g., history of depression, low social support; [8]), this period constitutes a major life transition for all postpartum women, including low-risk women, who can also experience symptoms of depression and anxiety [9,10].

Mental illness during the postpartum period has increasingly been considered a high-priority public health problem due to the long-term negative implications for maternal health, infant health and development [11,12] and economic costs [13,14]. Even the presence of subclinical symptoms of depression has been associated with increased psychosocial difficulties (poorer maternal self-esteem, more negative and less negative positive affect) [15]. Several efforts have targeted the treatment and prevention of psychological disorders during this period, particularly PPD [16,17]. With respect to preventive interventions, there is evidence that cognitive behavioral therapy (CBT) is effective in preventing depression both among women who present risk factors for PPD (selective/indicated prevention) and among all women in the community (universal prevention), although the effects of these preventive interventions may be more robust among groups at a higher risk of perinatal depression [16,18].

In addition to prevention, the promotion of positive mental health has been increasingly recognized as a priority [19,20], with research suggesting the need to address positive mental health directly since interventions that are effective in reducing psychopathological symptoms are not necessarily effective in enhancing levels of positive mental health [21,22]. However, previous research has tended to consider women's psychological adjustment to this period in terms of levels of depression and anxiety, and the promotion of positive mental health has been neglected in favor of a greater focus on the prevention and reduction of mental illness [23]. Positive mental health has received growing attention in recent years as research has shown that it is not simply the absence of mental illness [22,24]. Optimal levels of positive mental health involve the experience of high levels of emotional (positive feelings, e.g., feeling happy, satisfaction with life), psychological (optimal functioning in life, e.g., self-acceptance, purpose in life, personal growth) and social wellbeing (optimal social functioning, e.g., social integration and contribution) [24]. Keyes [24] conceptualized those with high levels of emotional, psychological and social wellbeing as flourishing individuals. Existing studies about the impact of flourishing underline the need for interventions that increase positive mental health. For instance, the presence of flourishing has been associated with better physical health and longevity [25,26], fewer health limitations of activities of daily living and fewer missed days of work [24] and may act as a buffer against future mental illness [27,28]. Although still rarely studied in the postpartum period, higher levels of positive mental health in mothers have been longitudinally associated with better development outcomes in children, specifically cognitive, communication and social development [29]. Thus, proactively addressing and assessing positive mental health in psychological interventions should be a complementary goal of psychological interventions in the postpartum period, including those targeting low-risk women.

Reaching all women in the postpartum period through traditional face-to-face interventions is difficult considering the high amount of human and economic costs involved [30]. Additionally, help-seeking rates for postpartum women with depressive symptoms range from 15% to 40% [31,32]. Suggested barriers that contribute to these low rates include feelings of shame, guilt and stigma and demands associated with infant care [33,34]. eHealth interventions have the potential to effectively address these barriers because they provide an opportunity to enhance the capacity and accessibility of mental health care and can be delivered at a very low cost and with privacy and convenience [35, 36]. Moreover, these interventions have been shown to have long-term positive outcomes beyond the reduction of psychopathological symptoms, such as improvements in personal empowerment, self-esteem and quality of life [37]. In a recent review, the role of eHealth in the perinatal period was also highlighted as having the potential to be revolutionary if integrated into standard care [38].

In line with this, *Be a Mom* was developed to be a short-term, fully self-guided web-based intervention for Portuguese postpartum women. It was primarily developed to prevent PPD among at-risk women, and a previous pilot trial demonstrated its efficacy in reducing depressive and anxiety symptoms among a sample at high risk for PPD [39]. Although *Be a Mom* addresses the minimization of psychosocial risk factors for PPD (e.g., lack of social support, poor marital relationship), it does not focus solely on the minimization of such risk factors. Rather, *Be a Mom* specifically targets the development and strengthening of psychological competences and resources, namely, acceptance- and compassion-based skills. *Be a Mom* has already proven its efficacy in promoting self-compassion and emotion regulation skills among a high-risk sample for PPD [40]. Because the enhancement of psychological resources could be useful to all women in the postpartum period, *Be a Mom* may also be effective in the promotion of mental health among postpartum women presenting low risk for PPD. *Be a Mom* is grounded in CBT principles applied to the postpartum context and includes content based on the third wave of CBT, namely, acceptance- and compassion-focused approaches. Third-wave CBT approaches aim not only to reduce psychopathology but also to promote flourishing [41].

There is evidence of web-based CBT interventions as well as acceptance and compassion-based approaches enhancing positive mental health in general population samples [42,43]. However, there is still a lack of studies assessing the efficacy of these interventions in increasing positive mental health in the postpartum period. One study using an eHealth compassion-based intervention found that postpartum women in the intervention group showed an improvement in positive mental health compared to the control group [44], although the effects were small and only significant among participants with lower levels of positive mental health at baseline. Another study using an intervention based on positive psychology and metacognitive therapy only found a significant effect of the intervention with regard to emotional well-being [45]. The majority of web-based intervention studies in the perinatal period focus on the treatment or prevention of psychopathological symptoms using mostly high-risk samples [46]. However, given the characteristics of eHealth interventions and the importance of maternal mental health in influencing lifelong health outcomes, low-risk women may also benefit from these interventions.

Therefore, the present study reports the results of a pilot randomized controlled trial of the *Be a Mom* web-based intervention compared to a waiting-list control (WLC) group. The aims of this study were (1) to explore the efficacy of *Be a Mom* in enhancing positive mental health among low-risk postpartum women; (2) to investigate *Be a Mom*'s efficacy considering secondary outcomes (depressive and anxiety symptoms, maternal self-efficacy, empowerment and relationship satisfaction); and (3) to test *Be a Mom*'s acceptability, adherence and pattern of usage.

2. Materials and Methods

2.1. Study Design

This study was a two-arm, open-label, pilot randomized controlled trial on the efficacy of *Be a Mom* vs. a WLC for postpartum women presenting low risk for PPD. This study is part of a wider research project assessing *Be a Mom*'s efficacy as a web-based program for the promotion of maternal mental health during the postpartum period. The study was conducted in accordance with the Declaration of Helsinki, and the protocol was approved by the Ethics Committee of the Faculty of Psychology and Educational Sciences, University of Coimbra and was registered on ClinicalTrials.gov (NCT04055974). The extensions of the CONSORT 2010 checklist for pilot trials [47] and CONSORT-EHEALTH [48] were used for study reporting.

2.2. Recruitment Procedure and Participants

Participants were recruited online between January 2019 and February 2020. In addition to unpaid cross-posting, paid advertisements were placed on social media websites (Facebook and Instagram) targeting women aged 18–45 years old with interests in maternity topics. The tagline to advertise the study was "Did you have a baby in the last three months? We want to know if *Be a Mom* is effective in promoting postpartum women's mental health, and you can help us! To know if you are eligible to participate in the study fill out the following form and we will contact you". Participants who clicked on the link were then given information about the study's goals and procedures, the participants' and researchers' roles, the voluntary nature of participation, and all aspects related to data protection (anonymity and confidentiality). Participants who gave online informed consent (by clicking the option "I understand and accept the conditions of the study") answered a set of questions to assess eligibility criteria and provided their contact information (email address and telephone number). The inclusion criteria to participate in this study were a) being in the early postpartum period (up to 3 months postpartum); b) being 18 years or older; c) presenting low risk for PPD (having a score lower than 5.5 on the Postpartum Depression Predictors Inventory-Revised; [49]); d) having internet access at home; e) being a resident of Portugal; and f) understanding Portuguese. Exclusion criteria were the presence of a serious medical condition (physical or psychiatric) in the mother or in the infant (self-reported). Participants who did not meet eligibility criteria were sent an email informing them of the reason they could not participate in this study and advising them to seek professional help if needed. Because this study was part of a wider research project, women who presented risk factors for PPD were contacted by the research team to take part in a separate study to assess *Be a Mom*'s efficacy in preventing postpartum depressive symptoms (i.e., the primary outcome was depressive symptoms).

A priori calculations indicated that a sample size of at least 200 participants at postintervention assessment was needed to assess preliminary evidence of efficacy for the primary outcome (detecting a small effect size [$d = 0.10$] with a statistical power of 0.80 in a two-tailed test, $p < 0.05$). Considering the dropout rate of approximately 35% in the pilot study of *Be a Mom* [39], at least 350 participants were needed for randomization.

2.3. Randomization

After completing the baseline assessment, eligible participants were randomly assigned (allocation ratio 1:1) to the intervention group (*Be a Mom*) or to the WLC group. Randomization was performed using a computerized random number generator. After randomization, participants received an email with information about their assigned group. The last author was responsible for randomization, and the first author was responsible for the enrollment and assignment of participants to either the *Be a Mom* group or the WLC group.

2.4. Interventions

Participants in the intervention arm were invited to a password-protected website that contained the *Be a Mom* intervention (beamom.pt). Access to the program was free of cost, and no compensation was given to participants. *Be a Mom* has five sequential modules (Changes and Emotional Reactions; Cognitions; Values and Social Support; Couple's Relationship (only presented to women in a relationship); PPD Alert Signs and Professional Help-seeking) and its contents are presented in an attractive format (simple text, animations, interactive exercises). The modules follow the structured and goal-oriented nature of CBT: first, the module's goals are presented, followed by the thematic content and, finally, a homework activity at the end to guarantee continued therapeutic practice. Each module has an approximate length of 30–45 min, and women can interrupt it whenever they need to and resume when they are available. Asynchronous communication channels (e.g., reminders, email contact for program-related support) are available. The formative evaluation process that informed the design and the intervention components of *Be a Mom* is detailed elsewhere [50].

Participants were given the instructions that they should complete one module per week, but they were allowed to complete the program at their own pace. Those who did not register on *Be a Mom* were sent two email reminders during the course of the eight weeks given to complete *Be a Mom*. Participants who registered on the program and who had a valid telephone number were contacted via telephone by the first author approximately two weeks after registration. This contact aimed to clarify any questions regarding the flow of the program or help with difficulties accessing the website. Email reminders were sent automatically by the *Be a Mom* website to the participants if they went three, seven and 13 days without accessing it. Approximately two days after completing *Be a Mom*, participants were sent an email with the postintervention assessment. Those who did not complete the program were sent an email with the postintervention assessment eight weeks after randomization.

Participants in the WLC arm were offered no intervention but were informed that they would receive access to *Be a Mom* at the end of the study. They were asked to complete the postintervention assessment protocol at the same time as the participants in the *Be a Mom* group (eight weeks after randomization). All participants could access usual care from their health services.

Outcome variables were assessed at baseline (Time 1—T1) and eight weeks after randomization (Time 2—T2) by self-report using the survey platform Limesurvey®. To reduce attrition, email and text message reminders were sent on an alternate basis each week for one month to women in both groups who failed to complete T1 and T2 online questionnaires.

2.5. Measures

Women's sociodemographic (e.g., age, marital status, number of children, employment status, educational level, household monthly income, and residence), clinical (psychopathology history) and infant-related data (e.g., infant's age, infant's sex and infant's gestational weeks at birth) were collected through a self-report questionnaire developed by the researchers.

To identify women presenting low risk for PPD, the Portuguese version of the Postpartum Depression Predictors Inventory-Revised (PDPI-R) was used [51]. This questionnaire comprises 39 items answered on a dichotomous scale (yes vs. no, except for the first two items in which participants report their marital and socioeconomic status). The PDPI-R total score ranges from 0 to 39. Higher scores indicate increased risk for PPD. In Portuguese validation studies, a score of 5 or lower is indicative of lower PPD risk [49].

2.5.1. Primary Outcome-Positive Mental Health

Positive mental health was assessed using the Mental Health Continuum Short Form (MHC-SF; [52]; Portuguese Version [PV]: [53]). The MHC-SF comprises 14 items divided into three dimensions: emotional (3 items; e.g., "During the past month, how often did you feel happy?"), social (five items; e.g., "During the past month, how often did you feel that you had something important to contribute to society?") and psychological wellbeing (six items; e.g., "During the past month, how often did you feel that your life has a sense of direction or meaning to it?"). Each item is rated on a six-point response scale from 0 (*never*) to 5 (*every day*) in reference to the last month. In Portuguese psychometric studies, only the use of the total score was recommended as no adequate support was found for the use of the subscales as measures of distinct dimensions. The MHC-SF can be scored continuously (scores range from 0 to 70, and higher scores indicate better positive mental health) or categorically considering mental health status (flourishing, moderate mental health, languishing). Using Keyes' criteria [52], women who answered *every day* or *almost every day* at least once in the emotional wellbeing subscale and at least six times in the psychological and social wellbeing subscales were categorized as flourishing. Women who answered *never* or *once or twice* for at least one item in the emotional wellbeing subscale and at least six items in the psychological and social wellbeing subscales were categorized as languishing. Finally, women who did not fit the criteria for either flourishing or languishing were considered moderately mentally healthy. In this study, we categorized participants as flourishing and not flourishing (including both languishers and those with moderate mental health). The Cronbach's alpha values in this study ranged from 0.90 (intervention group—T1) to 0.93 (intervention group—T2).

2.5.2. Secondary Outcomes

The Edinburgh Postnatal Depression Scale (EPDS; [54]; PV: [54]) was used to assess postpartum depressive symptoms. EPDS comprises 10 items (e.g., "I have blamed myself unnecessarily when things went wrong") that are rated with an individualized four-point response scale (ranging from 0 to 3). The total score ranges between 0 and 30, and higher scores are indicative of more severe depressive symptoms. In this study, the Cronbach's alpha values ranged from 0.80 (intervention group—T1) to 0.86 (control group—T2).

The Anxiety Subscale of the Hospital Anxiety and Depression Scale (HADS-A; [55]; PV: [56]) was used to assess anxiety symptoms. This widely used seven-item subscale (e.g., "Worrying thoughts go through my mind") employs a four-point response scale (ranging from 0 to 3) that assesses the presence of anxiety symptoms in the week prior to completion. Higher scores denote higher anxiety symptoms. In this study, the Cronbach's alpha values ranged from 0.76 (intervention group—T1) to 0.82 (intervention group—T2).

The Empowerment Scale (ES; [57]; PV: [58]) was used to assess empowerment. The ES is a self-reported questionnaire with 20 items (e.g., "I am usually confident about the decision I make") that are rated with a four-point scale ranging from 1 (*strongly agree*) to 4 (*strongly disagree*). Higher scores indicate higher levels of empowerment. The Cronbach's alpha values in this study ranged from 0.79 (control group—T2) to 0.89 (intervention group—T2).

Women's perception of self-efficacy in the mothering role was assessed using the Perceived Maternal Parenting Self-Efficacy (PMP S-E; [59]). This measure comprises 20 items (e.g., "I am good at understanding what my baby wants") rated with a four-point scale ranging from 1 (*strongly disagree*) to 4 (*strongly agree*). Higher scores indicate higher levels of perceived self-efficacy. In this study, the Cronbach's alpha values ranged from 0.91 (control group—T2) to 0.95 (intervention group—T2).

The Satisfaction subscale of the Investment Model Scale (IMS-S; [60]; PV: [61]) was used to assess satisfaction in the relationship with the woman's partner. This subscale comprises five items (e.g., "Our relationship makes me very happy") answered on nine-point scale ranging from 0 (*do not agree at all*) to 8 (*completely agree*). Higher scores indicate higher satisfaction with the relationship. In this study, the Cronbach's alpha values ranged from 0.81 (intervention group—T1) to 0.83 (control group—T2).

2.5.3. Be a Mom's Web System Data

Data were collected through the *Be a Mom* website regarding the number of completed modules and pages accessed in each module, number of logins, average minutes spent on the website at each login, number of finished exercises and number of times each audio exercise was played.

2.5.4. Be a Mom's Acceptability and Experience

At the postintervention assessment, the intervention group completed an additional set of questions referring to *Be a Mom*'s acceptability. Participants were asked to answer questions with a two-point response scale (1 = *not applicable to me*; 2 = *applicable to me*) regarding their satisfaction with the help provided by the program, their intentions to use it again if needed and to recommend it to a friend, usefulness/relevance of the information learned and demandingness. Additional questions were presented about the participant's experience using *Be a Mom*; these were open-ended questions regarding the presence of others when accessing the program and reasons for not completing all modules of *Be a Mom*, when applicable.

2.6. Data Analysis

Statistical analyses were conducted in accordance with the intention-to-treat principles following the CONSORT statement [62] so that all participants who completed baseline assessment were included even if they did not complete postintervention assessment. Data were analyzed using the Statistical Package for Social Sciences (IBM SPSS, version 23.0 (IBM Corp., Armonk, NY, USA)). Descriptive statistics and comparison tests (t-tests and chi-squared tests) were computed for sample characterization and to examine *Be a Mom*'s usage and acceptability. Comparison analyses were also conducted between completers and dropouts and completers and non-completers. Dropout was defined as not completing the postintervention assessment regardless of the number of modules completed, and non-completers were defined as not completing the intervention.

Linear mixed models (LMMs) were used to determine the effects of the intervention over time on primary and secondary outcomes. LMMs are particularly helpful in longitudinal studies with missing data because they allow incomplete cases to be included in the analysis. All available data are used to obtain parameter estimates with small bias in the presence of data missing completely at random or missing at random [63]. Group, time and time by group interaction and covariates (variables presenting statistically significant differences between intervention and control groups at T1 and between completers and dropouts at T2: previous history of psychopathology, infant's age and category of positive mental health) were fitted as fixed effects. Participants were included as a random intercept. An LMM with an autoregressive covariance matrix was conducted for each outcome with the assumption of data missing completely at random (Little's MCAR test $\chi^2 = 415.21$, $p = 0.938$). Missing endpoints at posttest ranged from 119/367 (32.4%) on the MHC-SF to 127/367 (34.6%) on the IMS-S.

Additionally, chi-squared tests were used to examine differences in the proportion of patterns of change as a function of group (intervention vs. control group) considering the primary outcome. Based on the cutoff scores of the MHC-SF, participants were categorized as flourishing or not flourishing at both T1 and T2. Participants were then classified in accordance with their pattern of change from T1 to T2: (a) maintenance—flourishing (if they were flourishing at both T1 and T2); (b) maintenance—not flourishing (if they were not flourishing at both T1 and T2); (c) deterioration (if they were flourishing at T1 and not flourishing at T2); and (d) improvement (if they were not flourishing at T1 and flourishing at T2).

3. Results

3.1. Participant Characteristics

Figure 1 shows the flow diagram of the participants throughout the study period. Of the 1657 women who were screened for eligibility, 72.5% (n = 1202) were excluded due to not meeting eligibility criteria (mostly because they presented risk for PPD; n = 1030, 85.7%). Of the 455 eligible participants, 367 completed the baseline assessment and were randomized and allocated to the intervention group (n = 191) or to the WLC group (n = 176).

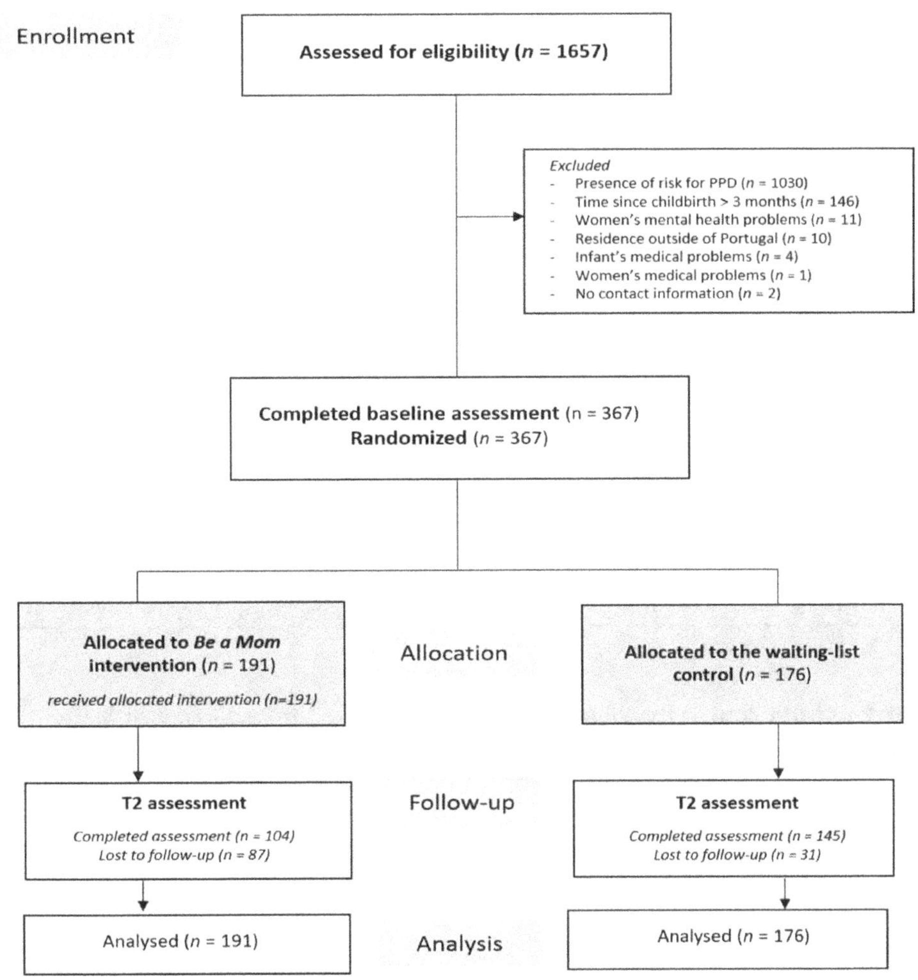

Figure 1. Flowchart of the participants in the study.

Table 1 summarizes the baseline sociodemographic and clinical characteristics of the intervention and control groups. There were no significant differences in most sociodemographic and clinical characteristics. However, a significantly higher proportion of participants in the intervention group had a previous history of psychopathology than in the control group (25.1% vs. 14.2%, $\chi^2 = 6.86$, $p = 0.009$). The control group also had a significantly higher proportion of participants who were flourishing (67% vs. 57.1%, $\chi^2 = 3.86$, $p = 0.049$).

Table 1. Participants' sociodemographic and clinical characteristics at baseline.

Variables	Intervention Group (n = 191) M (SD)/n (%)	Control Group (n = 176) M (SD)/n (%)	t/χ^2
Age	33 (4.04)	33 (4.43)	−0.14
Marital status			0.53
Married/co-habiting	183 (95.8)	170 (96.6)	
Single	4 (2.1)	2 (1.1)	
In a relationship (without living together)	4 (2.1)	4 (2.3)	
Primiparous	140 (73.3)	122 (69.3)	0.71
Employment status			3.35
Employed	176 (92.1)	170 (96.6)	
Not currently working	15 (7.9)	6 (3.4)	
Educational level			5.66
Up to the 9th grade	2 (1.0)	4 (2.3)	
10th to 12th grade	30 (15.7)	26 (14.8)	
Bachelor's degree	83 (43.5)	58 (33)	
Master's or Doctorate	76 (39.8)	88 (50)	
Household monthly income			4.92
Less than 580€	8 (4.2)	9 (5.1)	
580–1000€	88 (46.1)	80 (45.5)	
1000–2000€	87 (45.5)	70 (39.8)	
More than 2000€	8 (4.2)	17 (9.7)	
Residence			1.06
Urban	141 (73.8)	138 (78.4)	
Rural	50 (26.2)	38 (21.6)	
Psychopathology history			6.86 *
Yes	48 (25.1)	25 (14.2)	
No	143 (74.9)	151 (85.8)	
Positive mental health			3.86 *
Flourishing	109 (57.1)	118 (67)	
Not flourishing	82 (42.9)	58 (33)	
Infant's age (in months)	1.89 (0.94)	1.87 (1.32)	0.16
Infant's sex			0.43
Male	98 (51.3)	93 (53.1)	
Infant's gestational weeks (at birth)	38.89 (1.64)	38.95 (1.77)	−0.33

Note. * $p < 0.05$.

The overall retention rate at the postintervention assessment was 67.8%. The intervention arm had significantly higher loss to follow-up than the control arm (intervention group: $n = 87$, 45.5% vs. control group: $n = 31$, 17.6%, $\chi^2 = 32.77$, $p < 0.001$). Potential differences between completers and dropouts on baseline sociodemographic and clinical characteristics were explored but did not reveal any significant differences. The only exception was infant age, with infants of the participants who dropped out of the study being older than the infants of those who completed the postintervention assessment ($M = 2.11$ months, $SD = 0.97$ vs. $M = 1.77$ months, $SD = 1.20$, $t = -2.68$, $p = 0.008$). The proportion of women who had psychological/psychiatric treatment after the baseline assessment was also similar in both groups (intervention group: $n = 8$, 7.7% vs. control group: $n = 7$, 4.9%, $\chi^2 = 0.85$, $p = 0.356$).

3.2. *Be a Mom's Preliminary Evidence of Efficacy: Comparison with the Control Group*

Table 2 presents the estimated marginal means of all outcome measures and fixed effects for time, group and time × group interaction as well as for covariates (psychopathology history, infant's age and category of positive mental health at baseline).

Table 2. Estimated marginal means and fixed effects for primary and secondary outcome measures.

Variables	Group	Time 1 M (SE)	Time 2 M (SE)	Effect	B (SE)	95% CI	*p*
MHC-SF	Intervention	51.17 (0.54)	53.94 (0.69)	Time	−2.77 (0.69)	[−4.13, −1.40]	<0.001
	Control	50.47 (0.57)	51.19 (0.61)	Group	−2.74 (0.93)	[−4.56, −0.92]	0.003
				Time × Group	2.05 (0.93)	[0.22, 3.87]	0.028
				Psychopathology history	0.43 (0.88)	[−1.31, 2.16]	0.630
				MHC-SF baseline category	13.75 (0.73)	[12.31, 15.18]	<0.001
				Infant's age	−0.10 (0.31)	[−0.70, 0.50]	0.748
EPDS	Intervention	6.38 (0.26)	5.26 (0.33)	Time	1.12 (0.34)	[0.45, 1.80]	0.001
	Control	6.72 (0.27)	6.19 (0.29)	Group	0.93 (0.45)	[−0.06, 1.81]	0.036
				Time × Group	−0.60 (0.46)	[−1.50, 0.31]	0.194
				Psychopathology history	−1.43 (0.42)	[−2.25, −0.61]	0.001
				MHC-SF baseline category	−2.75 (0.34)	[−3.42, −2.08]	<0.001
				Infant's age	−0.05 (0.14)	[−0.33, 0.23]	0.739
HADS-A	Intervention	4.40 (0.22)	3.88 (0.28)	Time	0.53 (0.29)	[−0.04, 1.09]	0.069
	Control	4.54 (0.23)	4.72 (0.25)	Group	0.84 (0.38)	[0.09, 1.59]	0.028
				Time × Group	−0.71 (0.38)	[−1.46, 0.05]	0.067
				Psychopathology history	−2.02 (0.36)	[−2.73, −1.31]	<0.001
				MHC-SF baseline category	−1.62 (0.30)	[−2.20, −1.04]	<0.001
				Infant's age	0.05 (0.12)	[−0.20, 0.29]	0.710
PMPS-E	Intervention	69.06 (0.48)	73.09 (0.59)	Time	−4.11 (0.58)	[−5.14, −2.92]	<0.001
	Control	67.87 (0.50)	72.57 (0.53)	Group	−0.56 (0.81)	[−2.09, 1.05]	0.517
				Time × Group	−0.63 (0.77)	[−2.15, 0.81]	0.375
				Psychopathology history	−0.80 (0.79)	[−2.41, 0.72]	0.285
				MHC-SF baseline category	3.84 (0.65)	[2.54, 5.10]	<0.001
				Infant's age	0.94 (0.27)	[0.40, 1.47]	0.001
ES	Intervention	61.05 (0.38)	61.52 (0.46)	Time	−0.47 (0.40)	[−1.27, 0.32]	0.244
	Control	61.32 (0.40)	61.05 (0.42)	Group	−0.47 (0.63)	[−1.70, 0.76]	0.454
				Time × Group	0.74 (0.54)	[−0.32, 1.79]	0.170
				Psychopathology history	0.73 (0.65)	[−0.55, 2.01]	0.264
				MHC-SF baseline category	4.29 (0.53)	[3.24, 5.34]	<0.001
				Infant's age	−0.22 (0.22)	[−0.66, 0.22]	0.331
IMS-S	Intervention	6.54 (0.09)	6.36 (0.11)	Time	0.19 (0.09)	[0.00, 0.37]	0.046
	Control	6.48 (0.09)	6.30 (0.10)	Group	−0.05 (0.14)	[−0.33, 0.23]	0.718
				Time × Group	−0.02 (0.12)	[−0.26, 0.23]	0.901
				Psychopathology history	0.20 (0.15)	[−0.08, 0.49]	0.166
				MHC-SF baseline category	0.57 (0.12)	[0.33, 0.81]	<0.001
				Infant's age	−0.11 (0.05)	[−0.21, −0.02]	0.024

Note. MHC-SF—Mental Health Continuum-Short Form; EPDS—Edinburgh Postnatal Depression Scale; HADS-A—Hospital Anxiety and Depression Scale-Anxiety; ES—Empowerment Scale; PMPSE - Perceived Maternal Parenting Self-Efficacy; IMS-S—Investment Model Scale-Satisfaction.

Regarding the primary outcome, the LMM revealed a significant effect of time × group interaction, with women in the intervention group reporting a greater increase in positive mental health levels than participants in the control group (see Figure 2).

Regarding the secondary outcomes, significant effects of group were found for depressive and anxiety symptoms. Specifically, we found that these symptoms were higher overall in the control group. Although no significant time × group interactions were found, Figure 2 shows that a greater decrease in depressive and anxiety symptoms was found from T1 to T2 in the intervention group.

Regarding the remaining secondary outcomes, no interaction effects of time × group were found. For maternal self-efficacy and relationship satisfaction, significant effects of time were found. In both the intervention and control groups, there was a decrease in satisfaction in the relationship with the partner and an increase in maternal self-efficacy from T1 to T2, but there were no significant differences between the *Be a Mom* group and the WLC group.

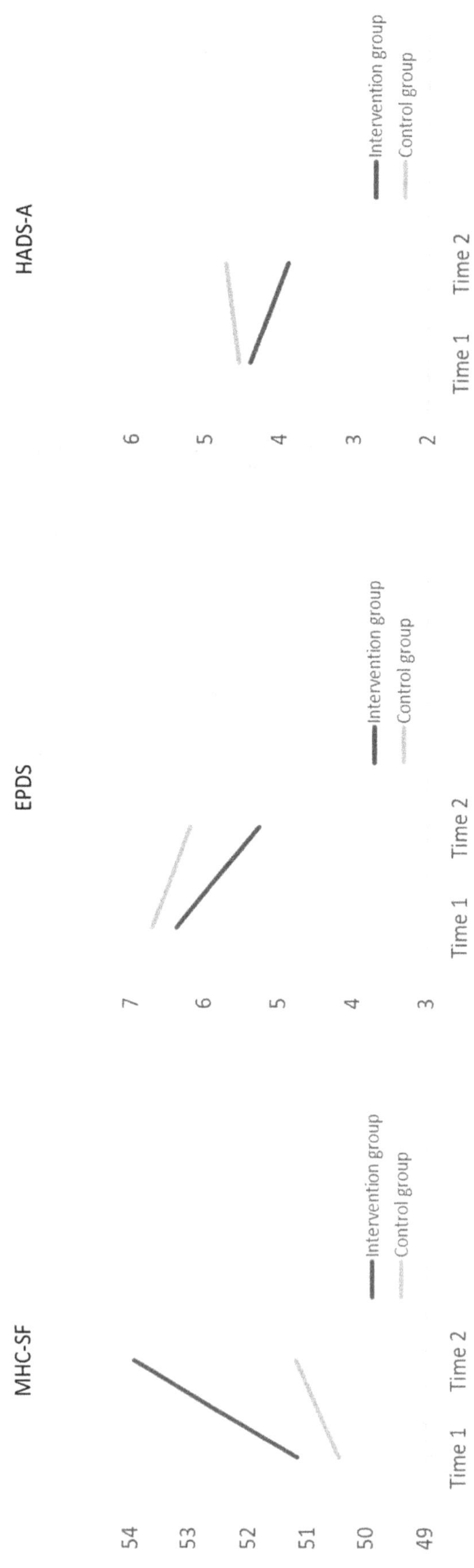

Figure 2. Intervention and control group trajectories for the Mental Health Continuum-Short Form, the Edinburgh Postnatal Depression Scale and the Anxiety subscale of the Hospital Anxiety and Depression Scale from T1 to T2 (based on mean estimates from linear mixed models).

Figure 3 shows that a significantly higher proportion of women in the intervention group had an improvement trajectory (from not flourishing at T1 to flourishing at T2) compared to women in the control group ($n = 21$, 20.2% vs. $n = 14$, 9.7%, $\chi^2 = 10.59$, $p = 0.014$). Additionally, a higher proportion of women in the control group had a deterioration trajectory (from flourishing at T1 to not flourishing at T2) compared to women in the intervention group ($n = 18$, 12.4% vs. $n = 4$, 3.8%).

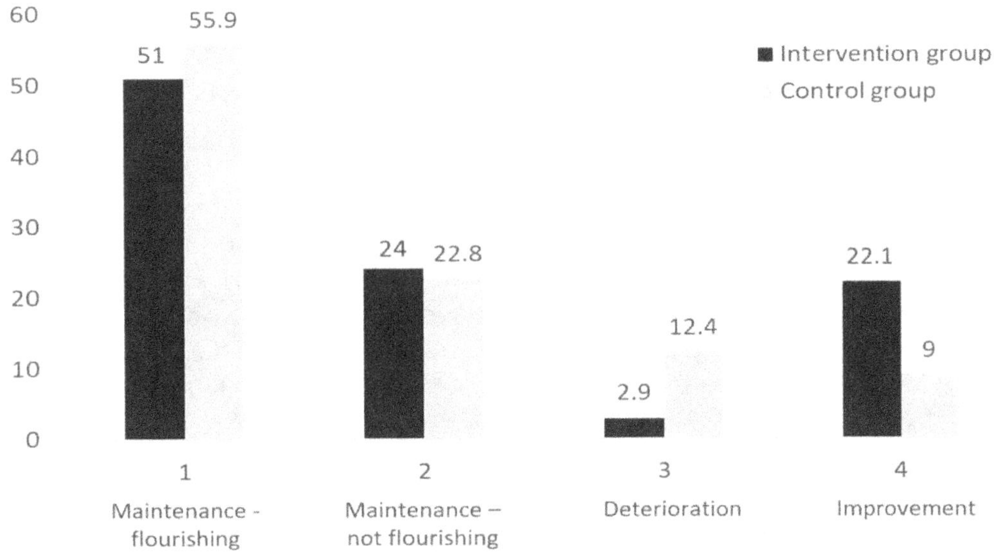

Figure 3. Trajectory of participants in the intervention and control groups from Time 1 to Time 2 regarding category of positive mental health. Maintenance—flourishing: flourishing at both T1 and T2; Maintenance—not flourishing: not flourishing at both T1 and T2; Deterioration: flourishing at T1 and not flourishing at T2; Improvement: not flourishing at T1 and flourishing at T2.

3.3. *Adherence to the Intervention, Be a Mom's Usage and Acceptability*

A total of 191 participants received an email invite to access the *Be a Mom* website. Of these, 62 (32.5%) completed the intervention, 23 (12%) completed half of the program, and 20 (10.5%) did not register on the website and initiate the intervention. Of the participants who registered on the *Be a Mom* website, 29 (17%) participants did not complete any module.

Considering all 171 participants who registered on the *Be a Mom* website, the average number of logins was 6 ($SD = 3.78$, range: 1–20) and the average number of minutes spent on the website in each login was 16 ($SD = 11.80$, range: 0–73). The majority of participants finished all four exercises of module 1 ($n = 128$, 74.9%) and the two exercises of module 2 ($n = 103$; 60.2%). Considering the participants who completed modules three, four and five, most of them finished all exercises proposed (four in module three, two in modules four and five; $n = 73/80$, 91.3%; $n = 58/60$, 96.7%; $n = 30/59$, 50.8%, respectively). Most of the participants who completed module 2 listened to the two audio exercises provided (observing thoughts and distancing of thoughts) ($n = 78/103$, 75.7% and $n = 48/103$, 46.6%, respectively).

Moreover, 113 participants in the intervention group answered a questionnaire about their experience using *Be a Mom* and its acceptability. Of these, 55 (48.7%) did not complete the intervention. Regarding the reasons for not completing *Be a Mom*, 53 (96.4%) participants highlighted lack of time, one (1.8%) participant answered that it was due to personal issues and one (1.8%) answered that *Be a Mom* was not useful in her case. Most women accessed *Be a Mom* on their own ($n = 102$; 90.3%). The remaining 11 participants accessed *Be a Mom* with their partners ($n = 10$; 90.9%) and other family members ($n = 1$; 9.1%), and all considered it beneficial for them and for the other person.

Of the 113 participants who answered the acceptability questionnaire, 65.5% ($n = 74$) were satisfied with the help provided by *Be a Mom*, 85% ($n = 96$) would recommend it to a friend, and 72.6% ($n = 82$) would use it again if needed. Moreover, 92% ($n = 104$) of participants rated the quality of *Be a Mom* as good/excellent. Additionally, 74.3% ($n = 84$) felt that they had learned relevant information with *Be a Mom*. Finally, 21 women (5.7%) considered participating in *Be a Mom* to be too demanding.

When comparing completers and non-completers of *Be a Mom*, a higher proportion of completers was satisfied with the help provided by *Be a Mom* ($n = 43$, 74.1% vs. $n = 31$, 56.4%, $\chi^2 = 3.95$, $p = 0.047$). Moreover, when compared to non-completers, a higher proportion of completers would recommend *Be a Mom* to a friend ($n = 54$, 93.1% vs. $n = 42$, 76.4%, $\chi^2 = 6.19$, $p = 0.013$), would use it again if they needed ($n = 48$, 82.8% vs. $n = 34$, 61.8%, $\chi^2 = 6.22$, $p = .013$) and felt that they learned relevant information with the program ($n = 49$, 84.5% vs. $n = 35$, 63.6%, $\chi^2 = 6.43$, $p = 0.011$). A higher proportion of non-completers considered participating in the *Be a Mom* program to be too demanding compared to completers ($n = 17$, 30.9% vs. $n = 4$, 6.9%, $\chi^2 = 10.76$, $p = 0.001$).

4. Discussion

The current study examined the efficacy of a web-based intervention, *Be a Mom*, in increasing positive mental health among postpartum women presenting low risk for PPD compared to a waiting-list condition. The efficacy of *Be a Mom* on secondary outcomes (depressive and anxiety symptoms, maternal self-efficacy, empowerment and relationship satisfaction) was also examined. The results of our study suggest that *Be a Mom* was superior to the WLC in increasing positive mental health. Additionally, there was a decreasing trend over time in depressive and anxiety symptoms in the *Be a Mom* group. *Be a Mom* was also shown to be an acceptable web-based intervention among low-risk postpartum women with satisfactory adherence and usage.

The significant improvement of positive mental health in the *Be a Mom* group is in line with previous evidence supporting the efficacy of web-based CBT interventions to promote positive mental health [42,43]. However, this is one of the first trials to successfully demonstrate this in the postpartum period. Additionally, our results showed that *Be a Mom* increased the proportion of flourishers over time. Conversely, a higher proportion of women in the control group had a deterioration trajectory (from flourishing at baseline to not flourishing at postintervention assessment). This is an important finding given the demonstrated importance of flourishing in protecting against future adversities and mental disorders, such as anxiety and depression [27,28], as well as its association with several health and psychosocial outcomes [24,64]. Thus, *Be a Mom* could have an important impact on mental health outcomes in the long term and, as such, enhance public mental health. Future studies using long-term assessments could test this hypothesis.

Regarding the secondary outcomes, the interaction effects of time and group failed to reach statistical significance. However, regarding depressive and anxiety symptoms, we found significant group effects (these symptoms were higher in the control group) as well as a trend of a greater decrease in the intervention group, particularly for anxiety symptoms. When looking at mean estimates, we found that from T1 to T2, there was an increase in anxiety symptoms in the control group contrasting with a reduction in the intervention group. This suggests that participants who received the *Be a Mom* program had greater benefits than those in the control group. However, although the efficacy of *Be a Mom* in reducing depressive and anxiety symptoms was previously demonstrated [39], it is important to note that *Be a Mom* seems to not have a substantial impact on such symptoms among low-risk postpartum women. A possible explanation may be the relatively low levels of depressive and anxiety symptoms at baseline, which leaves limited space for improvement.

Moreover, we found an increase over time in maternal self-efficacy in both study groups. This is consistent with the existing literature [65,66]: infants' demands become more predictable as they grow older, providing the opportunity to increase the mother's ability to successfully perform childcare tasks. However, we found that *Be a Mom* did not have a significant impact on the maternal self-efficacy of low-risk women. Although *Be a Mom* does not target caregiving behaviors, we expected that the emotional state of participants would influence the assessment of their self-efficacy, in line with Bandura's self-efficacy theory [67] and previous studies associating depressive symptoms with lower maternal self-efficacy [68]. This result is consistent with those previously found on the efficacy of *Be a*

Mom among a high-risk sample [39] and provides further evidence that *Be a Mom* may not be a suitable intervention to contribute to maternal confidence and self-efficacy, at least in the short term.

With respect to the results on empowerment, small, nonsignificant differences were found between the groups over time. Looking at mean estimates, the results suggest an increase in empowerment in the *Be a Mom* group compared with a decrease in the control group. A previous trial in the general population highlighted the significant impact of a web-based intervention on empowerment levels [37], suggesting that individuals who access the intervention may feel that they are more informed and involved in managing their own health outcomes. However, this was not found for *Be a Mom*. Future trials with follow-up assessments could provide more information on the pattern of this finding.

Finally, we found that both groups presented a decline in relationship satisfaction over time. Previous studies have emphasized that the arrival of an infant can strain the romantic relationship and produce changes in the couple, with a decline in satisfaction [69]. Although *Be a Mom* has a module that focuses on the changes that can happen within the couple during this period, most participants (90.3%) accessed *Be a Mom* on their own. The strategies that are presented (e.g., acknowledging the difficulties experienced by the other member of the couple, assertive and open communication skills, accepting differences in backgrounds and parental values) should ideally be implemented in a joint effort by the two members of the couple. In the future, further efforts and instructions to involve partners when accessing *Be a Mom* could help clarify its impact on relationship satisfaction.

In addition to the results on the efficacy of *Be a Mom*, our study provided results on *Be a Mom*'s acceptability as well as its usage and adherence. Extending on previous acceptability results among postpartum women presenting risk factors for PPD [39], *Be a Mom* appears to also be an acceptable option for low-risk postpartum women. However, adherence to the intervention was relatively low (only 32.5% women completed *Be a Mom*). This result is congruent with those found by previous research with web-based interventions applied to universal samples during the perinatal period [44,45] and could be explained by the hectic and challenging period women are experiencing, which leaves them with limited time for themselves. Additionally, *Be a Mom* is a fully self-guided intervention that was delivered to a low-risk sample with relatively good levels of overall mental health at baseline. It is possible that participants perceived that they did not need to complete the intervention and prioritized their limited time with other tasks. Nevertheless, those who completed the intervention or accessed half of the modules adhered to most of the exercises that were proposed.

Overall, the results of our study are very encouraging: they support mental health promotion strategies in the postpartum period and highlight the important role of web-based CBT interventions in achieving this. First, the postpartum represents an appropriate period to implement mental health promotion strategies given the pervasive consequences of mental health problems during this period and how they might shape children's development and health outcomes in the long term [11]. Second, the finding that low-risk women may significantly benefit from *Be a Mom* gives strength to the argument that mental health promotion strategies at a population level are needed. Growing research has emphasized that it is not sufficient to target only groups suffering from mental disorders or at-risk groups as new cases of mental illness will emerge [70,71]. A small change in the average level of positive mental health per individual could lead to significant benefits in population terms and shift the population distribution of positive mental health [70], with a possible impact on the prevalence and burden of mental disorders. Finally, *Be a Mom*'s brief and unguided format provides the opportunity to be delivered with low costs and to be easily disseminated at a population level. If implemented in healthcare, *Be a Mom* could be used as an early intervention of a stepped-care model, which is highly recommended by international guidelines [72], and could consequently provide a more efficient use of resources.

Although the results of our study are innovative and may add important input to public health policies, some limitations should be considered when interpreting our findings. First, the generalizability of the results is limited because the participants in the current study were self-selected, and it is possible that women with an interest in the topic were more likely to participate.

Moreover, one criterion to be included in this study was having internet access and this could also represent a selection bias. Additionally, our sample was mainly composed of highly educated and employed women. Future studies could build on current findings by investigating the efficacy of *Be a Mom* in more heterogeneous and representative samples. Second, there was a high attrition rate and low adherence in the intervention group. This is in line with previous intervention studies in the perinatal period [46] and, as previously mentioned, could be explained by the demanding nature of the early postpartum period. The lower attrition rate in the control group could be explained by the added incentive of gaining access to *Be a Mom* by continuing participation in the study. Future intervention studies during the postpartum period need to take into account the challenging and time-restricted period women are experiencing when designing research. Brief assessment protocols could help improve attrition rates. Additionally, future studies using the *Be a Mom* program must be mindful of this study's low adherence. Although a great proportion of participants answered that they did not complete the program due to lack of time, it is important to understand the reasons underlying this low rate and how much does it reflect the demandingness of the early postpartum period or the intervention's structure, length and contents. Third, the lack of an active control group does not allow us to rule out the possibility that the effects found were due to social desirability or placebo effects. Fourth, while the present study found evidence of the efficacy of *Be a Mom* in enhancing positive mental health, the observed effect was only a short-term improvement. Thus, the results presented are best interpreted as providing promising evidence. Future RCTs with follow-up assessments are needed to test *Be a Mom*'s efficacy in producing enduring positive effects. Examining the long-term impact of this approach with added input from a cost-effectiveness analysis could meaningfully inform public health policies. Finally, the mechanisms that explain the participants' response to treatment were not directly explored in this study. Because *Be a Mom* was developed to mainly target psychological resources such as self-compassion and emotion regulation, further studies exploring whether these mechanisms are involved in explaining the increase in levels of positive mental health are needed.

5. Conclusions

The promotion of positive mental health in the perinatal period has received very little attention to date. This is one of the first trials to test a web-based CBT intervention for this purpose among postpartum women presenting low risk for PPD. Given our findings, *Be a Mom* could be considered a new mental health promotion strategy among Portuguese postpartum women. The results of this pilot trial support its preliminary efficacy in increasing positive mental health to a flourishing mental health status with the potential to reduce depressive and anxiety symptoms among a nonclinical population. As an unguided web-based intervention, *Be a Mom* offers an accessible intervention option that could easily be disseminated among all postpartum women. Further research with a larger sample and long-term follow-up assessments is required to consolidate our findings and significantly inform public health policies.

Author Contributions: Conceptualization, F.M. and A.F.; Formal analysis, F.M. and A.F.; Investigation, F.M.; Methodology, F.M., M.P. and A.F.; Supervision, M.P., M.C.C. and A.F.; Writing—original draft, F.M.; Writing—review & editing, M.P., M.C.C. and A.F. All authors have read and agreed to the published version of the manuscript.

Acknowledgments: This study is part of the research project "Promoting maternal mental health: Applicability and effectiveness of an eHealth intervention for Portuguese postpartum women", integrated in the research group Relationships, Development & Health of the R&D Unit Center for Research in Neuropsychology and Cognitive Behavioral Center Intervention (CINEICC) of the Faculty of Psychology and Educational Sciences, University of Coimbra.

References

1. Winson, N. Transition to motherhood. In *The Social Context of Birth*, 3rd ed.; Squire, C., Ed.; Routledge: London, UK, 2017. [CrossRef]
2. Kanotra, S.; D'Angelo, D.; Phares, T.M.; Morrow, B.; Barfield, W.D.; Lansky, A. Challenges faced by new

mothers in the early postpartum period: An analysis of comment data from the 2000 Pregnancy Risk Assessment Monitoring System (PRAMS) survey. *Matern. Child Health J.* **2007**, *11*, 549–558. [CrossRef] [PubMed]

3. Woolhouse, H.; Gartland, D.; Perlen, S.; Donath, S.; Brown, S.J. Physical health after childbirth and maternal depression in the first 12 months post partum: Results of an Australian nulliparous pregnancy cohort study. *Midwifery* **2014**, *30*, 378–384. [CrossRef] [PubMed]
4. Woolhouse, H.; McDonald, E.; Brown, S. Women's experiences of sex and intimacy after childbirth: Making the adjustment to motherhood. *J. Psychosom. Obstet. Gynaecol.* **2012**, *33*, 185–190. [CrossRef] [PubMed]
5. Grice, M.M.; Feda, D.; McGovern, P.; Alexander, B.H.; McCaffrey, D.; Ukestad, L. Giving birth and returning to work: The impact of work-family conflict on women's health after childbirth. *Ann. Epidemiol.* **2007**, *17*, 791–798. [CrossRef] [PubMed]
6. Nowak, M.J.; Naude, M.; Thomas, G. Returning to work after maternity leave: Childcare and workplace flexibility. *J. Ind. Relat.* **2013**, *55*, 118–135. [CrossRef]
7. Jevitt, C.M.; Groer, M.W.; Crist, N.F.; Gonzalez, L.; Wagner, V.D. Postpartum stressors: A content analysis. *Issues Ment. Health Nurs.* **2012**, *33*, 309–318. [CrossRef]
8. Norhayati, M.N.; Hazlina, N.H.; Asrenee, A.R.; Emilin, W.M. Magnitude and risk factors for postpartum symptoms: A literature review. *J. Affect. Disord.* **2015**, *175*, 34–52. [CrossRef]
9. Murphey, C.; Carter, P.; Price, L.R.; Champion, J.D.; Nichols, F. Psychological distress in healthy low-risk first-time mothers during the postpartum period: An exploratory study. *Nurs. Res. Pract.* **2017**, *2017*, 8415083. [CrossRef]
10. Weisman, O.; Granat, A.; Gilboa-Schechtman, E.; Singer, M.; Gordon, I.; Azulay, H.; Kuint, J.; Feldman, R. The experience of labor, maternal perception of the infant, and the mother's postpartum mood in a low-risk community cohort. *Arch. Womens Ment. Health* **2010**, *13*, 505–513. [CrossRef]
11. Slomian, J.; Honvo, G.; Emonts, P.; Reginster, J.Y.; Bruyere, O. Consequences of maternal postpartum depression: A systematic review of maternal and infant outcomes. *Womens Health (Lond.)* **2019**, *15*, 1745506519844044. [CrossRef]
12. Wen, D.J.; Poh, J.S.; Ni, S.N.; Chong, Y.S.; Chen, H.; Kwek, K.; Shek, L.P.; Gluckman, P.D.; Fortier, M.V.; Meaney, M.J.; et al. Influences of prenatal and postnatal maternal depression on amygdala volume and microstructure in young children. *Transl. Psychiatry* **2017**, *7*, e1103. [CrossRef] [PubMed]
13. Bauer, A.; Knapp, M.; Parsonage, M. Lifetime costs of perinatal anxiety and depression. *J. Affect. Disord.* **2016**, *192*, 83–90. [CrossRef] [PubMed]
14. Ladd, C.; Rodriguez McCullough, N.; Carmaciu, C. Perinatal mental illness. *InnovAiT* **2017**, *10*, 653–658. [CrossRef]
15. Weinberg, M.K.; Tronick, E.Z.; Beeghly, M.; Olson, K.L.; Kernan, H.; Riley, J.M. Subsyndromal depressive symptoms and major depression in postpartum women. *Am. J. Orthopsychiatry* **2001**, *71*, 87–97. [CrossRef]
16. Sockol, L.E. A systematic review of the efficacy of cognitive behavioral therapy for treating and preventing perinatal depression. *J. Affect. Disord.* **2015**, *177*, 7–21. [CrossRef]
17. Lin, P.Z.; Xue, J.M.; Yang, B.; Li, M.; Cao, F.L. Effectiveness of self-help psychological interventions for treating and preventing postpartum depression: A meta-analysis. *Arch. Womens Ment. Health* **2018**, *21*, 491–503. [CrossRef]
18. Dennis, C.L.; Creedy, D. Psychosocial and psychological interventions for preventing postpartum depression. *Cochrane Database Syst. Rev.* **2004**. [CrossRef]
19. Barry, M.M.; Clarke, A.M.; Petersen, I.; Jenkins, R. *Implementing Mental Health Promotion*; SpringerNature Switzerland: Cham, Switzerland, 2019.
20. Forsman, A.K.; Wahlbeck, K.; Aaro, L.E.; Alonso, J.; Barry, M.M.; Brunn, M.; Cardoso, G.; Cattan, M.; de Girolamo, G.; Eberhard-Gran, M.; et al. Research priorities for public mental health in Europe: Recommendations of the ROAMER project. *Eur. J. Public Health* **2015**, *25*, 249–254. [CrossRef]
21. Newnham, E.A.; Hooke, G.R.; Page, A.C. Progress monitoring and feedback in psychiatric care reduces depressive symptoms. *J. Affect. Disord.* **2010**, *127*, 139–146. [CrossRef]
22. Trompetter, H.R.; Lamers, S.M.A.; Westerhof, G.J.; Fledderus, M.; Bohlmeijer, E.T. Both positive mental health and psychopathology should be monitored in psychotherapy: Confirmation for the dual-factor model in acceptance and commitment therapy. *Behav. Res. Ther.* **2017**, *91*, 58–63. [CrossRef]

23. Smith, V.; Daly, D.; Lundgren, I.; Eri, T.; Benstoem, C.; Devane, D. Salutogenically focused outcomes in systematic reviews of intrapartum interventions: A systematic review of systematic reviews. *Midwifery* **2014**, *30*, e151–e156. [CrossRef] [PubMed]
24. Keyes, C.L. Mental illness and/or mental health? Investigating axioms of the complete state model of health. *J. Consult. Clin. Psychol.* **2005**, *73*, 539–548. [CrossRef] [PubMed]
25. Howell, R.T.; Kern, M.L.; Lyubomirsky, S. Health benefits: Meta-analytically determining the impact of well-being on objective health outcomes. *Health Psychol. Rev.* **2007**, *1*, 83–136. [CrossRef]
26. Keyes, C.L.; Simoes, E.J. To flourish or not: Positive mental health and all-cause mortality. *Am. J. Public Health* **2012**, *102*, 2164–2172. [CrossRef] [PubMed]
27. Schotanus-Dijkstra, M.; Keyes, C.L.M.; de Graaf, R.; Ten Have, M. Recovery from mood and anxiety disorders: The influence of positive mental health. *J. Affect. Disord.* **2019**, *252*, 107–113. [CrossRef]
28. Keyes, C.L.; Dhingra, S.S.; Simoes, E.J. Change in level of positive mental health as a predictor of future risk of mental illness. *Am. J. Public Health* **2010**, *100*, 2366–2371. [CrossRef]
29. Phua, D.Y.; Kee, M.; Koh, D.X.P.; Rifkin-Graboi, A.; Daniels, M.; Chen, H.; Chong, Y.S.; Broekman, B.F.P.; Magiati, I.; Karnani, N.; et al. Positive maternal mental health during pregnancy associated with specific forms of adaptive development in early childhood: Evidence from a longitudinal study. *Dev. Psychopathol.* **2017**, *29*, 1573–1587. [CrossRef]
30. Kazdin, A.E.; Blase, S.L. Rebooting Psychotherapy Research and Practice to Reduce the Burden of Mental Illness. *Perspect. Psychol. Sci.* **2011**, *6*, 21–37. [CrossRef]
31. McGarry, J.; Kim, H.; Sheng, X.; Egger, M.; Baksh, L. Postpartum depression and help-seeking behavior. *J. Midwifery Womens Health* **2009**, *54*, 50–56. [CrossRef]
32. Fonseca, A.; Gorayeb, R.; Canavarro, M.C. Womens help-seeking behaviours for depressive symptoms during the perinatal period: Socio-demographic and clinical correlates and perceived barriers to seeking professional help. *Midwifery* **2015**, *31*, 1177–1185. [CrossRef]
33. Moore, D.; Ayers, S.; Drey, N. A Thematic Analysis of Stigma and Disclosure for Perinatal Depression on an Online Forum. *JMIR Ment. Health* **2016**, *3*, e18. [CrossRef] [PubMed]
34. Dennis, C.L.; Chung-Lee, L. Postpartum depression help-seeking barriers and maternal treatment preferences: A qualitative systematic review. *Birth* **2006**, *33*, 323–331. [CrossRef] [PubMed]
35. Lal, S.; Adair, C.E. E-mental health: A rapid review of the literature. *Psychiatr. Serv.* **2014**, *65*, 24–32. [CrossRef] [PubMed]
36. Andersson, G.; Titov, N. Advantages and limitations of Internet-based interventions for common mental disorders. *World Psychiatry* **2014**, *13*, 4–11. [CrossRef] [PubMed]
37. Crisp, D.; Griffiths, K.; Mackinnon, A.; Bennett, K.; Christensen, H. An online intervention for reducing depressive symptoms: Secondary benefits for self-esteem, empowerment and quality of life. *Psychiatry Res.* **2014**, *216*, 60–66. [CrossRef] [PubMed]
38. van den Heuvel, J.F.; Groenhof, T.K.; Veerbeek, J.H.; van Solinge, W.W.; Lely, A.T.; Franx, A.; Bekker, M.N. eHealth as the Next-Generation Perinatal Care: An Overview of the Literature. *J. Med. Internet Res.* **2018**, *20*, e202. [CrossRef]
39. Fonseca, A.; Alves, S.; Monteiro, F.; Gorayeb, R.; Canavarro, M.C. Be a Mom, a Web-Based Intervention to Prevent Postpartum Depression: Results From a Pilot Randomized Controlled Trial. *Behav. Ther.* **2019**. [CrossRef]
40. Fonseca, A.; Monteiro, F.; Alves, S.; Gorayeb, R.; Canavarro, M.C. Be a Mom, a web-based intervention to prevent postpartum depression: The enhancement of self-regulatory skills and its association with postpartum depressive symptoms. *Front. Psychol.* **2019**, *10*, 265. [CrossRef]
41. Ciarrochi, J.; Kashdan, T.B. (Eds.) The foundations of flourishing. In *Mindfulness, Acceptance and Positive Psychology*; New Harbinger Press: Oakland, CA, USA, 2013; pp. 1–29.
42. Powell, J.; Hamborg, T.; Stallard, N.; Burls, A.; McSorley, J.; Bennett, K.; Griffiths, K.M.; Christensen, H. Effectiveness of a web-based cognitive-behavioral tool to improve mental well-being in the general population: Randomized controlled trial. *J. Med. Internet Res.* **2012**, *15*, e2. [CrossRef]
43. Rasanen, P.; Lappalainen, P.; Muotka, J.; Tolvanen, A.; Lappalainen, R. An online guided ACT intervention for enhancing the psychological wellbeing of university students: A randomized controlled clinical trial. *Behav. Res. Ther.* **2016**, *78*, 30–42. [CrossRef]
44. Gammer, I.; Hartley-Jones, C.; Jones, F.W. A Randomized Controlled Trial of an Online, Compassion-Based

Intervention for Maternal Psychological Well-Being in the First Year Postpartum. *Mindfulness* **2020**, *11*, 928–939. [CrossRef]

45. Haga, S.M.; Kinser, P.; Wentzel-Larsen, T.; Lisøy, C.; Garthus-Niegel, S.; Slinning, K.; Drozd, F. Mamma Mia—A randomized controlled trial of an internet intervention to enhance subjective well-being in perinatal women. *J. Posit. Psychol.* **2020**. [CrossRef]
46. Lee, E.W.; Denison, F.C.; Hor, K.; Reynolds, R.M. Web-based interventions for prevention and treatment of perinatal mood disorders: A systematic review. *BMC Pregnancy Childbirth* **2016**, *16*, 38. [CrossRef] [PubMed]
47. Eldridge, S.M.; Chan, C.L.; Campbell, M.J.; Bond, C.M.; Hopewell, S.; Thabane, L.; Lancaster, G.A. PAFS consensus group (2016) CONSORT 2010 statement: Extension to randomised pilot and feasibility trials. *BMJ* **2016**, *355*, i5239. [CrossRef] [PubMed]
48. Eysenbach, G.; Group, C.-E. CONSORT-EHEALTH: Improving and standardizing evaluation reports of Web-based and mobile health interventions. *J. Med. Internet Res.* **2011**, *13*, e126. [CrossRef]
49. Alves, S.; Fonseca, A.; Canavarro, M.C.; Pereira, M. Predictive validity of the Postpartum Depression Predictors Inventory-Revised (PDPI-R): A longitudinal study with Portuguese women. *Midwifery* **2019**, *69*, 113–120. [CrossRef]
50. Fonseca, A.; Pereira, M.; Araújo-Pedrosa, A.; Gorayeb, R.; Ramos, M.M.; Canavarro, M.C. Be a Mom: Formative evaluation of a web-based psychological intervention to prevent postpartum depression. *Cogn. Behav. Pract.* **2018**, *25*, 473–495. [CrossRef]
51. Alves, S.; Fonseca, A.; Canavarro, M.C.; Pereira, M. Preliminary Psychometric Testing of the Postpartum Depression Predictors Inventory-Revised (PDPI-R) in Portuguese Women. *Matern. Child Health J.* **2018**, *22*, 571–578. [CrossRef]
52. Keyes, C.L.; Wissing, M.; Potgieter, J.P.; Temane, M.; Kruger, A.; van Rooy, S. Evaluation of the Mental Health Continuum-Short Form (MHC-SF) in Setswana-speaking South Africans. *Clin. Psychol. Psychother.* **2008**, *15*, 181–192. [CrossRef]
53. Monteiro, F.; Fonseca, A.; Pereira, M.; Canavarro, M.C. Measuring positive mental health in the postpartum period: The bifactor structure of the Mental Health Continuum-Short Form in Portuguese women. *Assessment* **2020**. [CrossRef]
54. Areias, M.E.; Kumar, R.; Barros, H.; Figueiredo, E. Comparative incidence of depression in women and men, during pregnancy and after childbirth. Validation of the Edinburgh Postnatal Depression Scale in Portuguese mothers. *Br. J. Psychiatry* **1996**, *169*, 30–35. [CrossRef] [PubMed]
55. Zigmond, A.S.; Snaith, R.P. The hospital anxiety and depression scale. *Acta Psychiatr. Scand.* **1983**, *67*, 361–370. [CrossRef] [PubMed]
56. Pais-Ribeiro, J.; Silva, I.; Ferreira, T.; Martins, A.; Meneses, R.; Baltar, M. Validation study of a Portuguese version of the Hospital Anxiety and Depression Scale. *Psychol. Health Med.* **2007**, *12*, 225–235. [CrossRef] [PubMed]
57. Rogers, E.S.; Chamberlin, J.; Ellison, M.L.; Crean, T. A consumer-constructed scale to measure empowerment among users of mental health services. *Psychiatr. Serv.* **1997**, *48*, 1042–1047. [CrossRef] [PubMed]
58. Jorge-Monteiro, M.F.; Ornelas, J.H. Properties of the Portuguese version of the empowerment scale with mental health organization users. *Int. J. Ment. Health Syst.* **2014**, *8*, 48. [CrossRef]
59. Barnes, C.R.; Adamson-Macedo, E.N. Perceived Maternal Parenting Self-Efficacy (PMP S-E) tool: Development and validation with mothers of hospitalized preterm neonates. *J. Adv. Nurs* **2007**, *60*, 550–560. [CrossRef]
60. Rusbult, C.E.; Martz, J.M.; Agnew, C.R. The Investment Model Scale: Measuring commitment level, satisfaction level, quality of alternatives, and investment size. *Pers. Relatsh.* **1998**, *5*, 357–387. [CrossRef]
61. Rodrigues, D.; Lopes, D. The Investment Model Scale (IMS): Further studies on construct validation and development of a shorter version (IMS-S). *J. Gen. Psychol.* **2013**, *140*, 16–28. [CrossRef]
62. Schulz, K.F.; Altman, D.G.; Moher, D.; Group, C. CONSORT 2010 statement: Updated guidelines for reporting parallel group randomised trials. *BMJ* **2010**, *340*, c332. [CrossRef]
63. Siddiqui, O.; Hung, H.M.; O'Neill, R. MMRM vs. LOCF: A comprehensive comparison based on simulation study and 25 NDA datasets. *J. Biopharm. Stat.* **2009**, *19*, 227–246. [CrossRef]
64. Dyrbye, L.N.; Harper, W.; Moutier, C.; Durning, S.J.; Power, D.V.; Massie, F.S.; Eacker, A.; Thomas, M.R.; Satele, D.; Sloan, J.A.; et al. A multi-institutional study exploring the impact of positive mental health on

medical students' professionalism in an era of high burnout. *Acad. Med.* **2012**, *87*, 1024–1031. [CrossRef] [PubMed]

65. Zheng, X.; Morrell, J.; Watts, K. Changes in maternal self-efficacy, postnatal depression symptoms and social support among Chinese primiparous women during the initial postpartum period: A longitudinal study. *Midwifery* **2018**, *62*, 151–160. [CrossRef]
66. Law, K.H.; Dimmock, J.; Guelfi, K.J.; Nguyen, T.; Gucciardi, D.; Jackson, B. Stress, Depressive Symptoms, and Maternal Self-Efficacy in First-Time Mothers: Modelling and Predicting Change across the First Six Months of Motherhood. *Appl. Psychol. Health Well Being* **2019**, *11*, 126–147. [CrossRef] [PubMed]
67. Bandura, A. Regulation of cognitive processes through perceived self-efficacy. *Dev. Psychol.* **1989**, *25*, 729–735. [CrossRef]
68. Bornstein, M.H.; Hendricks, C.; Hahn, C.-S.; Haynes, O.M.; Painter, K.M.; Tamis-LeMonda, C.S. Contributors to Self-Perceived Competence, Satisfaction, Investment, and Role Balance in Maternal Parenting: A Multivariate Ecological Analysis. *Parent. Sci. Pract.* **2003**, *3*, 285–326. [CrossRef]
69. Dyrdal, G.M.; Roysamb, E.; Nes, R.B.; Vitterso, J. Can a Happy Relationship Predict a Happy Life? A Population-Based Study of Maternal Well-Being During the Life Transition of Pregnancy, Infancy, and Toddlerhood. *J. Happiness Stud.* **2011**, *12*, 947–962. [CrossRef] [PubMed]
70. Huppert, F.A. A New Approach to Reducing Disorder and Improving Well-Being. *Perspect. Psychol. Sci.* **2009**, *4*, 108–111. [CrossRef]
71. Herrman, H.; Saxena, S.; Moodie, R. *Promoting Mental Health: Concepts, Emerging Evidence, Practice. A WHO Report in Collaboration with the Victoria Health Promotion Foundation and the University of Melbourne*; World Health Organization: Geneva, Switzerland, 2005.
72. National Institute for Health and Excellence. *Antenatal and Postnatal Mental Health: Clinical Management and Service Guidance*. Updated February 2020. 2014. Available online: https://www.nice.org.uk/guidance/cg192/resources/antenatal-and-postnatal-mental-health-clinical-management-and-service-guidance-pdf-35109869806789 (accessed on 8 May 2020).

7

How are Information and Communication Technologies Supporting Routine Outcome Monitoring and Measurement-Based Care in Psychotherapy?

Patricia Gual-Montolio [1], Verónica Martínez-Borba [1], Juana María Bretón-López [1], Jorge Osma [2] and Carlos Suso-Ribera [1,*]

1 Department of Basic and Clinical Psychology and Psychobiology, Jaume I University, Avda. Vicent Sos Baynat s/n, 12071 Castellon de la Plana, Spain; al384421@uji.es (P.G.-M.); borba@uji.es (V.M.-B.); breton@uji.es (J.M.B.-L.)

2 Department of Psychology and Sociology, Universidad de Zaragoza and Instituto de Investigación Sanitaria de Aragón, Ciudad Escolar s/n, 44003 Teruel, Spain; osma@unizar.es

* Correspondence: susor@uji.es

Abstract: Psychotherapy has proven to be effective for a wide range of mental health problems. However, not all patients respond to the treatment as expected (not-on-track patients). Routine outcome monitoring (ROM) and measurement-based care (MBC), which consist of monitoring patients between appointments and using this data to guide the intervention, have been shown to be particularly useful for these not-on-track patients. Traditionally, though, ROM and MBC have been challenging, due to the difficulties associated with repeated monitoring of patients and providing real-time feedback to therapists. The use of information and communication technologies (ICTs) might help reduce these challenges. Therefore, we systematically reviewed evidence regarding the use of ICTs for ROM and MBC in face-to-face psychological interventions for mental health problems. The search included published and unpublished studies indexed in the electronic databases PubMed, PsycINFO, and SCOPUS. Main search terms were variations of the terms "psychological treatment", "progress monitoring or measurement-based care", and "technology". Eighteen studies met eligibility criteria. In these, ICTs were frequently handheld technologies, such as smartphone apps, tablets, or laptops, which were involved in the whole process (assessment and feedback). Overall, the use of technology for ROM and MBC during psychological interventions was feasible and acceptable. In addition, the use of ICTs was found to be effective, particularly for not-on-track patients, which is consistent with similar non-ICT research. Given the heterogeneity of reviewed studies, more research and replication is needed to obtain robust findings with different technological solutions and to facilitate the generalization of findings to different mental health populations.

Keywords: information and communication technologies; outcome monitoring; therapist feedback; measurement-based care; mental health

---

1. Introduction

The effectiveness of psychotherapy for the treatment of mental disorders has been supported by an impressive amount of evidence. However, some patients do not respond to treatment as expected, either because they do not show an improvement during the intervention or they discontinue it, or because they show a deterioration [1,2]. There might be several reasons explaining individual differences in response to psychological treatments, including unchallengeable patient characteristics (e.g., age), their personality and behavioral profiles, treatment characteristics and context, and patient physical health status and life context, to name some examples [3]. While acknowledging the previous, an increased number of studies have pointed to methodological deficits, namely, in how patients are monitored during treatments, as key factors influencing current treatment effectiveness [4,5].

Specifically, it has been proposed that a paradigm shift in the practice of psychotherapy towards an ecological momentary assessment (EMA) is necessary in order to monitor patients repeatedly and frequently in their natural environment [6,7]. However, simply monitoring the patient does not appear to be enough to improve the patient's outcomes [8,9]. In this sense, therapist (and patient) feedback has been argued to be a fundamental aspect if patient monitoring during therapy is to be effective [1,10].

The aforementioned procedure is known by different terms in the literature, such as routine outcome monitoring, with outcome or continuous feedback; progress monitoring; or, probably the most popular, measurement-based care (MBC) [9,11]. For simplicity and readability, the latter will be preferred throughout this text.

MBC is defined as a periodic and recurrent assessment of the patient's status over the course of an intervention using standardized measures. Importantly, the evaluation is followed by immediate, frequent, and systematic feedback of the patient's information to the therapist [12,13]. This procedure has been argued to help therapists to assess actual patient progress, suggest necessary adjustments to the treatment, and identify patient deterioration or improvement trajectories, thus enhancing the patient's response to the intervention [1,14–16]. According to the American Psychological Association's (APA) Division 28 Task Force on Empirically Supported Relationships, MBC may also lead to an improvement in the therapeutic alliance and may avoid premature treatment termination, because MBC encourages collaboration between patients and therapists, thus promoting engagement, dialogue and discussion of real-life, daily patient difficulties during sessions. Furthermore, giving feedback to patients raises awareness of their progress and makes them become more mindful of their symptoms, which may also enhance the quality of psychological interventions and the patient–therapist alliance [14].

Several studies have shown the efficacy of this systematic patient monitoring with progress feedback to the therapist in psychological interventions [10,17]. Research also indicates that feedback from outcome measures enhances treatment effectiveness, particularly in not-on-track patients (i.e., those who do not make the expected changes) or when it is provided both to clinicians and patients [8,10,13,14,17,18]. Specifically, providing the therapists with immediate feedback about the patient's symptoms appears to reduce the number of early dropouts and improve several treatment outcomes (depressive and anxiety symptoms, psychosocial functioning, psychosis, quality of life, therapeutic alliance, etc.) when compared against usual treatment [17,19]. Overall, medium effect sizes have been reported when using MBC [1,14].

What the existent literature suggests is that MBC is a promising methodology to enhance the effectiveness of psychological treatments. However, there are a number of flaws into the literature on MBC that might have limited the impact and dissemination of this procedure [20,21]. Traditionally, MBC has been conducted with self-report, paper-and-pencil questionnaires that patients complete before or after therapy sessions. Additionally, assessments are mostly retrospective and based on the patient's recalled experiences during the past week [11]. With this information, the therapist examines and discusses the results during the actual therapy session [22]. As noted earlier, while this practice has been shown to provide some relevant information, relying on paper-and-pencil retrospective reports only, where daily experiences are not reported, might result in recall bias, thus making it difficult to understand patient fluctuations over time [23,24]. Furthermore, focusing on self-reports exclusively is problematic, as more objective data (e.g., actual number of steps taken or time spent out of the home) is ignored or based on patient appraisal only.

Currently, the rapid growth of new technologies in our society has changed the way psychotherapy is conducted. For example, information and communication technologies (ICT) have been argued to allow therapists to evaluate and receive patient progress feedback in real time, thus minimizing patient recall bias [25]. Additionally, the use of ICT allows obtaining objective data of patient changes in natural settings, for example, using sensors (accelerometers, positioning system, or pedometers, among others) [22]. Therefore, the use of handheld ICT devices such as smartphones, tablets, or laptops might increase the effectiveness of MBC by facilitating EMA before, during, and after treatment, providing the information immediately to therapists and researchers, and making it easier to combine collection of objective and subjective patient data [11,21,25].

In order to investigate to what extent ICTs are being implemented to enhance psychological interventions and how their application is effectively improving outcomes, we have conducted a systematic review to explore how ICT is being used for MBC in face-to-face psychological treatments. In doing so, we have investigated: 1. what the different technologies and procedures used for MBC during psychological interventions are and 2. to what extent the use of ICT for MBC is feasible, acceptable, and effective.

2. Materials and Methods

2.1. Search Strategy

The search was conducted in accordance with the Preferred Reporting Items for Systematic Reviews and Meta-Analyses [26]. The search was conducted in February 2020 and included published and unpublished studies from the electronic databases PubMed, PsycINFO, and SCOPUS. In addition, reference mining was performed by searching through bibliographies of relevant articles. The selection of these databases was motivated by previous research showing that PsycINFO has high sensitivity and specificity when retrieving intervention studies and is especially suitable for psychology research, and that SCOPUS offers about 20% more coverage than other important databases such as Web of Science. Additionally, it has been argued that Google Scholar provides inaccurate results, and PubMed is one of the preferred tools for biomedical research [27,28].

The search strategy included variations of the terms "psychological treatment", "progress monitoring", and "technology" (See Appendix A for the complete list of search terms and combinations). Due to the diversity of terms, a broad search strategy of terms was used. Synonyms, abbreviations, and spelling variations were identified for the three concepts and combined in the search using the "OR" Boolean operator, with non-synonymous concepts combined using "AND". These terms were searched in titles and abstracts. The references of included studies and relevant systematic reviews were searched to identify studies that were missed during the literature search. There were no restrictions regarding language or publication period, but the search was only conducted in English.

2.2. Inclusion Criteria

Included studies were psychological treatments enhanced by MBC using technology systems. Specifically, included studies 1. were clinical trials (either feasibility, case studies, and both randomized or non-randomized investigations); 2. included the use of technology during MBC (both for monitoring and feedback provision) while undergoing a face-to-face psychological intervention; and 3. involved feedback to the therapist or to both therapists and patients based on standardized measures.

To be considered MBC, the intervention must satisfy the following components: 1. routine assessment of a symptom, an outcome, or a process measure; 2. therapist review of data; and 3. therapist use of data to inform clinical decisions. Therefore, the study population can include patients with any mental disorder from all ages who are routinely monitored via validated outcome measures using technologies over the course of a face-to-face psychological treatment.

2.3. Exclusion Criteria

Studies in which technology systems were not used in the whole MBC process, including the assessment and feedback parts, or where only patients but not therapists were provided with feedback, were excluded. In addition, studies were excluded if they did not include a face-to-face psychological intervention.

2.4. Search and Screening

Initially, 193 publications were identified from database searches and screening of reference lists (see Figure 1 for the study diagram flow). After excluding duplicates ($n = 63$), 130 publications were retained for screening. After initial screening of titles and abstracts, 84 of these documents were excluded due to eligibility reasons. For the remaining 46 publications, full texts were retrieved. After eligibility assessment of the full texts, 28 publications were excluded. The majority of publications were excluded because they did not meet the eligibility criteria, resulting in a final sample that comprised 18 publications.

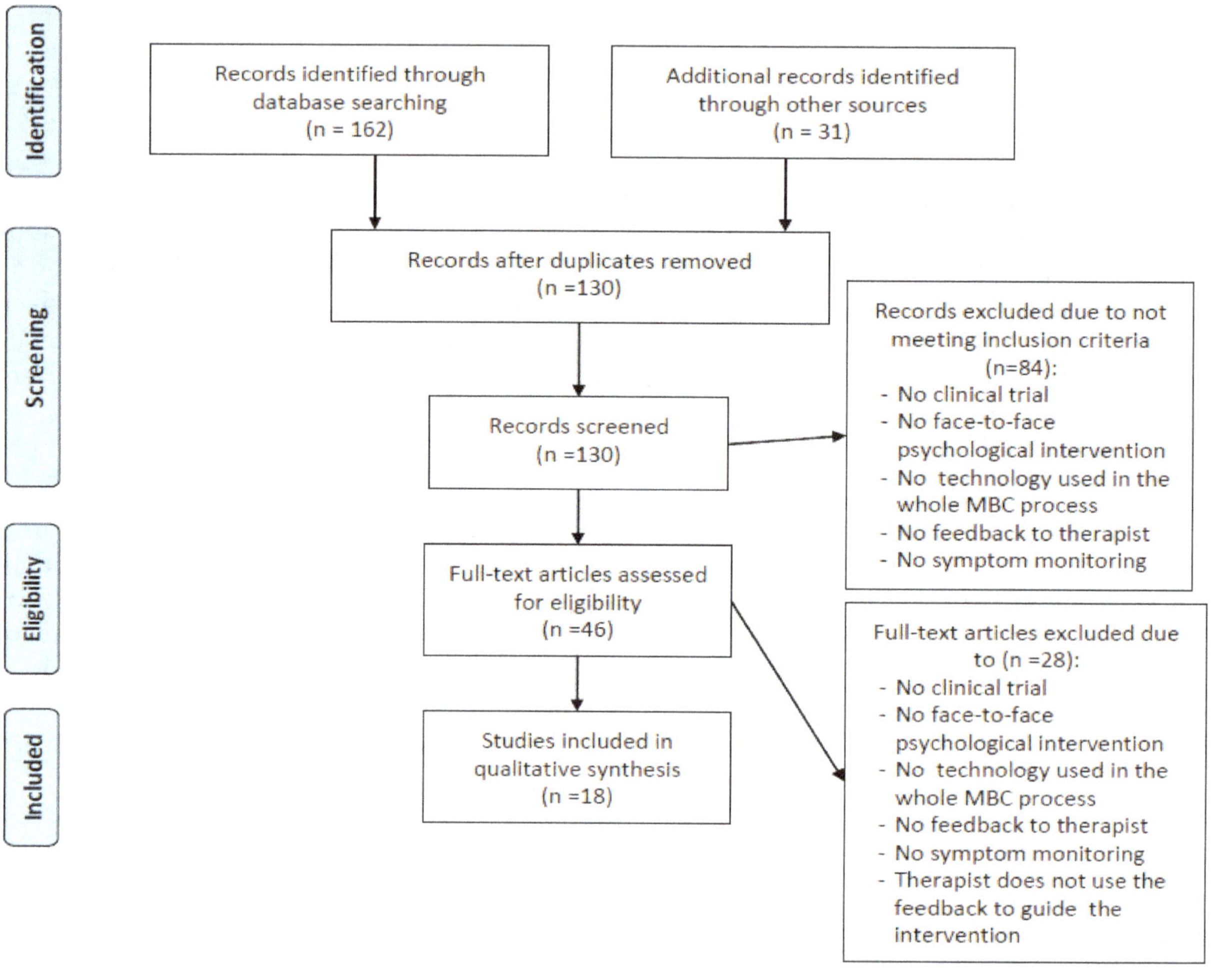

Figure 1. Flow diagram of study selection following PRISMA guidelines [26].

The search, screening process, and data extraction were conducted independently by the first two authors (PGM and VMB). When in doubt, study eligibility was discussed with a third author (CSR). After the phase of study eligibility assessment, inter-rater agreement was calculated (Cohen's kappa). This coefficient showed a substantial overall agreement, represented by a kappa of 0.908 ($SD = 0.064$; 95% CI, 0.781, 1.000).

2.5. Data Extraction

The following data were extracted from each included study, using a standardized data-extraction form developed a priori: authors, study setting (geographical setting and type of clinic), sample size, study design, study participants (demographics and type of mental disorder), type of psychological intervention, assessment characteristics (frequency and setting), primary outcomes, feedback characteristics (to whom, frequency, and setting), type of technology used, technology feasibility, and clinical effectiveness. Data was extracted from all full texts by the first author (PGM) and then discussed with another author (VMB) before it was reviewed by all co-authors.

2.6. *Risk of Bias Assessment*

All studies included in this review were independently rated for quality by two reviewers (PGM and VMB). If the rating differed, reviewers discussed the articles to reach consensus with a third reviewer (CSR). The Study Quality Assessment Tools from the National Heart Lung and Blood Institute [29] were used to assess study quality and risk of bias. This tool was preferred because it includes six types of studies and specific criteria according to the study design (i.e., controlled intervention studies; systematic reviews and meta-analyses; observational cohort and cross-sectional studies; case-control studies; before–after studies with no control group; and case series studies). This tool allows reviewers to rate studies as "good", "fair", or "poor". Total quality scores ranged from 9 to 14 points depending on the study design.

2.7. *Synthesis of Results*

Frequency tables were used to summarize the characteristics of individual studies. We conducted a systematic review and not a meta-analysis, because the emphasis was not on effect sizes, but on how MBC with technology was being conducted. Additionally, we anticipated that included studies would be very heterogeneous, because the review includes any form of psychological intervention, all types of technologies, several trial designs, and different types of mental disorders and outcomes. Thus, we performed a narrative synthesis only.

2.8. *Additional Analyses*

Factors affecting study heterogeneity included variations in the type of mental disorder (e.g., major depressive disorder or anxiety disorders), outcomes included, treatment characteristics (type, format, and duration), measures used (clinician-rated versus self-rated), study design, and differences in the means by which MBC was delivered. The description of the findings was sensitive about the aforementioned subgroups when possible.

3. Results

3.1. *Characteristics of Included Studies*

The characteristics of included studies are shown in Table 1. Of the 18 studies included in the systematic review, eight were published in the USA [30–37], with the remaining studies being published in Australia (n = 3 [38–40]), the United Kingdom (n = 3 [41–43]), Austria (n = 2 [44,45]), Greece (n = 1 [46]), and the Netherlands (n = 1 [47]). Most studies took place in outpatient settings (n = 15, 83.33%) such as mental health services (n = 3 [33,34,47]), specialist clinics (n = 4 [36,38,39,43]), hospital clinics (n = 7 [31,35,37,41,42,45,46]), and university clinics (n = 1 [32]); only three of them were conducted in inpatient settings [30,40,44]. In terms of design, six studies were feasibility pilot investigations (single group) [30,31,34,36,37,44]; four studies were case studies [32,39,45,46]; four studies were randomized controlled trials (RCTs) [35,38,42,47]; two of them were non-randomized controlled trials [33,40]; and two were pre–post investigations [41,43]. The sample sizes of the included investigations ranged from 1 to 2233 participants.

Table 1. Characteristics of the included studies.

Reference	Country	Setting	Psychological Disorder	Sample size	Study Design	Type of Psychological Intervention
[30]	California (USA)	Specialist inpatient treatment center	PTSD	27 Tx	SG (feasibility study)	Residential group psychotherapy (4–5 months)
[31]	Pittsburgh (USA)	Outpatient Psychiatric Institute and Clinic	Anxiety disorders (children from 9 to 14 years old)	9 Tx (3 received 16-sessions CBT, 6 received 8-sessions Brief CBT)	SG (feasibility pilot trial)	"Coping Cat": 16 CBT sessions"Brief Coping Cat": 8 CBT sessions
[32]	Evanston, Illinois (USA)	Outpatient clinic at the Family Institute at Northwestern University	Couple problems	1 Tx	Case study	Four Couple Multisystemic Psychotherapy sessions
[33]	California University: Berkeley (USA)	Outpatient behavioural health clinic	Depression	85 (40 cont. + 45 Tx)	nRCT (not blinded)	16 weeks of weekly group CBT therapy
[34]	California (USA)	4 Outpatient Early Psychosis clinics	Psychotic disorder	61 Tx	SG (feasibility study)	Early Psychosis Program (up to 5 months)
[35]	New York (USA)	Outpatient primary care	Substance use	240 (83 cont. + 77 Tx + 80 Tx HealthCall)	Three-arm RCT (1:1:1 allocation ratio)	Brief (25–30 min) individual (motivational interview) psychoeducation (3 sessions: every 30 days)
[36]	California University (USA)	Outpatient specialist clinic	Psychotic disorder (adolescent and young)	76 Tx	SG (feasibility pilot trial)	Early Psychosis Program (minimum 3 months)
[37]	Washington University (USA)	Outpatient primary care clinic affiliated with the Washington University	Depression and Anxiety	17 Tx	SG (feasibility and acceptability pilot study)	Collaborative care program (over 6 months)
[38]	Melbourne (Australia)	Outpatient Specialist Voices Clinic and clinical services	Schizophrenia	34 (17 cont. + 17 Tx)	A single-blind, parallel group, pilot RCT (1:1 allocation ratio)	Brief CBT (four in-person therapy sessions) + EMA + EMI
[39]	Melbourne (Australia)	Outpatient Specialist Voices clinic	Schizophrenia	1 Tx	Case study	Brief CBT (four in-person therapy sessions) + EMA+ EMI
[40]	Perth (Australia)	Private inpatients and day-patients psychiatric hospital	Mood and Anxiety	1308 (408 Tx Fb +, 439 nFb + 461 cont.)	nRCT	10 days of intensive CBT group

Table 1. *Cont.*

Reference	Country	Setting	Psychological Disorder	Sample size	Study Design	Type of Psychological Intervention
[41]	Leeds (England)	Outpatient clinic	Depression and Anxiety	594 (349 cont. + 245 Tx)	Quasi-experimental pre-post study	Low-intensity guided self-help CBT or High-intensity CBT, interpersonal psychotherapy and counselling
[42]	England	8 outpatient clinics	Depression and Anxiety	2233 (1057 cont. + 1176 Tx)	Multisite, open-label, cluster RCT	Low-intensity guided self-help CBT or High-intensity CBT, interpersonal psychotherapy and counselling
[43]	Oxford (UK)	Outpatient specialist mental health	Bipolar disorder	19 Tx	SG (pre-post)	five sessions of psychoeducational intervention (FIMM) + pharmacotherapy
[44]	Salzburg (Austria)	Inpatient and a day-treatment clinic	Mood disorders; Psychoactive substance use mental disorders; Schizophrenia, schizotypal, and delusional disorders; Neurotic, stress-related, and somatoform disorders; Personality disorders, and others	151 Tx	SG (feasibility pilot trial)	Psychotherapy (8 weeks in the day-treatment clinic and 12 weeks in the inpatient clinic)
[45]	Salzburg (Austria)	Outpatient clinic	Bulimia nervosa	1 Tx	Case study	six Rogerian person-centred psychotherapy sessions
[46]	Thessaloniki (Greece)	Alzheimer day care centre (at home)	Dementia	4 Tx	Case study	15 Individual psychotherapy sessions (psychosocial intervention, CBT, relaxation techniques, etc.)
[47]	The Netherlands	Outpatient mental health institutions or private practices	Mood disorder, Adjustment disorder, Anxiety disorder, Relational problems, Personality disorders, and others	475 (159 Tx FbT; 172 Tx FbTP; 144 cont. nFb)	RCT	Long and short psychotherapy (CBT, client-centered, psychodynamics)

Note: Cont., control group; Tx, treatment group; nRCT, non-randomized controlled trial; CBT, Cognitive-Behavioural Therapy; RCT, randomized controlled trial; EMA, ecological momentary assessment; EMI, ecological momentary intervention; FbT, feedback to the therapist; FbTP, feedback to the therapist and the patient; Fb, feedback; nFb, no-feedback; FIMM, Facilitated Integrated Mood Management; SG, single group design.

The included studies targeted very heterogeneous diagnoses. However, depression and anxiety disorders were the most frequent (n = 6, 33.33% of studies [31,33,37,40–42]). The remaining disorders were schizophrenia spectrum disorders (n = 4, 22.22% of studies [34,36,38,39]), bulimia nervosa (n = 1, 5.6% of studies [45]), substance use (n = 1, 5.6% of studies [35]), dementia (n = 1, 5.6% of studies [46]), post-traumatic stress (n = 1, 5.6% of studies [30]), bipolar disorder (n = 1, 5.6% of studies [43]), couple problems (n = 1, 5.6% of studies [32]), and combinations of heterogeneous disorders together (n = 2, 11.11% of studies [44,47]). The majority of treatments were addressed to adult populations (n = 16) and only two investigations (n = 2 [34,36]) aimed at treating mental health problems in younger populations (i.e., adolescents and young adults).

Regarding the treatments offered in the included studies, different face-to-face interventions were provided across studies. However, cognitive behavioral therapy (CBT) was the most frequent (n = 13). Other therapeutic options were client-centered psychotherapy (n = 1 [45]), collaborative care (n = 1 [37]), an early psychosis program (n = 2 [34,36]), and couple multisystemic psychotherapy (n = 1 [32]). The format of the intervention was mainly individual (n = 15), but some studies included group treatments (n = 3 [30,33,40]). Finally, the intensity (i.e., frequency) of the intervention also differed across investigations. Some studies implemented a low-intensity treatment plan (i.e., less than eight sessions; n = 6 [32,35,38,39,43,45]), while others applied a higher-intensity intervention (i.e., more than eight sessions; n = [30,33,34,36,37,40,44,46]) or both a low- and a high-intensity treatment (n = 4 [31,41,42,47]).

3.2. *MBC Characteristics*

3.2.1. Assessment Procedure Used to Track the Patient's Status

The characteristics of studies included in the review are described in Table 2. Most studies (n = 9 [30,31,33,35,38–40,44,46]) monitored their patients daily. The remaining studies monitored their patients weekly (n = 4 [32,41,42,47]), before every therapy session, or both daily and weekly (n = 5 [34,36,37,43,45]). In the latter studies conducting assessments both daily and weekly, daily assessments usually included shorter questionnaires that evaluated therapeutic process outcomes, mood, or medication adherence, while longer outcome scales (i.e., measures of depressive or anxiety symptoms) were administered weekly. Treatment effectiveness was assessed most commonly with the primary outcome measures of interest for the investigation, which most often were the Patient Health Questionnaire-9 for depressive symptoms and the Generalised Anxiety Disorder-7 for anxiety symptoms (n = 4 [33,37,41,42]). Other outcomes included the frequency and amount of drug use (n = 1 [35]); the Subjective Experiences of Psychosis Scale, the Auditory Hallucinations subscale of the Psychotic Symptom Rating Scales for psychotic symptoms, and the Depression Anxiety Stress Scale for negative emotional symptoms (n = 2 [38,39]); the Outcome Questionnaire-45 (n= 1 [47]); the Therapy Process Questionnaire (n = 1 [44]); the World Health Organization's Wellbeing Index (n = 1 [40]) for well-being; the Symptom Checklist-90 for bulimia symptoms and the Intersession Experience Questionnaire for the psychotherapy process (n = 1 [45]); the Altman Self-Rating Mania scale and the 16-item Quick Inventory of Depressive Symptoms-Self Report scale (n = 1 [43]); and other clinical measures related to sleep, mood, medication use, or daily functioning (n = 6 [30–32,34,36,46]).

Table 2. Measurement-based care characteristics.

Reference	Assessment Frequency and Setting	Primary Outcome Measures	Feedback to	Feedback Frequency and Setting	Type of Technology Used
[30]	Daily at a random time	Adapted questionnaire from Symptom Checklist-6, the BriefCOPE and Beck Depression Inventory-II	T and P	P: T regularly shared P progress in order to incorporate strategies in therapy sessions and treatment plan.T: They got patient information several times a week in a graph format to discuss with them during sessions, to encourage them and monitor them.	EMA and Text messages
[31]	Daily questions about recent emotional events (e.g., emotions, scenario, somatic symptoms, automatic thoughts) + answers on demand by the participant	Skills entries and satisfaction with the treatment.	P and T	P: They received personalized feedback from therapists.T: Information and graphs from the portal about patients' progress were discussed in weekly CBT sessions with the patients.	Smartphone app: SmartCAT app + SmartCAT therapist portal..
[32]	Online before every session	STIC: set of questionnaires	T and clinicians stakeholders	T: On-demand graphs of patient progress were provided to the therapist through STIC	STIC online
[33]	Once daily mood monitoring messages at random between 8 a.m. and 8 p.m.	Attendance to therapy, duration of therapy and PHQ-9	P and T	P: They received feedback about their mood responsesT: T reviewed information from an online dashboard were patient progress is shown. T can periodically review the graphs, identify key aspects and address any important event during or between sessions.	Automated text messages and Web-based platform (HealthySMS)
[34]	Daily and weekly surveys (between 5 p.m. and 10:30 p.m.)	Mood, medication use, socialization and conflict	P and T	P: They discussed their feedback with the T at every session.T: They reviewed and discussed patient information (plots of symptoms over time, etc.) on the dashboard with P during sessions and between sessions.	Smartphone app: RealLife Exp + web-based platform
[35]	Once daily call (HealthCall) for self-monitoring	Primary drug use (frequency and amount), use of other drugs, medication adherence, and mood	P and T	P: They received the feedback at 30 and 60 days, where their information was discussed with the T.T: At 30 and 60 days, T discussed with P the generated graphs based on HealthCall about their drug use, moods and health behaviors.	Phone IVR system
[36]	Daily surveys (at 5 p.m. until 11:55 p.m.), weekly surveys (Sundays at 10 a.m. until Monday 11:55) and monthly in-person psychosocial assessments with research staff	Daily surveys assessing mood, medication adherence, and social interaction, weekly surveys assessing symptoms, sleep, and medication adherence	T	T: They received alerts from the dashboard when P scores were clinically significant and took the proper decisions according to the patient demand.	Ginger.io (software) = Smartphone app + Clinician dashboard
[37]	3/4 times daily, weekly; 8/12 weeks	PHQ-9 and GAD-7	P and T	P: P received notifications about their progress in the app, becoming more aware of their symptoms.T: T reviewed patient-reported information via an online dashboard and visualized patient progress graphs.	Smartphone app + online platform
[38]	Session 1 and 2: 10 daily evening EMA for 6 days. Session 3 and 4: 8 evening daily EMA (monitor changes in voices and coping strategies)	SEPS, PSYRATS-AH, and DASS-21	P and T	P: In session 2, P received a summary sheet with their EMA progress.T: In session 2, EMA feedback was discussed with the P in order to guarantee understanding, detect predictors and avoid causation.	Smartphone app: MovisensXS + web-based platform

Table 2. *Cont.*

Reference	Assessment Frequency and Setting	Primary Outcome Measures	Feedback to	Feedback Frequency and Setting	Type of Technology Used
[39]	Session 1 and 2: 10 daily evening EMA for 6 days. Session 3 and 4: 8 evening daily EMA (monitor changes in voices and coping strategies)	SEPS, PSYRATS-AH, and DASS-21	P and T	P: In session 2, P received a summary sheet with their EMA progress.T: In session 2, EMA feedback was discussed with the P in order to guarantee understanding, detect predictors and avoid causation.	Smartphone app: RealLife Exp + web-based platform
[40]	Daily self-reported measures of well-being	Well-being (WHO-5)	P and T	P: They received routinely individualized information about their progress in group discussion with the therapist.T: T received daily automatic plots of each patient's outcomes within trajectories.	Touch-screen technology in therapy rooms
[41]	Weekly (session-by-session)	PHQ-9 and GAD-7	P and T	P: They received their feedback in session with the therapist, where the information was reviewed, discussed and used to guide the treatment plan.T: They had access to patient progress graphs and response curves from the monitoring system, and they were warned automatically when a P was not-on-track.	Computer PCMIS
[42]	Weekly (session-by-session)	PHQ-9 and GAD-7	P and T	P: They received their feedback in session with the therapist, where the information was reviewed, discussed and used to guide the treatment plan.T: They had access to patient progress graphs and response curves from the monitoring system, and they were warned automatically when a P was not-on-track.	Computer PCMIS
[43]	Twice a day (only during psychoeducation sessions) and once a week	Daily: mood and sleepWeekly: QIDS, ASRM and mood management strategies questionnaire	P and T	P: P received their feedback at every session with the T.T: T reviewed patient progress from daily mood rating and weekly scales from the previous week and discussed with the P the relationship between his/her mood changes and stressors.	Phone text messages or e-mails (True Colours mood monitoring system)
[44]	Daily process monitoring (during evenings).	TPQ	T	T: On demand. Feedback was used for individualizing therapeutic decisions.	SNS
[45]	Daily measures of psychotherapy process. Weekly measure of therapy outcome.	IEQ daily, weekly SCL-90 (Bulimia)	P, T and researchers	P: They viewed their progress and estimated their moods and symptoms during the past day.T: They had access to P data from the system in order to adapt the intervention delivered.	Smartphone: DynAMo web app
[46]	Daily monitoring	Sleep patterns, physical activity, and activities of daily living	P, T and caregivers	P and caregiver: They could see a proportionate share of the information adapted to their needs.T: Information collected was available at all times in order to design personalized interventions.	Tablet app (assistive technology: wearable, sleep, movement, presence sensors)
[47]	Once a week just before therapy session (at waiting room)	OQ-45	P and T, or only T	P: P can access the feedback via email or into their portal system.T: T could access the feedback via email or in their portal system and could discuss the feedback information (progress charts and a message) with the P based on the OQ-45 patient's scores.	Computer: Web-based monitoring app

Note: PHQ-9, Patient Health Questionnaire-9; P, patient; T, therapist; GAD-7, Generalised Anxiety Disorder-7; EMA, Ecological Momentary Assessment; SEPS, Subjective Experiences of Psychosis Scale; PSYRATS-AH, Auditory Hallucinations subscale of the Psychotic Symptom Rating Scales; DASS-21, Depression Anxiety Stress Scale; OQ-45, Outcome Questionnaire; IEQ, Intersession Experience Questionnaire; SCL-90, Symptom Checklist-90; QIDS, Quick Inventory of Depressive Symptomatology; ASRM, Altman Self Rating Mania Scale; WHO-5, World Health Organization's Wellbeing Index; STIC, Systemic Therapy Inventory of Change System; CBT, Cognitive Behavioral Therapy; TPQ, Therapy Process Questionnaire; IVR, interactive voice response; App, mobile application; STIC, Systemic Therapy Inventory of Change System; SNS, Synergetic Navigation System; PCMIS, Patient Case Management Information System.

3.2.2. Feedback Procedure

The majority of studies provided feedback to both therapists and patients (n = 15). The remaining studies gave feedback to therapists only (n = 3 [32,36,44]). Most studies used feedback to track the patients' progress focusing on key aspects during treatment and to monitor responses in-between sessions. Even when the feedback was not directly provided to the patient, this information was used to discuss patient progress during treatment sessions or to take clinical decisions (e.g., emphasize a specific content during session).

Feedback included information about treatment evolution in progress charts, summary sheets, graphs of scores and curves, and plots of scores within trajectories. Feedback information was either sent periodically to the therapist in response to patient assessments or on-demand (weekly or daily). In some studies, feedback to the therapist appeared when the patients' responses were considered clinically significant according to pre-established criteria.

3.3. Technology Characteristics

The technology characteristics of included studies are presented in Table 2. Most studies included handheld technology, such as smartphone apps (n = 7 [31,34,36–39,45]), touch-screen technologies (n = 2 [40,46]), or laptops (n = 5 [32,41,42,44,47]), together with a web-based platform for the therapist. The remaining studies used phone text messages (n = 2 [30,33]), e-mail (n = 1 [43]), or a phone interactive voice response system (n = 1 [35]). For example, in one study, automated text messages and a web-based platform (e.g., HealthySMS) were used [33]. In other investigations, authors implemented an Internet-based system, such as the Patient Case Management Information System (PCMIS), or an electronic clinical record system which includes outcome-monitoring graphs that chart depression and anxiety scores at every session [41,42]. A similar example was the Synergetic Navigation System, an Internet-based device for data collection (with web-compatible devices such as PCs, tablets, or smartphones) and data analysis that allows for the implementation of questionnaires at any chosen interval [44]. Another Internet-based system was the DynAMo web app, a piece of software that combines algorithm-based treatment planning, process monitoring, and outcome monitoring, which can be used by both researchers and clinicians to plan treatments and monitor psychotherapeutic processes [45]. One investigation used the Systemic Therapy Inventory of Change System, an online system that assesses and tracks changes in the patients' interpersonal system, as well as in the therapeutic alliance, and also feeds these data back to the therapists on demand [32]. A final example of an Internet-based system used in one of the included investigations was Ginger.io, an mHealth software program comprising a therapist dashboard and an app which can collect data from self-report surveys sent to the participant in addition to "passive" data from the participant's phone, such as number of calls and SMS messages, and movement patterns based on Global Positioning System data [36].

3.3.1. Technology Feasibility

Because of the large differences in sample sizes across investigations (Table 3), case studies with one to four participants [32,39,45,46] have been described in previous sections but will not be considered in the feasibility and effectiveness summaries. The remaining studies included at least 17 participants, and therefore will be discussed in detail here and in Table 3. Overall, the results demonstrated that enhancing MBC in psychological therapy with technology was generally feasible and acceptable (Table 3). This statement is supported by the high average response rate for daily (mean = 63.3%, range = 40%–81% [34,36,43]), weekly (mean = 73.0%, range = 39%–88% [34,36,37,43]), and monthly (92.7% [30]) symptom monitoring across studies, low average missing data rates amongst patients (13% [44]), and high completion rates (mean = 77.8%; range = 64.1%–90% [31,35,38,40,44]). In addition, several studies reported satisfaction with the technology used to improve MBC in the intervention delivered, and most of them revealed that patients and therapists would recommend the technology used as part of the treatment [31,34,38].

Table 3. Usability, acceptability, and effectiveness of technology-supported measurement-based care.

Reference	Sample Size	Feasibility of Technology	Clinical Effectiveness
[30]	27 Tx	Monthly: 92.7%	NA
[31]	9 Tx	Completion rate was 82.8%. Patients reported the app being easy to use. All parents report treatment satisfaction and would recommend the program.	NA
[33]	85 (40 cont. + 45 Tx)	NA	Technology-supported MBC significantly increased treatment adherence (median of 13.5 weeks before dropping out) compared to traditional CBT (median of 3 weeks before dropping out). Effect sizes of technology-supported MBC CBT on depressive symptoms' severity (z = −5.80) were larger than for traditional CBT (z = −3.12), but differences were not significant
[34]	61 Tx	Moderate survey completion (daily = 40%; weekly = 39%). In general, both T (66%) and P (85%) reported they would continue using the app as part of the treatment.	NA
[35]	240 (83 cont. + 77 Tx + 80 Tx)	HealthCall shows a great retention rate and response rate (64.1%), supporting feasibility, patient acceptability and generalizability.	At 12-month follow-up, reductions in non-injection drug use were comparable in traditional and technology-supported MBC motivational interviewing and superior than in the control condition. In the subset of patients with drug dependence, drug use was significantly lower in the technology-supported MBC condition at 12 months post-treatment. At 60 days, treatment retention in the technology-supported MBC group (88.8%) was superior than in the motivational intervention only condition (81.8%) and the control condition (78.3%)
[36]	76 Tx	Feasibility and acceptability of the smartphone app as an adjunct treatment tool is supported by the high response rate sate (weekly surveys: 77%; daily surveys: 69%)	NA
[37]	17 Tx	The feasibility and acceptability of the mobile platform is supported by the high early response rate (weekly = 88%).	NA
[38]	34 (17 cont. + 17 Tx)	High completion rates (74%) of EMA questionnaires and good satisfaction of participants support the feasibility and acceptability of the study, respectively.	Compared with the usual treatment, the technology-supported MBC treatment resulted in large improvements in confidence in coping with voices (Hedges g = 1.45) and medium improvements in understanding of voices (Hedges g = 0.61) and in psychotic symptoms (Hedges g = 0.51). Both groups showed similar changes in the impact of psychosis.
[40]	1308 (408 Tx Fb +, 439 nFb + 461 cont.)	High rates of touch-screen questionnaire completion (over 90%).	Technology-supported MBC for NOT patients was more effective than traditional CBT or monitoring without feedback in reducing depressive symptoms and the impact of emotions on functioning, as well as on increasing vitality. By contrast, changes in well-being, anxiety, and stress were comparable across conditions.
[41]	594 (349 cont. + 245 Tx)	MBC technology was generally acceptable and feasible to integrate in routine practice.	Technology-supported MBC achieved comparable reductions in depression and anxiety compared to controls, but with significantly less time (adjusted mean = 10.25, SE = 0.45 vs. adjusted mean = 6.59, SE = 0.51) and cost (between £65.88 and £129.20 cost reductions per treatment). Cases in the control condition were twice as likely to become not-on-track patients compared to those in the technology-supported MBC.

Table 3. *Cont.*

Reference	Sample Size	Feasibility of Technology	Clinical Effectiveness
[42]	2233 (1057 cont. + 1176 Tx)	NA	NOT patients in the technology-enhanced MBC condition obtained significantly larger reductions in depressive ($d = 0.23$) and anxiety symptom severity ($d = 0.19$), as well as improved work and social adjustment ($d = 0.19$) compared with active controls (traditional CBT).
[43]	19 Tx	High response rate (daily = 81%, weekly = 88%)	NA
[44]	151 Tx	High average compliance rates (78.3%) and low average missing data rates (13%) amongst the inpatients support the feasibility.	NA
[47]	475 (159 Tx FbT; 172 Tx FbTP; 144 cont. nFb)	NA	In short-term interventions (less than 35 weeks), receiving feedback was protective of negative outcomes in NOT cases ($d = 1.28$). No significant differences between conditions were found for on-track patients, but there was a trend for the technology-supported MBC group to be more effective ($d = 0.24$ at 35 weeks and $d = 0.29$ at 78 weeks) and to have lower deterioration rates ($z = 1.3$), especially when feedback was provided to both patient and therapist.

Note: Cont., Control Group; Tx, Treatment Group; FbT, Feedback to The Therapist; FbTP, Feedback to The Therapist and The Patient; Fb, Feedback; nFb, No Feedback; NA, Not Applicable/Not Specified; IVR, Interactive Voice Response; App, Mobile Application; EMA, Ecological Momentary Assessment; MBC, Measurement-Based Care; NOT, Not-on-Track patients; T, Therapist; P, Patient. The feasibility and effectiveness reports are not provided for case studies due to the reduced number of patients ($n \leq 4$).

3.3.2. Clinical Effectiveness

As summarized in Table 3, data about clinical effectiveness was described in seven studies, including four RCTs [35,38,42,47], two nRCTs [33,40], and a quasi-experimental pre–post investigation [41]. All RCTs included active controls (i.e., traditional face-to-face psychological treatment) without MBC. According to these investigations, the use of technology-supported MBC appears to significantly reduce symptom severity, and changes are sometimes larger than with traditional interventions [38], especially in patients at risk of poor response to treatment (i.e., not-on-track cases) [35,40,42,47], which is consistent with previous research [42,46]. Furthermore, one study showed that although traditional CBT and technology-enhanced MBC CBT were comparable in terms of treatment effectiveness, the latter significantly reduced therapy duration and cost of treatment [41]. Also in favor of technology-assisted MBC, another investigation revealed that patients stayed in therapy longer (i.e., higher adherence) in the experimental condition, that is, when MBC was supported by technology (group CBT with a text messaging adjunct) as opposed to traditional MBC without technology (group CBT without the text messaging adjunct) [33]. In sum, most studies suggest that technology-supported MBC has the potential to improve the efficacy and cost-effectiveness of psychotherapy, especially for not-on-track individuals.

3.4. Risk of Bias Assessment

As observed in Tables 4–7, studies included in this review could be placed in four of the categories proposed by the National Heart Lung and Blood Institute [29], namely, case studies, before-after studies; observational cohort and cross-sectional studies; and controlled intervention studies. Overall, the four studies classified as case studies had a "good" quality, with total scores ranging from 5 to 7 points out of a maximum of 9 points [32,39,45,46]. Even so, none of them had follow-up sessions, or these were not reported, and two studies did not include a complete case definition [32,45]. Secondly, the two before–after studies could also be rated as "good" quality investigations, as both obtained 9 points of a maximum of 12 [41,43]. The main issue with one of the studies was related to sample size, although this concern was justified, as this was a pilot study and authors reported the previous in the limitation section [43]. The six studies classified as observational, cohort and cross-sectional studies correspond to feasibility and acceptability studies, and some quality criteria, such as numbers 7, 8, 12, and 14, were not applicable [30,31,34,36,37,44]. Overall, feasibility and acceptability studies did not meet most criteria required in observational and cross-sectional studies (they met only seven or eight criteria of a maximum of 14), so their quality could only be rated as "fair". It is important to note that just two studies maintained 80% of the sample [30,31] and four studies did not meet the participation rate of 50% from eligible participant criteria [30,31,37,44]. Finally, two of the controlled intervention studies [33,40] were rated as "poor" quality as they were non-randomized and did not follow most of the criteria for controlled studies (i.e., randomization, blind allocation, or assessment). These two studies met, respectively, only two [40] and eight [33] criteria of a maximum of 14. The remaining four controlled intervention studies [35,38,42,47] were "good" quality investigations despite the lack of blinded allocation and assessment [35,42,47] and relatively high drop-out rates [42,47].

Table 4. Quality assessment of case studies.

	[32]	[39]	[45]	[46]
1. Was the study question or objective clearly stated?	Yes	Yes	Yes	Yes
2. Was the study population clearly and fully described, including a case definition?	No	Yes	No	Yes
3. Were the cases consecutive?	NA	NA	NA	No
4. Were the subjects comparable?	NA	NA	No	Yes
5. Was the intervention clearly described?	Yes	Yes	Yes	Yes
6. Were the outcome measures clearly defined, valid, reliable, and implemented consistently across all study participants?	Yes	Yes	Yes	Yes
7. Was the length of follow-up adequate?	NR	No	No	NR
8. Were the statistical methods well-described?	Yes	Yes	Yes	Yes
9. Were the results well-described?	Yes	Yes	Yes	Yes
Total score (maximum 9 points)	5	6	5	7

Note: CD, Cannot Determine; NA, Not Applicable; NR, Not Reported.

Table 5. Quality assessment of before–after studies.

	[41]	[43]
1. Was the study question or objective clearly stated?	Yes	Yes
2. Were eligibility/selection criteria for the study population prespecified and clearly described?	Yes	Yes
3. Were the participants in the study representative of those who would be eligible for the test/service/intervention in the general or clinical population of interest?	NR	Yes
4. Were all eligible participants that met the prespecified entry criteria enrolled?	NR	No
5. Was the sample size sufficiently large to provide confidence in the findings?	Yes	No
6. Was the test/service/intervention clearly described and delivered consistently across the study population?	Yes	Yes
7. Were the outcome measures prespecified, clearly defined, valid, reliable, and assessed consistently across all study participants?	Yes	Yes
8. Were the people assessing the outcomes blinded to the participants' exposures/interventions?	No	NA
9. Was the loss to follow-up after baseline 20% or less? Were those lost to follow-up accounted for in the analysis?	Yes/Yes	Yes/Yes
10. Did the statistical methods examine changes in outcome measures from before to after the intervention? Were statistical tests done that provided p values for the pre-to-post changes?	Yes	Yes
11. Were outcome measures of interest taken multiple times before the intervention and multiple times after the intervention (i.e., did they use an interrupted time-series design)?	Yes	Yes
12. If the intervention was conducted at a group level (e.g., a whole hospital, a community, etc.) did the statistical analysis take into account the use of individual-level data to determine effects at the group level?	Yes	Yes
Total score (maximum 12 points)	9	9

Note: CD, Cannot Determine; NA, Not Applicable; NR, Not Reported.

Table 6. Quality assessment of observational cohort and cross-sectional studies.

	[30]	[31]	[34]	[36]	[37]	[44]
1. Was the research question or objective in this paper clearly stated?	Yes	Yes	Yes	Yes	Yes	Yes
2. Was the study population clearly specified and defined?	Yes	Yes	Yes	Yes	Yes	Yes
3. Was the participation rate of eligible persons at least 50%?	NR	NR	Yes	Yes	No	NR
4. Were all the subjects selected or recruited from the same or similar populations? Were inclusion and exclusion criteria for being in the study prespecified and applied uniformly to all participants?	Yes	Yes	Yes	Yes	Yes	Yes
5. Was a sample size justification, power description, or variance and effect estimates provided?	NR	NR	NR	NR	NR	NR
6. For the analyses in this paper, were the exposure(s) of interest measured prior to the outcome(s) being measured?	Yes	Yes	Yes	NA	Yes	Yes
7. Was the timeframe sufficient so that one could reasonably expect to see an association between exposure and outcome if it existed?	NA	NA	NA	NA	NA	NA
8. For exposures that can vary in amount or level, did the study examine different levels of the exposure as related to the outcome (e.g., categories of exposure, or exposure measured as continuous variable)?	NA	NA	NA	NA	NA	NA
9. Were the exposure measures clearly defined, valid, reliable, and implemented consistently across all study participants?	Yes	Yes	Yes	Yes	Yes	Yes
10. Was the exposure(s) assessed more than once over time?	Yes	Yes	Yes	Yes	Yes	Yes
11. Were the outcome measures clearly defined, valid, reliable, and implemented consistently across all study participants?	Yes	Yes	Yes	Yes	Yes	Yes
12. Were the outcome assessors blinded to the exposure status of participants?	NA	NA	NA	NA	NA	NA
13. Was loss to follow-up after baseline 20% or less?	Yes	Yes	No	No	No	No
14. Were key potential confounding variables measured for their impact on the relationship between exposure(s) and outcome(s)?	NA	NA	NA	NA	NA	NA
Total score (maximum 14 points)	8	8	8	7	7	7

Note: CD, Cannot Determine; NA, Not Applicable; NR, Not Reported.

Table 7. Quality assessment of controlled intervention studies.

	[33]	[35]	[38]	[40]	[42]	[47]
1. Was the study described as randomized, a randomized trial, a randomized clinical trial, or an RCT?	No	Yes	Yes	No	Yes	Yes
2. Was the method of randomization adequate (i.e., use of randomly generated assignment)?	NA	Yes	Yes	NA	Yes	Yes
3. Was the treatment allocation concealed (so that assignments could not be predicted)?	NA	Yes	Yes	NA	Yes	Yes
4. Were study participants and providers blinded to treatment group assignment?	No	No	No	No	No	No
5. Were the people assessing the outcomes blinded to the participants' group assignments?	No	NA	Yes	No	No	NA
6. Were the groups similar at baseline on important characteristics that could affect outcomes (e.g., demographics, risk factors, co-morbid conditions)?	Yes	Yes	Yes	Yes	Yes	No
7. Was the overall drop-out rate from the study at endpoint 20% or lower of the number allocated to treatment?	Yes	Yes	Yes	NR	No	No
8. Was the differential drop-out rate (between treatment groups) at endpoint 15 percentage points or lower?	Yes	Yes	Yes	NR	Yes	Yes
9. Was there high adherence to the intervention protocols for each treatment group?	Yes	Yes	Yes	NR	Yes	Yes
10. Were other interventions avoided or similar in the groups (e.g., similar background treatments)?	Yes	NR	Yes	NR	Yes	NR
11. Were outcomes assessed using valid and reliable measures, implemented consistently across all study participants?	Yes	Yes	Yes	No	Yes	Yes
12. Did the authors report that the sample size was sufficiently large to be able to detect a difference in the main outcome between groups with at least 80% power?	No	Yes	No	NR	Yes	Yes
13. Were outcomes reported or subgroups analyzed prespecified (i.e., identified before analyses were conducted)?	Yes	Yes	Yes	Yes	Yes	Yes
14. Were all randomized participants analyzed in the group to which they were originally assigned, i.e., did they use an intention-to-treat analysis?	Yes	No	Yes	NR	Yes	Yes
Total score (maximum 14 points)	8	10	12	2	11	9

Note: CD, Cannot Determine; NA, Not Applicable; NR, Not Reported.

4. Discussion

The aim of the present study was to systematically review evidence on how ICT is being used for MBC in psychological treatments. To the best of our knowledge, this is the first attempt to systematically examine the different technologies that have been used so far for MBC during psychological interventions and to explore to what extent the use of ICT for MBC is feasible, acceptable, and effective.

One important finding was that only 18 studies met our inclusion criteria, which suggests that this is a field that requires more research. Additionally, the included studies varied greatly in terms of study design, diagnoses, MBC characteristics, and technology used, which again suggests that more investigation and replication will be needed to obtain robust findings about different technological solutions for MBC and to facilitate the generalization of the results to different populations. Future research should also examine the implication of technology systems for MBC in specific populations (e.g., children and adolescents, who are more familiar with technology systems). Furthermore, most of the included studies focused on mood and anxiety disorders, so it would be interesting to investigate the effects of technology used for MBC in other mental disorders.

As noted in the results section, the included technologies to support MBC were frequently handheld ICTs, such as smartphone apps, tablets, or laptops, which were involved both in the patient monitoring process and in the feedback to the therapists. In this sense, while tablets and laptops might be more difficult to use for EMA, it is encouraging that smartphone apps, which might facilitate EMA to a greater extent than other technologies, are also being used as supporting technologies for MBC.

An important finding regarding technology was that, overall, the use of technology for MBC during psychological interventions appears to be feasible and acceptable. In addition, technology in MBC was found to be effective [38] and cost-effective [41], particularly for not-on-track patients [35,40,42,47], as revealed in previous studies using MBC without technology [1]. Importantly, treatment engagement (i.e., time until dropout) was also enhanced with technology-supported MBC [33]. While these findings should be interpreted with caution, due to the limited number of existing investigations and the reduced number of controlled trials comparing technology-supported and non-supported MBC, the results suggest that the use of ICT to support MBC should continue to be tested in the future.

It is important to acknowledge that technology-supported EMA for MBC is different to a similar concept, which is ecological momentary intervention (EMI). Specifically, while in EMI a given intervention is provided in response to EMA in a timely manner (e.g., providing therapeutic skills with an app based on patient responses), in MBC EMA is only used to enhance face-to-face psychological interventions.

It is also important to note that some studies were excluded from this systematic review for several reasons which should be mentioned here. For instance, in some investigations, the monitoring process was not used to guide therapeutic decisions, even though technology was used for monitoring (thus, this would not be considered MBC). Conversely, in other studies, the technology was only used in one part of the MBC process, most frequently during the feedback part, but not for EMA (e.g., assessments were made in a paper-and-pencil approach, but then the information was introduced in a computer and presented in graphs or charts to the therapists and/or patients) [16,48–50].

4.1. Limitations

Some limitations should also be considered when interpreting the results of the present systematic review. As in previous similar reviews [13,18], the heterogeneity of studies with respect to sample size, measures used, and methodology, to name some examples, made it difficult to piece together the results and restricted the implementation of a meta-analysis which affects the generalizability and robustness of findings. Moreover, the majority of included studies were feasibility pilot studies, case studies, or non-RCTs. Although these designs can yield valuable information, RCTs, which have been rarer, are considered superior because of their higher internal validity and, therefore, higher robustness of the evidence indicating a (causal) relationship. Additionally, some factors might have biased the present systematic review findings, including the fact that only three databases were used for the search, and the possibility that studies where ICT was not feasible or did not add any value have not been published. Finally, it is important to note that this systematic review is limited to the interpretations of the authors who conducted the systematic review.

4.2. Conclusions

To conclude, this systematic review found preliminary support for the use of technology in MBC during psychological interventions. The use of ICTs in MBC has brought some encouraging contributions to the evolution of psychotherapy and its inclusion in routine care might significantly change the way psychotherapists work. Particularly, the provision of real-time information on symptom progress over the course of psychological interventions might help therapists detect and rapidly react to problems that might occur during treatment (e.g., exacerbation in symptomatology or low adherence to recommended practices). This would make current interventions more flexible and personalized [22] and should favor the psychotherapeutic relationship during face-to-face interventions. Additionally, this might increase the patients' awareness of their own progress.

In addition, technology was generally found to be a feasible and acceptable add-on tool for the MBC process. Therefore, the use of technology for improving the MBC process is mostly supported, as it might facilitate EMA and offer some potential for improving psychotherapy thanks to the real-time connection between patient assessment and therapist and patient feedback [32]. While the presented results are, overall, encouraging, especially for not-on-track patients, more research is required in this field, especially RCTs comparing technology-supported MBC with traditional MBC without technology.

Author Contributions: Conceptualization, P.G.-M., V.M.-B., J.M.B.-L., J.O., and C.S.-R.; Methodology, P.G.-M., V.M.-B., J.M.B.-L., J.O., C.S.-R.; Validation, J.M.B.-L. and C.S.-R.; Formal Analysis, P.G.-M. and V.M.-B.; Investigation, P.G.-M. and V.M.-B.; Resources, J.M.B.-L. and C.S.-R.; Data Curation, P.G.-M., V.M.-B., and C.S.-R.; Writing Original Draft Preparation, P.G.-M., V.M.-B., and C.S.-R.; Writing Review & Editing, P.G.-M., V.M.-B., J.M.B.-L., J.O., and C.S.-R.; Visualization, P.G.-M., V.M.-B., and C.S.-R.; Supervision, J.M.B.-L., J.O., and C.S.-R.; Project Administration, J.M.B.-L., J.O., and C.S.-R. All authors have read and agreed to the published version of the manuscript.

Appendix A. Complete List of Search Terms and Combinations

The first set of search terms were related to psychological treatment: "psychotherapy" OR "psychological treatment" OR "psychological intervention" OR "CBT" OR "cognitive-behavioral therapy" OR "cognitive behavioral therapy" OR "cognitive-behavioural therapy" OR "cognitive behavioural therapy". The second set of search terms were related to progress monitoring: "outcome feedback" OR "ecological momentary", OR "outcome monitoring" OR "enhanced treatment" OR "enhanced assessment" OR "enhanced monitoring". The last set of search terms were related to the use of technology through diverse devices: "mHealth" OR "eHealth" OR "technology" OR "app" OR "smartphone" OR "phone". These sets of search terms were linked with the Boolean operator AND.

References

1. Shimokawa, K.; Lambert, M.J.; Smart, D.W. Enhancing treatment outcome of patients at risk of treatment failure: Meta-analytic and mega-analytic review of a psychotherapy quality assurance system. *J. Consult. Clin. Psychol.* **2010**, *78*, 298–311. [CrossRef] [PubMed]
2. Lambert, M.J.; Hansen, N.B.; Finch, A.E. Patient-focused research: Using patient outcome data to enhance treatment effects. *J. Consult. Clin. Psychol.* **2001**, *69*, 159–172. [CrossRef] [PubMed]
3. Kaplan, S.H.; Billimek, J.; Sorkin, D.H.; Ngo-Metzger, Q.; Greenfield, S. Who can respond to treatment? *Med. Care* **2010**, *48*, S9–S16. [CrossRef] [PubMed]
4. McDevitt-Murphy, M.E.; Luciano, M.T.; Zakarian, R.J. Use of ecological momentary assessment and intervention in treatment with adults. *Focus (Madison)* **2018**, *16*, 370–375. [CrossRef]
5. Suso-Ribera, C.; Mesas, Á.; Medel, J.; Server, A.; Márquez, E.; Castilla, D.; Zaragozá, I.; García-Palacios, A.; Mesas, A.; Medel, J.; et al. Improving pain treatment with a smartphone app: Study protocol for a randomized controlled trial. *Trials* **2018**, *19*, 145. [CrossRef]
6. Colombo, D.; Fernández-Álvarez, J.; Suso-Ribera, C.; Cipresso, P.; Valev, H.; Leufkens, T.; Sas, C.; Garcia-Palacios, A.; Riva, G.; Botella, C. The need for change: Understanding emotion regulation antecedents and consequences using ecological momentary assessment. *Emotion* **2020**, *20*, 30–36. [CrossRef]
7. Beute, F.; De Kort, Y.; Ijsselsteijn, W. Restoration in its natural context: How ecological momentary assessment can advance restoration research. *Int. J. Environ. Res. Public Health* **2016**, *13*, 420. [CrossRef]
8. Kendrick, T.; Moore, M.; Gilbody, S.; Churchill, R.; Stuart, B.; El-Gohary, M. Routine use of patient reported outcome measures (PROMs) for improving treatment of common mental health disorders in adults. *Cochrane Database Syst. Rev.* **2014**, *2014*. [CrossRef]
9. Canadian Psychological Association. *Outcomes and Progress Monitoring in Psychotherapy*; A Report of the Canadian Psychological Association, Prepared by the Task Force on Outcomes and Progress Monitoring in Psychotherapy; Canadian Psychological Association: Ottawa, ON, Canada, 2018.
10. Knaup, C.; Koesters, M.; Schoefer, D.; Becker, T.; Puschner, B. Effect of feedback of treatment outcome in specialist mental healthcare: Meta-analysis. *Br. J. Psychiatry* **2009**, *195*, 15–22. [CrossRef]
11. Scott, K.; Lewis, C.C. Using measurement-based care to enhance any treatment. *Cogn. Behav. Pract.* **2015**, *22*, 49–59. [CrossRef]

12. Lambert, M.J.; Whipple, J.L.; Smart, D.W.; Vermeersch, D.A.; Nielsen, S.L.; Hawkins, E.J. The effects of providing therapists with feedback on patient progress during psychotherapy: Are outcomes enhanced? *Psychother. Res.* **2001**, *11*, 49–68. [CrossRef] [PubMed]
13. Goldberg, S.B.; Buck, B.; Raphaely, S.; Fortney, J.C. Measuring psychiatric symptoms remotely: A systematic review of remote measurement-based care. *Curr. Psychiatry Rep.* **2018**, *20*, 81. [CrossRef] [PubMed]
14. Reese, R.J.; Norsworthy, L.A.; Rowlands, S.R. Does a continuous feedback system improve psychotherapy outcome? *Psychotherapy* **2009**, *46*, 418–431. [CrossRef] [PubMed]
15. Lambert, M.J.; Harmon, C.; Slade, K.; Whipple, J.L.; Hawkins, E.J. Providing feedback to psychotherapists on their patients' progress: Clinical results and practice sugges tions. *J. Clin. Psychol.* **2005**, *61*, 165–174. [CrossRef] [PubMed]
16. Bickman, L.; Kelley, S.D.; Breda, C.; De Andrade, A.R.; Riemer, M. Effects of routine feedback to clinicians on mental health outcomes of youths: Results of a randomized trial. *Psychiatr. Serv.* **2011**, *62*, 1423–1429. [CrossRef]
17. Carlier, I.V.E.; Meuldijk, D.; Van Vliet, I.M.; Van Fenema, E.; Van Der Wee, N.J.A.; Zitman, F.G. Routine outcome monitoring and feedback on physical or mental health status: Evidence and theory. *J. Eval. Clin. Pract.* **2012**, *18*, 104–110. [CrossRef]
18. Gondek, D.; Edbrooke-Childs, J.; Fink, E.; Deighton, J.; Wolpert, M. Feedback from outcome measures and treatment effectiveness, treatment efficiency, and collaborative practice: A systematic review. *Adm. Policy Ment. Health Ment. Health Serv. Res.* **2016**, *43*, 325–343. [CrossRef]
19. Imel, Z.E.; Caperton, D.D.; Tanana, M.; Atkins, D.C. Technology-enhanced human interaction in psychotherapy. *J. Couns. Psychol.* **2017**, *64*, 385–393. [CrossRef]
20. Aboraya, A.; Nasrallah, H.A.; Elswick, D.E.; Elshazly, A.; Estephan, N.; Aboraya, D.; Berzingi, S.; Chumbers, J.; Berzingi, S.; Justice, J.; et al. Measurement-based care in psychiatry—Past, present, and future. *Innov. Clin. Neurosci.* **2018**, *15*, 13–26.
21. Hallgren, K.A.; Bauer, A.M.; Atkins, D.C. Digital technology and clinical decision making in depression treatment: Current findings and future opportunities. *Depress. Anxiety* **2017**, *34*, 494–501. [CrossRef]
22. Bauer, S.; Moessner, M. Technology-enhanced monitoring in psychotherapy and e-mental health. *J. Ment. Health* **2012**, *21*, 355–363. [CrossRef] [PubMed]
23. Silk, J.S.; Forbes, E.E.; Whalen, D.J.; Jakubcak, J.L.; Thompson, W.K.; Ryan, N.D.; Axelson, D.A.; Birmaher, B.; Dahl, R.E. Daily emotional dynamics in depressed youth: A cell phone ecological momentary assessment study. *J. Exp. Child Psychol.* **2011**, *110*, 241–257. [CrossRef] [PubMed]
24. Suso-Ribera, C.; Castilla, D.; Zaragozá, I.; Ribera-Canudas, M.V.; Botella, C.; García-Palacios, A. Validity, reliability, feasibility, and usefulness of Pain Monitor. A multidimensional smartphone app for daily monitoring of adults with heterogeneous chronic pain. *Clin. J. Pain* **2018**, *34*, 900–908. [CrossRef] [PubMed]
25. Hegland, P.A.; Aasprang, A.; Hjelle Øygard, S.; Nordberg, S.; Kolotkin, R.; Moltu, C.; Tell, G.S.; Andersen, J.R. A review of systematic reviews on the effects of patient-reported outcome monitoring with clinical feedback systems on health-related quality of life-implications for a novel technology in obesity treatment. *Clin. Obes.* **2018**, *8*, 452–464. [CrossRef]
26. Moher, D.; Liberati, A.; Tetzlaff, J.; Altman, D.G.; Altman, D.G.; Antes, G.; Atkins, D.; Barbour, V.; Barrowman, N.; Berlin, J.A.; et al. Preferred reporting items for systematic reviews and meta-analyses: The PRISMA statement (Chinese edition). *J. Chin. Integr. Med.* **2009**, *7*, 889–896. [CrossRef]
27. Falagas, M.E.; Pitsouni, E.I.; Malietzis, G.A.; Pappas, G. Comparison of PubMed, Scopus, Web of Science, and Google Scholar: Strengths and weaknesses. *FASEB J.* **2008**, *22*, 338–342. [CrossRef]
28. Eady, A.M.; Wilczynski, N.L.; Haynes, R.B. PsycINFO search strategies identified methodologically sound therapy studies and review articles for use by clinicians and researchers. *J. Clin. Epidemiol.* **2008**, *61*, 34–40. [CrossRef]
29. National Heart Lung and Blood Institute (NHLBI). Study Quality Assessment Tools. Available online: https://www.nhlbi.nih.gov/health-topics/study-quality-assessment-tools (accessed on 1 May 2020).
30. Smith, B.; Harms, W.D.; Burres, S.; Korda, H.; Rosen, H.; Davis, J. Enhancing behavioral health treatment and crisis management through mobile ecological momentary assessment and SMS messaging. *Health Inform. J.* **2012**, *18*, 294–308. [CrossRef]
31. Pramana, G.; Parmanto, B.; Kendall, P.C.; Silk, J.S. The SmartCAT: An m-health platform for ecological momentary intervention in child anxiety treatment. *Telemed. e-Health* **2014**, *20*, 419–427. [CrossRef]

32. Pinsof, W.M.; Goldsmith, J.Z.; Latta, T.A. Information technology and feedback research can bridge the scientist–practitioner gap: A couple therapy example. *Couple Fam. Psychol. Res. Pract.* **2012**, *1*, 253–273. [CrossRef]
33. Aguilera, A.; Bruehlman-Senecal, E.; Demasi, O.; Avila, P. Automated Text messaging as an adjunct to cognitive behavioral therapy for depression: A clinical trial. *J. Med. Internet Res.* **2017**, *19*, e148. [CrossRef] [PubMed]
34. Kumar, D.; Tully, L.M.; Iosif, A.-M.; Zakskorn, L.N.; Nye, K.E.; Zia, A.; Niendam, T.A. A mobile health platform for clinical monitoring in early psychosis: Implementation in community-based outpatient early psychosis care. *JMIR Ment. Health* **2018**, *5*, e15. [CrossRef] [PubMed]
35. Aharonovich, E.; Sarvet, A.; Stohl, M.; DesJarlais, D.; Tross, S.; Hurst, T.; Urbina, A.; Hasin, D. Reducing non-injection drug use in HIV primary care: A randomized trial of brief motivational interviewing, with and without HealthCall, a technology-based enhancement. *J. Subst. Abuse Treat.* **2017**, *74*, 71–79. [CrossRef] [PubMed]
36. Niendam, T.A.; Tully, L.M.; Iosif, A.M.; Kumar, D.; Nye, K.E.; Denton, J.C.; Zakskorn, L.N.; Fedechko, T.L.; Pierce, K.M. Enhancing early psychosis treatment using smartphone technology: A longitudinal feasibility and validity study. *J. Psychiatr. Res.* **2018**, *96*, 239–246. [CrossRef]
37. Bauer, A.M.; Iles-Shih, M.; Ghomi, R.H.; Rue, T.; Grover, T.; Kincler, N.; Miller, M.; Katon, W.J. Acceptability of mHealth augmentation of Collaborative Care: A mixed methods pilot study. *Gen. Hosp. Psychiatry* **2018**, *51*, 22–29. [CrossRef]
38. Bell, I.H.; Rossell, S.L.; Farhall, J.; Hayward, M.; Lim, M.H.; Fielding-Smith, S.F.; Thomas, N. Pilot randomised controlled trial of a brief coping-focused intervention for hearing voices blended with smartphone-based ecological momentary assessment and intervention (SAVVy): Feasibility, acceptability and preliminary clinical outcomes. *Schizophr. Res.* **2019**. [CrossRef]
39. Bell, I.H.; Fielding-Smith, S.F.; Hayward, M.; Rossell, S.L.; Lim, M.H.; Farhall, J.; Thomas, N. Smartphone-based ecological momentary assessment and intervention in a blended coping-focused therapy for distressing voices: Development and case illustration. *Internet Interv.* **2018**, *14*, 18–25. [CrossRef]
40. Newnham, E.A.; Hooke, G.R.; Page, A.C. Progress monitoring and feedback in psychiatric care reduces depressive symptoms. *J. Affect. Disord.* **2010**, *127*, 139–146. [CrossRef]
41. Delgadillo, J.; Overend, K.; Lucock, M.; Groom, M.; Kirby, N.; McMillan, D.; Gilbody, S.; Lutz, W.; Rubel, J.A.; De Jong, K. Improving the efficiency of psychological treatment using outcome feedback technology. *Behav. Res. Ther.* **2017**, *99*, 89–97. [CrossRef]
42. Delgadillo, J.; De Jong, K.; Lucock, M.; Lutz, W.; Rubel, J.; Gilbody, S.; Ali, S.; Aguirre, E.; Appleton, M.; Nevin, J.; et al. Feedback-informed treatment versus usual psychological treatment for depression and anxiety: A multisite, open-label, cluster randomised controlled trial. *Lancet Psychiatry* **2018**, *5*, 564–572. [CrossRef]
43. Miklowitz, D.J.; Price, J.; Holmes, E.A.; Rendell, J.; Bell, S.; Budge, K.; Christensen, J.; Wallace, J.; Simon, J.; Armstrong, N.M.; et al. Facilitated Integrated Mood Management for adults with bipolar disorder. *Bipolar Disord.* **2012**, *14*, 185–197. [CrossRef] [PubMed]
44. Schiepek, G.; Aichhorn, W.; Gruber, M.; Strunk, G.; Bachler, E.; Aas, B. Real-time monitoring of psychotherapeutic processes: Concept and compliance. *Front. Psychol.* **2016**, *7*, 604. [CrossRef] [PubMed]
45. Kaiser, T.; Laireiter, A.R. DynAMo: A modular platform for monitoring process, outcome, and algorithm-based treatment planning in psychotherapy. *JMIR Med. Inform.* **2017**, *5*, e20. [CrossRef] [PubMed]
46. Lazarou, I.; Karakostas, A.; Stavropoulos, T.G.; Tsompanidis, T.; Meditskos, G.; Kompatsiaris, I.; Tsolaki, M. A novel and intelligent home monitoring system for care support of elders with cognitive impairment. *J. Alzheimer's Dis.* **2016**, *54*, 1561–1591. [CrossRef] [PubMed]
47. De Jong, K.; Timman, R.; Hakkaart-Van Roijen, L.; Vermeulen, P.; Kooiman, K.; Passchier, J.; Van Busschbach, J. The effect of outcome monitoring feedback to clinicians and patients in short and long-term psychotherapy: A randomized controlled trial. *Psychother. Res.* **2014**, *24*, 629–639. [CrossRef]
48. Amble, I.; Gude, T.; Stubdal, S.; Andersen, B.J.; Wampold, B.E. The effect of implementing the Outcome Questionnaire-45.2 feedback system in Norway: A multisite randomized clinical trial in a naturalistic setting. *Psychother. Res.* **2015**, *25*, 669–677. [CrossRef]

49. Janse, P.D.; De Jong, K.; Van Dijk, M.K.; Hutschemaekers, G.J.M.; Verbraak, M.J.P.M. Improving the efficiency of cognitive-behavioural therapy by using formal client feedback. *Psychother. Res.* **2017**, *27*, 525–538. [CrossRef]
50. Lucock, M.; Halstead, J.; Leach, C.; Barkham, M.; Tucker, S.; Randal, C.; Middleton, J.; Khan, W.; Catlow, H.; Waters, E.; et al. A mixed-method investigation of patient monitoring and enhanced feedback in routine practice: Barriers and facilitators. *Psychother. Res.* **2015**, *25*, 633–646. [CrossRef]

8

The Benefits of Emotion Regulation Interventions in Virtual Reality for the Improvement of Wellbeing in Adults and Older Adults

Jessica Isbely Montana [1,*], Marta Matamala-Gomez [1], Marta Maisto [1], Petar Aleksandrov Mavrodiev [1], Cesare Massimo Cavalera [2], Barbara Diana [1], Fabrizia Mantovani [1] and Olivia Realdon [1]

[1] Department of Human Sciences for Education, University of Milano-Bicocca, Piazza dell'Ateneo Nuovo 1, 20126 Milano, Italy; marta.matamalagomez@unimib.it (M.M.-G.); marta.maisto@unimib.it (M.M.); p.mavrodiev@campus.unimib.it (P.A.M.); barbara.diana@unimib.it (B.D.); fabrizia.mantovani@unimib.it (F.M.); olivia.realdon@unimib.it (O.R.)

[2] Department of Psychology, Catholic University of the Sacred Heart, Largo Gemelli 1, 20100 Milan, Italy; cesarem.cavalera@unicatt.it

* Correspondence: jessica.montana@unimib.it

Abstract: The impact of emotion regulation interventions on wellbeing has been extensively documented in literature, although only in recent years virtual reality (VR) technologies have been incorporated in the design of such interventions, in both clinical and non-clinical settings. A systematic search, following the Preferred Reporting Items for Systematic Reviews and Meta-Analysis (PRISMA) guidelines, was therefore carried out to explore the state of the art in emotion regulation interventions for wellbeing using virtual reality. The literature on this topic was queried, 414 papers were screened, and 11 studies were included, covering adults and older adults. Our findings offer an overview of the current use of VR technologies for the enhancement of emotion regulation (ER) and wellbeing. The results are promising and suggest that VR-based emotion regulation training can facilitate the promotion of wellbeing. An overview of VR-based training interventions is crucial for better understanding how to use these tools in the clinical settings. This review offers a critical debate on the structure of such intervention protocols. It also analyzes and highlights the crucial role played by the selection of the objective and subjective wellbeing assessment measures of said intervention protocols.

Keywords: emotion regulation; treatment; wellbeing intervention; adults; virtual reality; systematic review

1. Introduction

Emotion is a cultural and psychobiological adaptation mechanism that allows each individual to react flexibly and dynamically to environmental contingencies [1]. Emotions give meaning to our lives, intensify our connection with others, inform us about our needs and feelings and motivate us to make changes [2]. Emotions are multidimensional phenomena. A single emotion comprises of: a cognitive appraisal, a physical sensation, an intention, a subjective "feeling", a motor response and, in most cases, an interpersonal component [1,3]. Emotion Regulation (ER) denotes a set of mental processes that influences which emotions we have when we have them and how we experience and express them [4,5]. It is a dynamic process inherent to the mental functioning of human beings, aimed at down or up-regulating positive or negative emotions in order to reach desirable states [6,7]. Emotion dysregulation denotes the undesired intensification or deactivation given by the person's inability to manage or process emotions effectively [8,9]. Hence, dealing with emotionally rich experience is part of emotional regulation. A priori assumptions as to whether any particular form of emotion regulation is necessarily good or bad do not exist [10]. This is important because it aims to avoid a type of distinction that is made, for example, between coping strategies, as more or less adaptive regardless of the context [11,12]. The emotion regulation process is a mechanism may be used to make things either better or worse, depending on the context. Furthermore, in line with a functionalist perspective, regulatory strategies may accomplish desired goals but still be perceived by others as maladaptive [13], such as when a child cries loudly in order to get attention [7]. A notable contextually adaptive ER strategies is reappraisal. It changes the way one thinks about a potential emotion-eliciting event. Another one is suppression, which changes the behavioral response to an emotion-eliciting event [14]. Thus, an effective situation-based regulation of emotions is necessary for permanent and enduring change in a person's growth and their social functioning [14] and subjective wellbeing [15–17].

The growing development of new technologies and the interest in applying them in the field of psychology have led to the development of novel virtual reality (VR) systems for neuro-rehabilitation [18], or the treatment of different mental health disorders [19–22] with the aim of generating an engaging and realistic virtual world in line with the needs of the person [23]. Applying virtual reality in psychology has one major advantage. It allows researchers and clinicians to create life-like experiences in a safe environment such as a laboratory or a clinical setting [24,25]. VR-based assessment and treatment allows to keep complex variables under control while preserving the complexity of real-life experiences [26]. In this regard, the use of virtual reality is promising, because it allows real-time measurement of cognitive, emotional, physiological, and behavioral responses in a variety of "real-life" situations while allow for full experimental control [27,28]. In particular, concerning the application of VR in clinical psychology, virtual environments have been widely used to enhance the use of successful ER strategies [29]. Since we know that effective ER strategies have led to several important outcomes regarding mental health, subjective and psychological wellbeing, and relationship satisfaction [30]. Hence, positive changes in emotion regulation are an important outcome in the mental health interventions and the development of new technologies such as VR systems could facilitate and increase the positive outcomes of such ER strategies [29,31]. It has been demonstrated that VR systems can evoke emotional experiences that lead to psychologically valuable changes through an enhanced sense of presence in a virtual environment [32–34]. Hence, it is possible to create a sense of 'being there' in a virtual world by designing highly immersive VR experiences, which rely on multisensory feedback mechanisms [35].

Health and wellbeing are considered as indispensable resources for societies and human development [36]. The World Health Organization (WHO) has placed wellbeing on the "Health 2020: the European policy for health and well-being" agenda as an objective for social progress [37]. Following the WHO, the purpose of the present review is to investigate whether wellbeing can be enhanced using new technologies, such as virtual reality. Specifically, the present systematic review aims to better understand the efficacy of emotion regulation interventions for wellbeing, by using virtual reality systems in adults and older adults without psychopathological conditions.

2. Method

A systematic review of the scientific literature has been performed to identify studies that reported VR-based ER interventions for wellbeing in healthy and clinical adults and examined the structure of their protocols. The methodology is presented in the following paragraphs.

2.1. Search Methodology

Preferred Reporting Items for Systematic Reviews and Meta-Analysis (PRISMA) guidelines were followed [38]. Four high-profile databases (PubMed, Embase, Scopus, and Web of Science) were used to perform the computer-based research on the 30th of September 2019 (see Table 1 and Figure 1). According to the PICO format, we defined the review question as, "is VR training for emotion regulation, compared to treatment as usual, effective in improving wellbeing in adults (with psychological distress)." We then proceeded with the definition of keywords for the search strategy.

The string used to carry out the search strategy was ("virtual reality" OR "virtual environment*" OR "digital intervention*" OR "digital technologies") AND ("emotion regulation" OR "affect regulation" OR "wellbeing"). The initial searches on the databases yielded 530 results. Duplicates were removed leaving 414 articles for further evaluation. Table 1 shows the details of the results for each keyword on each database used.

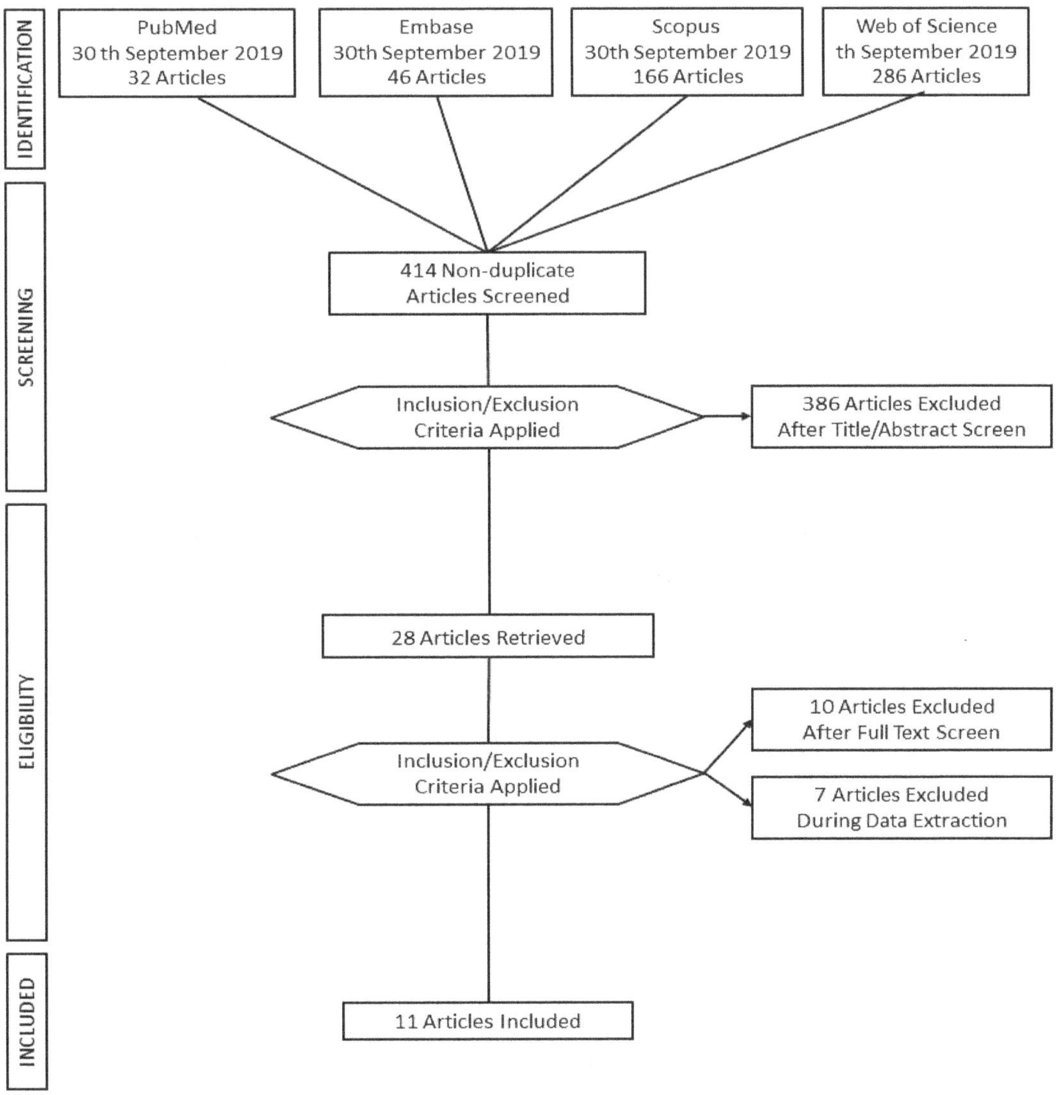

Figure 1. Flow Chart.

Table 1. Detailed search strategy.

"virtual reality" OR "virtual environment*" OR "digital intervention*" OR "digital technologies."						
AND	**PubMed**	**Embase**	**Scopus**	**Web of Science**		
"emotion regulation"	17	20	40	54		
"affect regulation"	1	1	2	104		
"wellbeing"	14	25	124	128		
Sub total	32	46	166	286	**Total**	530
					Without duplicates	414

2.2. *Study Selection and Inclusion Criteria*

This systematic review aims to evaluate the wellbeing and emotion regulation outcome of VR-based interventions in adults and older adults without psychopathological conditions. Given that the interest in VR continues to grow, researchers must focus on how the characteristics of VR systems and the different aspects of the training tasks could influence the intervention outcomes. The aim of this review is to provide knowledge and guide researchers in the selection of the most appropriate VR experience for ER interventions. The flow chart of the search strategy results, according to the PRISMA flow diagram, is shown in Figure 1.

The present systematic review considered randomized control trials, nonrandomized control trials, intervention studies, and case-control studies. Studies on emotion regulation for wellbeing with virtual reality (VR) devices in healthy or pathological adults and older adults presenting the following clinical conditions: traumatic brain injury, motor disabilities, tumor, chronic conditions (heart failure and chronic pain), were included. The review only includes studies in the English language, and which satisfied strict criteria for eligibility (research studies, interventions for adults and older adults, VR non-/semi-/immersive and immersive interventions, interventions for emotion regulation, interventions for wellbeing, healthy population and clinical patients but not psychopathological, wellbeing outcomes). Articles that treat psychopathological disorders such as post-traumatic stress disorder, phobias, substance abuse or psychosis, or lacked necessary information for review in the full-text or the abstract were excluded. Reviews, meeting abstracts, proceedings, poster presentations, notes, case reports, letters to the editor, assessment protocols, editorials, and other editorial materials were also excluded. Retrospective studies were not included because the area of interest requires post-intervention outcomes.

2.3. *Risk of Bias Assessment*

To assess the risk of bias, the reviewers followed the methods recommended by The Cochrane Collaboration Risk of Bias Tool [39] and the STROBE Statement [40]. Three reviewers (J.I.M., M.M.-G., and M.M.) independently assessed the risk of bias of each included study against key criteria: random sequence generation, allocation concealment, blinding of participants, personnel, and outcomes, incomplete outcome data, selective outcome reporting, and other sources of bias. The following judgments were used: low risk, high risk, or unclear (either lack of information or uncertainty over the potential for bias). Disagreements were resolved through consensus, and another author was consulted to resolve disagreements if necessary. In particular, the selected studies followed strict criteria in the methods, including presenting critical elements of study design, clearly defining all outcomes, describing the setting and relevant dates, including periods of recruitment and exposure, giving sources of data and details of methods of assessment (measurement).

3. Results

Of 414 non-duplicate studies, 386 did not fit the preliminary inclusion criteria; specifically, they did not present ER interventions for wellbeing using VR systems in adult and older adult populations. Subsequently, the full text of 28 articles was retrieved and the studies were evaluated for the specific inclusion criteria. Of 28 studies, only 11 passed the full-text screening phase, while 17 studies were excluded for the reasons that follow: Not interventions (= 4); Results not reported (= 7); Qualitative/descriptive study (= 6).

3.1. *Flow Chart of the Results*

The present flow chart (Figure 1) shows a summary of the research strategy (presented previously in Table 1), the methodology followed during the study selection process, and the final included studies according to PRISMA Guidelines.

3.2. Risk of Bias

The majority of the studies except one [41] exhibited a medium and high risk of bias across multiple dimensions. Table 2 shows the results for the risk of bias assessment. All the studies included in this review reported the sampling method [41–51], although the performance and the detection biases during blinding phase were unclear for all but one [41]. Concerning the outcomes, only two studies [45,47] presented high risk of bias for missing data handled appropriately or for missing a match between methods and results. Among other risks, we reported a high risk of bias for a small sample size with a range from eight to fifteen participants in three studies [44,47,51]. We considered important to report also a high risk of bias for lacking a control group for an experimental comparison [44,45,47–51]. Lastly, only one study addressed to patients have reported a high risk for no homogeneous clinical sample due to differences in clinical diseases and their specific characteristics [44] that might affect the interpretation of the outcomes. A clean sample is crucial for the comprehension of the ramification of disease on emotional functioning.

Table 2. Risk of bias assessment.

		Random Sequence Generation (Selection Bias)	Allocation Concealment (Selection Bias)	Blinding of Participants and Personal (Performance Bias)	Blinding of Outcome Assessment (Detection Bias)	Incomplete Outcome Data (Attrition Bias)	Selective Reporting (Reporting Bias)	Other Bias
Villani and Riva	2008	low	unclear	unclear	low	low	low	low
Tong et al.	2015	low	unclear	low	unclear	low	low	low
Cikajlo et al.	2016	high	high	unclear	unclear	low	low	high: small sample size/no control group/\no homogeneous clinical sample
Hasan et al.	2016	high	high	unclear	unclear	high	high	high: no control group
Konrad et al.	2016	low	low	low	low	low	low	low
Baez et al.	2017	low	low	unclear	low	low	low	low
Singh et al.	2017	high	high	unclear	unclear	high	high	high: small sample size/no control group
Weerdmeester et al.	2017	high	high	unclear	unclear	low	low	high: no control group
Bornioli et al.	2018	high	high	unclear	unclear	low	low	high: no control group
Lorenzetti et al.	2018	low	low	unclear	unclear	low	low	high: small sample size/no control group
Bornioli et al.	2019	high	high	unclear	unclear	low	low	high: no control group

NOTE: low (risk of bias); unclear (risk of bias); high (risk of bias).

3.3. Study Characteristics

Table 3 shows the studies' characteristics according to extraction parameters. Eleven studies were analyzed to understand the usefulness of interventions for emotion regulation and wellbeing using virtual reality (VR) systems. In order to accomplish the aims of the systematic review and to facilitate the understanding of the selected studies, the following clusters in Table 3 were considered: (1) Authors; (2) Year; (3) Sample (N); (4) Sample characteristics; (5) Mean age (SD or range); (6) VR Task; (7) VR Set-Up; (8) emotion regulation and/or wellbeing assessment; (9) Primary Outcomes.

Table 3. Study characteristics.

	Authors	Year	Sample (N)	Sample Characteristics	Mean Age (SD or Range)	VR Task	VR Set-Up	Emotion Regulation/Wellbeing Assessment	Primary Outcomes
1	Villani & Riva [42]	2008	60 healthy adults	Experimental Group (EG) for three conditions 45 persons (15 for each condition) Control Group (CG) without treatment 15 persons	Range 21–28 years old	relaxation environment + relaxing narrative	Immersive VR Condition: Sony Glastron PLM S-700 with a head-tracker: Intersense Intertrax2 and Semi-immersive DVD Condition: pc (Fujitsu Siemens AMILO Processor, Pentium 4	State-Trait Anxiety Inventory (STAI) and Positive And Negative Affect Scale (PANAS), Visual Analogue Scale (VAS), Coping Orientation to Problems Experienced Questionnaire (COPE) + Physiological Parameters: Respiration Rate, Respiration amplitude, Heart Rate, Heart Amplitude, Skin Conductance, Electromyography	Results show a significant reduction of anxiety and a significant improvement of positive emotional states—in particular, relaxation—measured through self-report questionnaires in all conditions. Physiological parameters showed some good changes related to respiration rate, heart rate, and skin conductance parameters, but less than expected.
2	Tong et al. [43]	2015	13 patients with chronic pain	EG, 7 patients (3 male, 4 female) CG, 6 patients (3 male, 3 female)	Range 35–55 years old (mean = 49, SD = 8.2)	The Virtual Meditative Walk (VMW) + biofeedback	Immersive environment stereoscopic VR display	Numerical Rating Scale (NRS) for Self-Report Pain Levels (values 0–10)	These findings indicate that the VMW (VR paired with biofeedback for MBSR training) was significantly more effective than MBSR alone at reducing reported pain levels among participants.
3	Cikajlo et al. [44]	2016	8 healthy adults and patients	EG, all participants (of which 4 patients with TBI, one with a brain tumor and 4 workers)	Healthy participants Range 27–40 years old; Patients participants Range 24–48 years old	Mindfulness-Based Stress Reduction VR	Immersive head-mounted display Samsung Gear + Samsung Smartphone S6 and Note4	Mindfulness Attention Awareness Scale (MASS) Satisfaction With Life Scale (SWLS) Mini-Mental State Examination Test (MMSE)	Patients achieved very high level of satisfaction (SWLS) at the end of the study. A slight increase in MASS score is also noticeable. All patients had MMSE score 30, except one; his score was 19 at the beginning, 29 at midterm and 26 at the end of the study.
4	Hasan et al. [45]	2016	27 older adults	Elderly group Seniors group	Older Range 70–98 years old; Seniors Range 50–70 years old	Weekly classes for developing ICT skills in aged-care facilities for 2 years	Non-immersive laptops and tablet	Social Care-Related Quality of Life (SCRQoL)	During the 2-year study, the participants developed various computing capabilities. The use of ICT appears to contribute positively to the wellbeing of the elderly: connection, self-worth/ esteem and personal development, productivity, occupation, self-sufficiency, being in control, and enjoyment.

Table 3. *Cont.*

	Authors	Year	Sample (N)	Sample Characteristics	Mean Age (SD or Range)	VR Task	VR Set-Up	Emotion Regulation/Wellbeing Assessment	Primary Outcomes
5	Konrad et al. [41]	2016	128 healthy adults	34 in the Incongruent Negative group, 34 in the Congruent Negative group, 30 in the Incongruent Positive and 30 in the Congruent Positive group	Range 18–62 years old (M = 24.56, SD = 8.87); 91 female and 37 male	MoodAdaptor—a technology-mediated reflection (TMR) application	Non-immersive mobile app	Subjective Happiness Scale, Satisfaction With Life Scale, Ryff Scales of Psychological Well-Being and Personal Emotion Scale Participants.	Autobiographical memory enhances positive mood through well-documented self-enhancement biases. Negative thoughts when in a positive mood reduced current mood, while positive thoughts, when in a negative mood, enhances it. Selecting incongruent memories is useful for mood-regulation and consequently for improving wellbeing.
6	Baez et al. [46]	2017	40 older adults	EG, 20 participants CG, 20 participants	Range 65–87 years old	OTAGO personalized exercise program for fall prevention	Non-immersive tablet-based application (10.1inch Sony Xperia tablet)	Physical Activity Enjoyment Scale (PACES), Wellbeing Scale of the Multidimensional Personality Questionnaire (MPQ), Trans Theoretical Model of Behavior Change (TTM), R-UCLA Loneliness Scale	In virtual group exercising, people with lesser physical skills improve to the level of the more fit participants. These results suggest that: the online group could overcome some of the major issues reported in the literature in terms of the negative effect of group-exercising in the motivation of heterogeneous groups; and it helped reduce the effect of the initial skill level and motivation levels of participants in comparison to the trainees complying with the group norm.
7	Singh et al. [47]	2017	15 patients with motor disabilities	EG	Mean age = 22.7, SD = 4.2	Physical activity task	Non-immersive Nintendo® Wii Fit	Depressive, Anxiety and Stress Scales (DASS)	The results of this study demonstrated that there was a significant difference in psychological well-being and reaction time after intervention using interactive VR games.
8	Weerdmeester et al. [48]	2017	72 healthy adults	EG	Range 18–30 (M = 21.5, SD = 2.7); 31% male, 69% female	DEEP VR a virtual reality biofeedback game	Immersive VR game + biofeedback	Trier Social Stress Test	These results provide a promising outlook for using biofeedback video games such as DEEP to help individuals learn how to regulate their physiological arousal engagingly.

Table 3. *Cont.*

	Authors	Year	Sample (N)	Sample Characteristics	Mean Age (SD or Range)	VR Task	VR Set-Up	Emotion Regulation/Wellbeing Assessment	Primary Outcomes
9	Bornioli et al. [49]	2018	269 healthy adults and older adults	EG, all participants see five different environments	Range 18–67 years old (M = 31.69, SD = 13.63; 30.9% male, 69.1% females	exposure urban walking task	Non-immersive laptop	University of Wales Institute of Science and Technology Mood Adjective Checklist (UWIST MACL scale), Russell's circumplex model of affect, Perceived Restorativeness Scale—Short Version (PRS scale)	This study sets out to investigate the immediate psychological wellbeing benefits of virtual exposure to different urban walking settings. The results suggest that walking in high-quality urban settings can have positive outcomes and highlight the negative role of traffic and the potential benefits of historical elements in the affective walking experience.
10	Lorenzetti et al. [51]	2018	8 healthy adults	EG	Range 23–28 years old	exposure to an autumnal nature environment	Non-Immersive virtual environments in a brain-computer interface (BCI) + rrtfMRI-NFB	Beck Depression Inventory (BDI), Trait Anxiety Inventory (STAI) and Positive And Negative Affect Scale (PANAS), Emotion Regulation Questionnaire (ERQ) and Satisfaction with Life Scale (SLS)	The study provides a novel proof of concept and demonstrates the feasibility of the implementation of rtfMRI-NFB using virtual environment and music to elicit the neural activity and measure the neural correlates of specific, complex emotional states. Real-time up-regulation of tenderness engaged the hypothalamic septum area and other regions previously implicated in positive affiliative emotions (i.e., medial frontal cortex and temporal pole, precuneus).
11	Bornioli et al. [50]	2019	384 healthy adults and older adults	EG, all participants see five different environments	Range 18–67 years old (M = 35.01, SD = 13.89)	exposure urban walking task	Non-immersive laptop	University of Wales Institute of Science and Technology Mood Adjective Checklist (UWIST MACL scale), Russell's Circumplex Model of Affect, Perceived Restorativeness Scale—Short Version (PRS scale)	Results show the crucial features that make walking positive for psychological wellbeing and encourage walking intentions are perceived safety, comfort, and moderate stimulation.

3.4. *Interventions for Adults and Older Adults*

3.4.1. Age Differences in Emotional Experience

Several investigations suggest that VR-based ER interventions in adults and older adults could improve quality of life, physical and mental health and delay the onset of health disorders [29,30]. We considered it appropriate to divide the discussion of the results according to the age of the participants. This choice was based on two reasons. Firstly, studies in the adult and elderly populations have different objectives. Secondly, emotional experience, expression and regulation, like all psychological phenomena, depend on physiological functioning [52]. In regard to the former, Gross et al. examine age differences in participants' reactions to negative events, showing that older people report better control over emotions compared to younger people [53]. In regard to the latter, studies observe how heart rate increases and epithelial cells lining the vasculature either constrict or dilate in response to an arousing stimulus. This overall pattern of reactivity is reduced among older adults [54,55].

In the following paragraphs we discuss the characteristics of the selected VR interventions. The examined studies focus on the use of virtual environments for intervening on emotion regulation processes, and for improving the wellbeing of healthy and clinical populations.

3.4.2. Interventions for Adults

The evaluated interventions for adults and older adults (specifically the VR characteristics, the VE content, and the aims) are summarized in Tables 4 and 5 respectively.

Table 4. Interventions for adults.

Study	Sample (Type of)	VE Characteristics	VE Content	Aim of the VR Task
		Virtual Environments for Healthy Participants		
Villani and Riva (2008) [42]	Healthy	Immersive	A waterfall and a beach of an island	Relaxation and enhancement of wellbeing
Konrad et al. (2016) [41]	Healthy	Non-immersive	Mood survey	Mood regulation and improvement wellbeing
Weerdmester et al. (2017) [48]	Healthy	Immersive	Underwater world	Regulation of physiological arousal
Bornioli et al. (2018) [49]	Healthy	Non-immersive	Five different pedestrian areas of a town	Enhancement of behavioral activation for wellbeing
Lorenzetti et al. (2018) [51]	Healthy	Non-immersive	A landscape of hills and cornfields	Regulation of physiological arousal
Bornioli et al. (2019) [50]	Healthy	Non-immersive	Five different pedestrian areas of a town	Enhancement of behavioral activation for wellbeing
		Virtual Environments for Patients		
Tong et al. (2015) [43]	Clinical	Immersive	Walk in the forest	Mindfulness-based stress reduction
Cikajlo et al. (2016) [44]	Clinical	Immersive	A river and a mountain landscape	Mindfulness-based stress reduction
Singh et al. (2017) [47]	Clinical	Non-immersive	Three different sports: tennis, bowling, and boxing	Enhancement of behavioral activation for wellbeing

Table 5. Interventions for older adults.

Study	Sample (Type of)	VE Characteristics	VE Content	Aim of the VR Task
Virtual Environments for healthy participants				
Hasan et al. (2016) [45]	Healthy	Non-immersive	Social networks, emails	Enhancement of ICT-skills for the improvement of social functioning and wellbeing
Baez et al. (2017) [46]	Healthy	Non-immersive	A gymnasium	Enhancement of behavioral activation for fall prevention and wellbeing
Bornioli et al. (2018) [49]	Healthy	Non-immersive	Five different pedestrian areas of a town	Enhancement of behavioral activation for wellbeing
Bornioli et al. (2019) [50]	Healthy	Non-immersive	Five different pedestrian areas of a town	Enhancement of behavioral activation for wellbeing

3.4.3. Virtual Environments (VE) for Healthy Participants

In what follows we examine studies conducted in a healthy population (see Table 4). Villani and Riva's used two virtual environments, one depicting a waterfall zone, and another an island, to induce relaxation and to enhance the wellbeing of participants [42]. The authors employed these scenarios in a way that maximizes the sense of presence in the virtual world, which enhances the quality of the relaxation experience [42]. Konrad et al. [41] used a web-based technology-mediated reflection (TMR) application, called the "Mood Adaptor," to enhance ER. It is a systematic process that reviews rich digital records of past personal experiences. According to the authors, such autobiographical memory approach increases general wellbeing. In their intervention, participants were instructed to write down a positive thought while experiencing a negative mood and, vice versa, write down a negative thought while in a positive mood [41]. Their explanation relies on the fact that recalling negative experiences while in a positive mood can update the emotional appraisal of the past experience and generate more adaptive perspectives of the past [41].

Weerdmeester et al. [48] have examined the role of self-efficacy in the context of biofeedback video games for ER. A pilot study was conducted with a VR videogame, called DEEP, which uses respiratory-based biofeedback to help individuals cope with stress and anxiety. Self-efficacy was found to be a significant predictor of physiological regulation, and a key factor in the improvement of mental wellbeing [48]. The biofeedback paradigm has been defined as a system in which physiological activity is continuously measured and fed back to the user in real-time [48]. In fact, in Weerdmeester's study, deep, calm breathing allows the player to stay afloat and move smoothly through the underwater world [48]. Lorenzetti et al. [51] have developed a neurofeedback game using a virtual environment as a medium to convey a real-time sensory feedback to participants, in association with ongoing tenderness, anguish, and neutral emotional states. Lorenzetti et al., used a BCI-based neurofeedback system in which neural activity was linked to the color of the virtual environment which allowed the real-time visualization of the fluctuation of emotional states. Orange denoted tenderness, purple—anguish, and natural light tones—neutral disposition [51]. Participants were instructed to experience tenderness or anguish as intensely as possible in the respective trials and to volitionally increase the intensity of their emotions [51].

Bornioli et al. [49,50] support the large amount of evidence concerning the benefits of walking in natural areas. In their two studies, participants had to walk, in five different, virtually recreate, sites: a pedestrianized historic environment in Bristol's Old Town, characterized by neoclassical buildings and cobbled paving; a pedestrianized modern environment in a complex of concrete and glass-fronted buildings; a pedestrianized environment with a mix of greenery and historic elements, framed by the Bristol Cathedral; a commercial road with high street retail outlets and cafés and a single-lane road with moderate moving traffic, constituted by cars and buses; and an urban park. The outcomes underline the crucial features that make walking positive for psychological wellbeing and encourage this activity [49,50].

3.4.4. Virtual Environments for Patients

Other studies have used interventions on patients with specific pathologies (see Table 4) using virtual environments to enhance ER and wellbeing. Two of these used Mindfulness-based Stress Reduction (MBSR) Meditation through virtual environments as a non-pharmacological approach to treating chronic disorders, such as chronic pain [43], and patients with traumatic brain injuries [44]. In both studies, virtual meditation was significantly more effective than MBSR alone in reducing reported levels of pain [43], and at making participants experience a higher level of satisfaction [44]. Singh et al. have examined the impact of VR games on psychological wellbeing, upper limb motor function and reaction time in adults with physical disabilities. In the latter study, wellbeing was a secondary outcome, as a positive consequence of the physical reactivation of the patient through the use of motor task games [47].

3.4.5. Virtual Reality Set-Up

The examined studies have used different types of virtual reality systems. Among the studies that have used immersive VR systems, two have selected a head-mounted display in combination with a smartphone and a head-tracker [42,44]. However, in the study conducted by Tong et al. [43], the authors used a Virtual Meditative Walk system that requires the use of a stereoscopic VR display. The display was mounted on a movable arm to ensure flexibility and to ease patient comfort. Furthermore, the authors used a sensor in order to track changing arousal levels, which are small clips put onto two of the patient's fingertips [43]. In the DEEP biofeedback game study, participants had to use deep diaphragmatic breathing in order to navigate in an immersive virtual environment through an enchanted underwater world [48]. The game used a customized controller belt that measures the expansion of the player's diaphragm and a head-mounted device. Other studies have used non-immersive devices, such as mobile applications [41]; Nintendo® Wii Fit [47]; tablet and laptop [45,46,49,50]; and computer-based interface (BCI) [51].

3.4.6. VR Interventions for Older Adults

Positive emotions have a significant influence on mental and physical health [56,57]. Their role in the wellbeing of the elderly has been established in numerous studies, so it is worthwhile exploring how older adults can improve the number of positive experiences in their daily lives [58]. Digital technologies are a powerful tool to enhance social inclusion [59], to support a more active and independent life in older adults and consequently to facilitate their wellbeing [60]. Among the presently investigated studies (see Table 5), Hasan et al. [45] and Baez et al. [46] proposed VR interventions focused on enhancing abilities for the maintenance of autonomy in older adults. Hasan et al. have carried out a two-year project on the social use of information and communications technologies (ICT) in older adults. The interventions consisted in the establishment of computer kiosks in aged-care facilities and weekly classes for developing ICT skills and enhancing wellbeing [45]. The study conducted by Baez et al. was a home-based intervention program to promote physical activity in older adults [46]. In this study, a web and a tablet application have been delivered to participants in order to enable and motivate them to participate in a home-based group training session, under the supervision of a human coach. After a period of eight weeks of training, participants presented a significant improvement of subjective wellbeing [46]. Moreover, in two studies conducted by Bornioli's and co-authors with older adults, the authors used a virtual walk intervention to enhance physical activity intentions and psychological wellbeing [49,50].

3.5. Outcome Measures for Wellbeing

3.5.1. Physiological Markers

A large number of studies among those evaluated in this systematic review use physiological markers as an objective measure to assess the effectiveness of VR interventions for ER. In this regard, the appraisal theory of Scherer allows us to explain the link between emotional states experienced by participants during interventions and their physiological responses [61,62]. In particular, this occurs due to the direct connections between stimulus evaluation check units and response modalities in the neuroendocrine system, autonomic nervous system, and somatic nervous system, independently from action tendencies [61]. A study by Villani and Riva (2008) [42] shows a significant reduction of anxiety, as well as a significant improvement of positive emotional states, in particular, relaxation, measured through physiological parameters that demonstrate good fluctuations of respiration rate, heart rate, and skin conductance. Tong et al. use a VR system that incorporates biofeedback mechanisms to support the learning of mindfulness practice [43]. This technological intervention may be an effective and long term non-pharmacological alternative to traditional pain management [43]. Furthermore, a biofeedback system has been used through the implementation of a belt for tracking the breathing rhythm of the participant during a VR relaxation-based game [48]. Biofeedback is an interesting mind-body therapy using electronic instruments to help individuals gain awareness and control over physiological processes [63]. Biofeedback is the process of measuring an individual's physiological activity such as brain activity, heart rate or breathing, and subsequently provide real-time information about this activity to the individual [64]. Through this feedback component, participants become more aware of their physiological activity, so they can learn how to gain control over it and improve their wellbeing [65,66].

In addition to the studies examined above, a neurofeedback (NFB) system had been used to enable the participants to regulate their brain activity, to enhance and recover emotional and cognitive capacity and to improve their underlying neurobiology [51]. Neurofeedback makes use of electroencephalography (EEG) biofeedback to guide participants in modifying their cortical activity, alter their states of consciousness, and affect cortically mediated physical and psychological functioning [67]. Novel forms of NFB, such as ones based on real-time functional magnetic resonance imaging (rtfMRI), hold a still vastly unexplored potential for complex technological applications, such as the currently discussed VR-based ER interventions [68].

3.5.2. Wellbeing Scales Outcomes

Given the primary objective of the present manuscript, in Table 6 we summarized an overview of the main wellbeing measures used in the evaluated studies. Several wellbeing measures were used as pre- and post-intervention measures: the State and Trait Anxiety Inventory (STAI) to evaluate anxiety levels [42,51]; the Beck Depression Inventory (BDI) to assess depression levels [51]; the Depressive, Anxiety and Stress Scales (DASS) to assess state anxiety and depression levels [47]; the Positive And Negative Affect Scale (PANAS) to measure the positive and negative affect through 10 positive and 10 negative moods/emotion adjectives [42,51]; the Coping Orientation to Problems Experienced Questionnaire (COPE) assessed the different strategies commonly activated in daily problem solving [42]. Results show a significant reduction of anxiety [42,47,51], and a significant improvement of positive emotional states [42,51]. Given that there is no universal measure of wellbeing, Konrad et al. include both hedonic (e.g., pleasure, satisfaction), and eudaimonic (e.g., meaning, personal growth) scales to triangulate different measurement perspectives: Subjective Happiness Scale, Satisfaction With Life Scale, and Ryff Scales of Psychological Wellbeing [41]. Moreover, positive intervention outcomes have been measured in both clinical and healthy populations with the Mindfulness Attention Awareness Scale (MASS), and the Satisfaction With Life Scale (SWLS) [44]. Tong et al., did not use a scale to monitor changes in mindfulness awareness, rather, they used the pain level and biofeedback data as an objective wellbeing measure [43]. However, there are no subjective wellbeing measures in that study [43]. Another interesting measure that has been used in the reviewed studies is the wellbeing scale of the Multidimensional Personality Questionnaire (MPQ) that underlined improvements in both groups with no significant difference between groups in social wellbeing outcomes [46].

Table 6. Wellbeing Measure Scales Description.

Scale	Description of Measure
State-Trait Anxiety Inventory (STAI)	A commonly used measure of trait and state anxiety. It can be used in clinical settings to diagnose anxiety and to distinguish it from depressive syndromes. Form Y, is its most popular version. It has 20 items for assessing trait anxiety and 20 for state anxiety. All items are rated on a 4-point scale (e.g., from "Almost Never" to "Almost Always"). Higher scores indicate greater anxiety.
Positive And Negative Affect Scale (PANAS)	A self-report questionnaire that consists of two 10-item scales to measure both positive and negative affect. Each item is rated on a 5-point scale of 1 (not at all) to 5 (very much).
Coping Orientation to Problems Experienced Questionnaire (COPE)	A self-reported questionnaire developed to assess a broad range of coping responses with a score on a 4-point scale (e.g., from "I usually don't do this at all" to "I usually do this a lot"). There are two main components to the COPE inventory: problem-focused coping and emotion-focused coping.
Mindfulness Attention Awareness Scale (MASS)	A 15-item scale designed to assess a core characteristic of mindfulness, namely, a receptive state of mind in which attention, informed by a sensitive awareness of what is occurring in the present, simply observes what is taking place.
Satisfaction With Life Scale (SWLS)	A 5-item scale designed to measure global cognitive judgments of one's life satisfaction (not a measure of either positive or negative affect). Participants indicate how much they agree or disagree with items on a 7-point scale (e.g., from 1 "strongly disagree" to 7 "strongly agree").
Subjective Happiness Scale	A 4-item self-report measure developed to assess an individual's overall happiness as measured through self-evaluation on a 7-point Likert-type scale.
Ryff Scales of Psychological Well-Being	A psychometric inventory in which respondents rate statements on a scale of 1 to 6 (e.g., from 1 "strong disagreement" to 6 "strong agreement"). It is based on six factors: autonomy, environmental mastery, personal growth, positive relations with others, purpose in life, and self-acceptance. Higher total scores indicate higher psychological well-being.
Wellbeing scale of the Multidimensional Personality Questionnaire (MPQ)	A personality test meant to measure personality that gives ratings on four broad traits: Positive Emotional Temperament, Negative Emotional Temperament, Constraint, and Absorption. High scorers on the specific wellbeing scale describe: having a cheerful happy disposition; feeling good about themselves; seeing a bright future ahead; being optimists; living interesting, exciting lives; enjoying the things they are doing.
Depressive, Anxiety and Stress Scales (DASS)	A 42-item self report instrument designed to measure the three related negative emotional states of depression, anxiety and tension/stress. The rating is based on a 0-3 point scale (e.g., from 0 "Did not apply to me at all" to 1 "Applied to me very much or most of the time").
Emotion Regulation Questionnaire (ERQ)	A 10-item scale designed to measure respondents' tendency to regulate their emotions in two ways: (1) Cognitive Reappraisal and (2) Expressive Suppression. Respondents answer each item on a 7-point Likert-type scale (e.g., from 1 "strongly disagree" to 7 "strongly agree").
University of Wales Institute of Science and Technology Mood Adjective Checklist (UWIST MACL scale)	A scale that measures self-reported mood in the dimensions of energetic arousal, tense arousal, and hedonic tone.

The Social Care-Related Quality of Life (SCRQoL) Scale was administered to track changes in the quality of life of older users to their daily routines, based on the outcome domains of social care-related quality of life identified in the Adult Social Care Outcomes Toolkit (ASCOT) [45]. Moreover, Weerdmester and colleagues selected the Trier Social Stress Test, a tool for investigating psychobiological stress responses [48]. Pre- and post-wellbeing assessments used the stress and hedonic tone measures based on the University of Wales Institute of Science and Technology Mood Adjective Checklist scale (UWIST MACL), to measure different stress-related states (nervous, tense, relaxed, calm), and the hedonic tone (happy, content, sad, sorry) [49,50].

4. Discussion

This review aimed to investigate how emotion regulation interventions using virtual reality (VR) systems can enhance the wellbeing in healthy and clinical adults and older adults, without presenting psychopathological conditions. In recent years there is a growing interest in the use of advanced technologies in supporting wellbeing and promoting health [34], following emerging evidence that technology can increase emotional, psychological and social wellbeing [69]. Technological approaches appear to be more advantageous in terms of intensity and duration of treatment, costs, and usefulness in the continuity-of-care [70,71]. Considering the multifaceted construct of wellbeing, in what follows, we strive to unpack the complex picture provided by the results of the hereby examined studies. This complexity emerges from the different functional aims of the studies, employed in pursuit of wellbeing enhancement. Three studies (27%) were developed for relaxation or following the Mindfulness-Based Stress Reduction (MBSR) protocol [42–44]; two studies (18%) used biofeedback or neurofeedback as peripherical technique for the regulation of physiological arousal [48,51]; one study (9%) used survey forms for a mood regulation and improvement wellbeing [41]; four studies (37%) intended to encourage a participants' behavioral and physical activation in order to enhance their subjective wellbeing through outdoor [49,50] or indoor activities [46,47]; one study (9%) aimed to enhance ICT-skills of elderly people in support of their social functioning and wellbeing [45].

In the examined studies, virtual reality has been used in different ways to promote wellbeing in healthy and clinical populations. Some authors used mindfulness as a non-pharmacological approach to manage participant's emotion regulation abilities and to enhance their wellbeing [43,44]. It has been demonstrated that immersive VR can be used as a powerful pain control technique to manage and modulate pain in healthy and clinical populations [72–75]. This is in line with the study conducted by Tong et al., in which the authors found that the use of an immersive VR combined with a biofeedback system, can be a helpful approach for managing chronic pain on a long-term scale [43].

In the present review, the combination of VR with biofeedback systems was particularly interesting. In recent years the development and use of game-based biofeedback to promote physical and mental wellbeing is growing [76–78]. An example, is the study of Weerdmester et al., in which an intervention based on the VR game "Deep", combined with a biofeedback system, highlighted positive and promising outcomes to help individuals cope with stress and anxiety [48]. This technique relies on visual and auditory feedback to guide participants in becoming more aware of their breathing and incentivizes the adoption of a more calm and relaxed breathing pattern [66,79,80]. Furthermore, promising results of game-based biofeedback have been found for emotion regulation and the treatment of stress and anxiety [81].

Neurofeedback (NFB) is a type of biofeedback which facilitates the real-time voluntary regulation of brain activity through a brain-computer interface [67,68]. Lorenzetti et al. [51] showed that NFB has promising effects on enhancing behavior, cognitive and emotional processes in healthy subjects. Performing exercises in an immersive VR environment is shown to decrease depression, anxiety, and stress [82]. Intervention outcomes, are in accordance with the literature, highlight a reduction in anxiety scales [42,47,51], and an improvement of positive emotional states [41,42,44,49–51].

For instance, Singh et al. [47] suggest that interactive VR games can be used as an exercise tool to improve psychological wellbeing and reaction time among adults with physical disabilities, for whom the use of technology may promote adherence, motivation, and participation in physical activity and exercise programs [46,47,49,50]. Positive results can also be seen in older adults, as demonstrated in the intervention program proposed by Baez et al. [46]. This intervention program was designed to promote physical activity in older adults, either in a group or in a home-based setting, showing equivalent health outcomes for both groups, but different results when considering adherence [46]. These interventions point out the importance of immediate wellbeing responses, in that, positive affect can be beneficial to long-term health [57,83]. A large number of studies have demonstrated the association of regular physical activity with positive outcomes for improving health and wellbeing conditions [84,85]. Moreover, home-based intervention programs aimed at promoting physical activity in older adults, either in a group or individually, have demonstrated the potential to improve health and functional performance [86]. The social wellbeing in the elderly is another issue that requires attention. Hasan et al. identified the complexity of this problem domain and engaged older adults through activities aimed at enhancing their ability to remain productive [45].

These results are an important outcome for wellbeing. The literature demonstrates that VR-based interventions are as effective as traditional ones in the treatment of different mental disorders, but can achieve positive outcomes in less time [87]. The difference between VR-based interventions and treatment as usual (TAU) remains to be clarified. Some of the currently examined studies, highlights a significative difference between the experimental and the control group [43,46], but further randomized controlled trials are required to achieve a better understanding of the effectiveness of VR compared to non-VR interventions.

Why are VR-based ER interventions important for wellbeing? To address this question, we have to consider several things. Emotions can be transient phenomena which emerge from momentary situational goals and subside with the short-term achievement of such goals [88]. Emotions can also derive from long-term goals and enduring values concerning health, close relationships, and important work-related projects [89]. Hence, knowing the specific antecedents of specific emotions is crucial to better understand the complexity and potential of technological ER interventions.

The present review underlines that virtual reality systems evoke a general positive emotion and could promote a healthy life [90] and an optimal state of functioning such as flow [91]. The sense of flow in VR is evoked when the user is immersed in a highly rewarding activity, accompanied by a high sense of control [92,93]. Flow can subsequently promote the feeling of immersion in the virtual environment [94]. Four studies among those investigated, have used an immersive VR system and have emphasized the importance of the immersion degree in a virtual environment. These studies used a head-mounted display (HMD) through which participants can be immersed in an interactive virtual reality scenario [19]. Through the HMD, the experimenter may provide different sensory input, as well as synchronize participants' movements with the generated virtual feedback (e.g., avatar movements, or reaching virtual objects) [20]. In order to increase the sense of immersion, feedback across different sensory channels is provided, such as, visual, acoustic, and tactile. This can also be achieved through the use of input tools such as trackers, gloves and other controllers, that allow to continuously monitor the position and movements of the users, and synchronize them with the VR interactions [32,95]. From a psychological point of view, at the basis of the feeling of immersion in VR is the sense of "presence," defined as the psychological sensation of "being there" in the virtual scene instead of in the physical and real environment [28,35,96]. The sense of presence has also been defined as the "feeling of being in a world that exists outside of self" [93,94]. The sense of presence in a virtual environment is given not only by the realism of its graphics but also by subjective characteristics, such as the potential of a given virtual scenario to elicit certain emotional responses [42]. In this way, a VR-based intervention can modify personal experiences by inspiring users to try new things [97] and allow them to modify habitual emotional responses to specific situations [7,98]. A VR system has the potential for a laboratory vs. everyday functioning rapprochement. Virtual environments allow to immerse participants in digitally recreated real-world activities which can be enacted in the safety of the laboratory setting [99]. The ability of VR systems to reproduce the complexity of real-life situations is a peculiar element for ER interventions. Due to this peculiarity, the user can be immersed in a complex virtual environment that requires the use of a complex set of ER strategies that form a dynamic pattern. An ER strategy does not have to be unique and universal, but in order to be useful and transferable to daily life, it must be adaptive and generalizable across situations [6,100]. In this sense, the use of virtual reality is promising, because it allows the user to learn complex ER strategies and, potentially, experience them in different environments similar to the real world. Lastly, a VR system provides experimental control and dynamic presentation of stimuli in ecologically valid scenarios [18,26,27,71,101]. This can be done by measuring the real-time cognitive, emotional, physiological and behavioural responses in a variety of life-like virtual situations [28].

The obtained results show that interventions using virtual reality systems allow people to change or improve their ER strategies. One such strategy is "situation selection" [4]. It is an antecedent-focused strategy that examines all the actions that we execute before the emotional response has become fully active and has modified behavioral or physiological responses and selects the best action [55]. Furthermore, technology can provide different options to appraise emotional stimuli, hence different cognitive appraisals pertaining to the same potential trigger and eventually different emotional responses [7]. In regard to patients with specific disorders, VR interventions can facilitate the approach to rehabilitation therapy by training more contextually adaptive ER strategies such as "reappraisal", which lead to better short-term affective, cognitive, and social consequences, compared to less adaptive strategies such as "suppression" [14]. VR systems improve patients ability to regulate the emotions that accompany their everyday experiences with their health condition [29]. Such targeted interventions that facilitate a reappraisal, can elicit a subsequent "cognitive change" [7,55]. This change refers to selecting what meaning people attach to the specific intervention [4,7]. External variables that are properties of the stimulus can influence the choice of emotion regulation strategy; in fact, reappraisal affordances, defined as the opportunities for re-interpretating a stimulus, which are inherent to the stimulus itself, can greatly shape such choices [13]. The personal meaning assigned to a specific situation is crucial for establishing habitual experiential, behavioral and physiological responses which repeat in that same situation [5].

One of the main aims of emotion regulation interventions is to modify the emotional responses of the subjects to one specific situation [102]. The outcome of the interventions reviewed in this article could be interpreted according to "The process model of emotion regulation" of Gross. According to Gross reappraisal-like processes could influence emotional responses. Efforts to down-regulate emotion through reappraisal alters the trajectory of the entire emotional response, leading to lesser experiential, behavioral, and physiological responses [7,102]. An example of this process is found in the studies that used Mindfulness-Based Stress Reduction (MBSR) protocol in virtual reality to minimize the negative emotional impact in patients with traumatic brain injuries [44] and the Meditative Virtual Walk for patients with chronic pain [43]. Mindfulness is a core skill of Dialectical Behavioral Therapy employed in the treatment of emotion dysregulation. It consists in observing, describing, and "allowing" emotions to flow without judging them or trying to inhibit them. Mindfulness is hypothesized to influence the habitual or automatic response to emotional behaviors and their associated appraisals. Hence, in comparison to Gross's Model, mindfulness may alter automatic response tendencies by altering the habitual approach or avoidance response to that of a non-judgemental awareness of the emerging emotions [103]. During the interventions the individual can reappraise the emotional responses to their health conditions. This type of reappraisal can also be seen in the intervention conducted by Konrad et al. [41]. In this intervention, subjects were asked to describe a negatively appraised past experience while in a positive mood. This was proven to update their emotional response to the past experience, encouraging the emergence of more adaptive perspectives [104,105]. Finally, virtual reality tools promote the sense of environmental mastery and the continued development of competence and self-knowledge, both in clinical and non-clinical populations [106,107]. However, there is a major difference between both populations. In a healthy population, an ER intervention can cultivate more adaptive, for daily life, ER strategies. In a clinical population, ER interventions are useful for increasing the patient's ability to handle their specific pathology.

In conclusion, the choice of wellbeing measures is essential to assessing the efficacy of the intervention. Humans do not act mechanically, but rather according to their subjective interpretation of the world. Hence, objective indicators alone may not be sufficient to hedge the several conceptualizations of wellbeing [108]. It is fundamental to gain knowledge about the subjective interpretations of emotional states. This can happen by directly asking people about their emotions, perceptions, and evaluations [108]. Currently, wellbeing is not a clearly defined concept and the present review shows that several ways to measure wellbeing exist [36]. Despite that difficulty, it is important for studies to clarify the theoretical framework of wellbeing in which the intervention intends to operate. The choice of the theoretical framework can better guide the design of the intervention and the choice of more adequate wellbeing measures.

5. Conclusions

In conclusion, the results of this systematic review show that technology can improve the ability of people to handle emotionally-rich life situations by training more contextually adaptive emotion regulation strategies.

The use of virtual reality in this sense is promising because it allows the user to learn complex ER strategies in the context of life-like digital environments. VR interventions can modify the user's ER by inspiring new actions, allowing for the modification of the emotional response across a reappraisal of emotional stimuli, and subsequently, memorizing the re-evaluated experience. Finally, virtual reality is a tool that fosters a sense of environmental mastery, and, a feeling of personal growth and autonomy.

The literature in this field is going in an interesting direction, and we recommend some future steps based on the findings of this systematic review, for future design, implementation, and evaluation of VR-based ER interventions in healthy adults and older adults. The results of this systematic review underly the importance of an appropriate assessment and highlight the positive effects of assessing both subjective and objective measures in future studies to fully evaluate the efficacy of VR interventions for ER. The results from both subjective and objective measures will provide an overall and complete frame of the efficacy of VR interventions for ER. Finally, future research should aim to investigate the underlying mechanisms and factors that may contribute to the effectiveness of biofeedback systems when using VR interventions for ER in order to maximize their positive therapeutic outcomes.

Author Contributions: Conceptualization O.R. and J.I.M.; methodology, J.I.M. and M.M.-G.; studies selection, J.I.M., M.M.-G. and M.M.; data curation, J.I.M., M.M.-G. and M.M.; writing—original draft preparation, J.I.M.; writing—review and editing, O.R., M.M.-G., B.D., C.M.C. and P.A.M.; final editing of English P.A.M.; supervision, O.R. and F.M.; project management F.M. All authors were involved in a critical revision of the manuscript for important intellectual content. All the authors approved the final version of the manuscript for submission. All authors have read and agreed to the published version of the manuscript.

References

1. Scherer, K.R. Emotions are emergent processes: They require a dynamic computational architecture. *Philos. Trans. R. Soc. B Biol. Sci.* **2009**, *364*, 3459–3474. [CrossRef] [PubMed]
2. Leahy, R.; Tirch, D.; Napolitano, L. Why is emotion regulation important? *Psychother. Aust.* **2012**, *19*, 68–81.
3. Beck, A.T. *Cognitive Therapy and the Emotional Disorders*, 1st ed.; International Universities Press: Madison, CT, USA, 1976.
4. Gross, J.J. The Emerging Field of Emotion Regulation: An Integrative Review. *Rev. Gen. Psychol.* **1998**, *2*, 271–299. [CrossRef]
5. Gross, J.J. Emotion regulation: Affective, cognitive, and social consequences. *Psychophysiology* **2002**, *39*, 281–291. [CrossRef] [PubMed]
6. Gross, J.J. Emotion regulation: Current status and future prospects. *Psychol. Inq.* **2015**, *26*, 1–26. [CrossRef]
7. Gross, J.J.; Thompson, R.A. Emotion Regulation: Conceptual Foundations. In *Handbook of Emotion Regulation*; The Guilford Press: New York, NY, USA, 2007; pp. 3–24.
8. Cole, P.M.; Michel, M.K.; Teti, L.O.D. The Development of Emotion Regulation and Dysregulation: A Clinical Perspective. *Monogr. Soc. Res. Child Dev. Dev. Emot. Regul. Biol. Behav. Consid.* **1994**, *59*, 73–100. [CrossRef]
9. Lazarus, R.S.; Folkman, S. *Stress, Appraisal, and Coping*; Springer Publishing Company: Berlin/Heidelberg, Germany, 1984.
10. Thompson, R.A.; Calkins, S.D. The double-edged sword: Emotional regulation for children at risk. *Dev. Psychopathol.* **1996**, *8*, 163–182. [CrossRef]
11. Parker, J.D.A.; Endler, N.S. Coping and defense: A historical overview. In *Handbook of Coping: Theory, Research, Applications*; John Wiley & Sons: Oxford, UK, 1996; pp. 3–23.
12. Folkman, S.; Lazarus, R.S. Coping as a Mediator of Emotion. *J. Personal. Soc. Psychol.* **1988**, *54*, 466–475. [CrossRef]
13. Suri, G.; Sheppes, G.; Young, G.; Abraham, D.; McRae, K.; Gross, J.J. Emotion regulation choice: The role of environmental affordances. *Cogn. Emot.* **2018**, *32*, 963–971. [CrossRef]
14. John, O.P.; Gross, J.J. Healthy and unhealthy emotion regulation: Personality processes, individual differences, and life span development. *J. Personal.* **2004**, *72*, 1301–1334. [CrossRef]
15. Greenberg, L.S. *Emotion-Focused Therapy*; Theories of Psychotherapy; American Psychological Association: Worcester, MA, USA, 2011.
16. Lucas, R.E.; Diener, E. Subjective Well-Being. In *Handbook of Emotion*; T.G. Press: New York, NY, USA, 2008; pp. 471–484.

17. Diener, E.; Suh, E.M.; Lucas, R.E.; Smith, H.L. Subjective Well-Being: Three Decades of Progress. *Psychol. Bull.* **1999**, *125*, 276–302. [CrossRef]
18. Montana, J.I.; Tuena, C.; Serino, S.; Cipresso, P.; Riva, G. Neurorehabilitation of Spatial Memory Using Virtual Environments: A Systematic Review. *J. Clin. Med.* **2019**, *8*, 1516. [CrossRef] [PubMed]
19. Mishkind, M.C.; Norr, A.M.; Katz, A.C.; Reger, G.M. Review of Virtual Reality Treatment in Psychiatry: Evidence Versus Current Diffusion and Use. *Curr. Psychiatry Rep.* **2017**, *19*. [CrossRef] [PubMed]
20. Clus, D.; Larsen, M.E.; Lemey, C.; Berrouiguet, S. The use of virtual reality in patients with eating disorders: Systematic review. *J. Med. Internet Res.* **2018**, *20*, 1–9. [CrossRef]
21. Wiederhold, B.K.; Riva, G.; Gutiérrez-Maldonado, J. Virtual Reality in the Assessment and Treatment of Weight-Related Disorders. *Cyberpsychol. Behav. Soc. Netw.* **2016**, *19*, 67–73. [CrossRef]
22. Rus-Calafell, M.; Garety, P.; Sason, E.; Craig, T.J.K.; Valmaggia, L.R. Virtual reality in the assessment and treatment of psychosis: A systematic review of its utility, acceptability and effectiveness. *Psychol. Med.* **2018**, *48*, 362–391. [CrossRef]
23. Riva, G.; Gaggioli, A.; Villani, D.; Preziosa, A.; Morganti, F.; Corsi, R.; Faletti, G.; Vezzadini, L. NeuroVR: An open source virtual reality platform for clinical psychology and behavioral neurosciences. *Stud. Health Technol. Inf.* **2007**, *125*, 394–399.
24. Riches, S.; Garety, P.; Rus-Calafell, M.; Stahl, D.; Evans, C.; Sarras, N.; Yeboah, K.; Valmaggia, L. Using Virtual Reality to Assess Associations Between Paranoid Ideation and Components of Social Performance: A Pilot Validation Study. *Cyberpsychol. Behav. Soc. Netw.* **2019**, *22*, 51–59. [CrossRef]
25. Valmaggia, L. The use of virtual reality in psychosis research and treatment. *World Psychiatry* **2017**, *16*, 245–246. [CrossRef]
26. Parsons, T.D.; Carlew, A.R.; Magtoto, J.; Stonecipher, K. The potential of function-led virtual environments for ecologically valid measures of executive function in experimental and clinical neuropsychology. *Neuropsychol. Rehabil.* **2017**, *27*, 777–807. [CrossRef]
27. Serino, S.; Baglio, F.; Rossetto, F.; Realdon, O.; Cipresso, P.; Parsons, T.D.; Cappellini, G.; Mantovani, F.; De Leo, G.; Nemni, R.; et al. Picture Interpretation Test (PIT) 360°: An Innovative Measure of Executive Functions. *Sci. Rep.* **2017**, *7*, 1–10. [CrossRef] [PubMed]
28. Bohil, C.J.; Alicea, B.; Biocca, F.A. Virtual reality in neuroscience research and therapy. *Nat. Rev. Neurosci.* **2011**, *12*. [CrossRef]
29. Colombo, D.; Fernández-álvarez, J.; Palacios, A.G.; Cipresso, P.; Botella, C.; Riva, G. New technologies for the understanding, assessment, and intervention of emotion regulation. *Front. Psychol.* **2019**, *10*. [CrossRef]
30. Villani, D.; Carissoli, C.; Triberti, S.; Marchetti, A.; Gilli, G.; Riva, G. Videogames for Emotion Regulation: A Systematic Review. *Games Health J.* **2018**, *7*, 85–99. [CrossRef] [PubMed]
31. Kompus, K. Virtual-reality-assisted therapy in patients with psychosis Title. *Lancet Psychiatry* **2018**, *5*, 189–191. [CrossRef]
32. Riva, G.; Baños, R.M.; Botella, C.; Mantovani, F.; Gaggioli, A. Transforming experience: The potential of augmented reality and virtual reality for enhancing personal and clinical change. *Front. Psychiatry* **2016**, *7*, 1–14. [CrossRef] [PubMed]
33. Baños, R.M.; Etchemendy, E.; Mira, A.; Riva, G.; Gaggioli, A.; Botella, C. Online positive interventions to promote well-being and resilience in the adolescent population: A narrative review. *Front. Psychiatry* **2017**, *8*. [CrossRef]
34. Schek, E.J.; Mantovani, F.; Realdon, O.; Dias, J.; Paiva, A.; Schramm-Yavin, R.; Pat-Horenczyk, S. Positive Technologies for Promoting Emotion Regulation Abilities in Adolescents. In *Lecture Notes of the Institute for Computer Sciences, Social Informatics and Telecommunications Engineering*; Springer: Berlin/Heidelberg, Germany, 2016; pp. 169–174.
35. Sanchez-Vives, M.V.; Slater, M. Opinion: From presence to consciousness through virtual reality. *Nat. Rev. Neurosci.* **2005**, *6*, 332–339. [CrossRef]
36. Feller, S.C.; Castillo, E.G.; Greenberg, J.M.; Abascal, P.; Van Horn, R.; Wells, K.B.; University of California, Los Angeles Community Translational Science Team. Emotional well-being and public health: Proposal for a model national initiative. *Public Health Rep.* **2018**, *133*, 136–141. [CrossRef]
37. Vik, M.H. Measuring subjective well-being for policy purposes: The example of well-being indicators in the WHO 'Health 2020' framework. *J. Scand. Public Health* **2018**, *46*, 279–286. [CrossRef]
38. Moher, D.; Liberati, A.; Tetzlaff, J.; Altman, D.G.; Grp, P. Preferred Reporting Items for Systematic Reviews

and Meta-Analyses: The PRISMA Statement (Reprinted from Annals of Internal Medicine). *Phys. Ther.* **2009**, *89*, 873–880. [CrossRef] [PubMed]

39. Higgins, J.; Green, S. *Cochrane Handbook for Systematic Reviews of Interventions*; Version 5; John Wiley & Sons: Hoboken, NJ, USA, 2011.
40. Von Elm, E.; Altman, D.G.; Egger, M.; Pocock, S.J.; Gøtzsche, P.C.; Vandenbroucke, J.P. The Strengthening the Reporting of Observational Studies in Epidemiology (STROBE) statement: Guidelines for reporting observational studies. *Lancet* **2007**, *370*, 1453–1457. [CrossRef]
41. Konrad, A.; Tucker, S.; Crane, J.; Whittaker, S. Technology and Reflection: Mood and Memory Mechanisms for Well-Being. *Psychol. Well Being* **2016**, *6*. [CrossRef] [PubMed]
42. Villani, D.; Riva, G. Presence and relaxation: A preliminary controlled study. *PsychNol. J.* **2008**, *6*, 7–26.
43. Tong, X.; Gromala, D.; Choo, A.; Amin, A.; Shaw, C. The Virtual Meditative Walk: An Immersive Virtual Environment for Pain Self-modulation Through Mindfulness-Based Stress Reduction Meditation. In Proceedings of the 7th International Conference, VAMR 2015, Held as Part of HCI International 2015, Los Angeles, CA, USA, 2–7 August 2015; Lecture Notes in Computer Science. Springer Int. Publ.: Cham, Switzerland, 2015; pp. 388–397. [CrossRef]
44. Cikajlo, I.; Čižman-Štaba, U.; Vrhovac, S.; Larkin, F.; Roddy, M. Recovr: Realising collaborative virtual reality for wellbeing and self-healing. In Proceedings of the 3rd IASTED International Conference Telehealth Assistive Technology TAT 2016, Zurich, Switzerland, 5–7 October 2016; pp. 11–17. [CrossRef]
45. Hasan, H.; Linger, H. Enhancing the wellbeing of the elderly: Social use of digital technologies in aged care. *Educ. Gerontol.* **2016**, *42*, 749–757. [CrossRef]
46. Baez, M.; Far, I.K.; Ibarra, F.; Ferron, M.; Didino, D.; Casati, F. Effects of online group exercises for older adults on physical, psychological and social wellbeing: A pilot trial Marcos. *J. Chem. Inf. Model.* **2017**, *53*, 1689–1699. [CrossRef]
47. Singh, D.K.A.; Rahman, N.N.A.; Seffiyah, R.; Chang, S.Y.; Zainura, A.K.; Aida, S.R.; Rajwinder, K.H.S. Impact of virtual reality games on psychological well-being and upper limb performance in adults with physical disabilities: A pilot study. *Med. J. Malays.* **2017**, *72*, 119–121.
48. Weerdmeester, J.; van Rooij, M.; Harris, O.; Smit, N.; Engels, R.C.M.E.; Granic, I. Exploring the role of self-efficacy in biofeedback video games. In Proceedings of the CHI Play 2017 Ext. Abstr.—Ext. Abstr. Publ. Annu. Symp. Comput. Interact. Play, Amsterdam, The Netherlands, 15–18 October 2017; pp. 453–461. [CrossRef]
49. Bornioli, A. Psychological Wellbeing Benefits of Simulated Exposure to Five Urban Settings: An Experimental Study from the Pedestrian's Perspective. *Transp. Res. Part A Policy Pract.* **2019**, *123*, 200–215. [CrossRef]
50. Bornioli, A.; Parkhurst, G.; Morgan, P.L. Affective experiences of built environments and the promotion of urban walking. *Transp. Res. Part. A Policy Pract.* **2019**, *123*, 200–215. [CrossRef]
51. Lorenzetti, V.; Bruno, M.; Rodrigo, B.; Chao, S.; Murat, Y.; Carlos, J.T.-C.; Jorge, M. Emotion regulation using virtual environments and real-time fMRI neurofeedback. *Front. Neurol.* **2018**, *9*, 1–15. [CrossRef]
52. Turk, C.S.; Carstensen, L.L. Emotion Regulation and Aging. In *Handbook of Emotion Regulation*; Guilford: New York, NY, USA, 2007; pp. 307–325.
53. Gross, J.J.; Carstensen, L.L.; Pasupathi, M.; Tsai, J.; Skorpen, C.G.; Hsu, A.Y.C. Emotion and aging: Experience, expression, and control. *Psychol. Aging* **1997**, *12*, 590–599. [CrossRef] [PubMed]
54. Cacioppo, J.T.; Berntson, G.G.; Klein, D.J.; Poehlmann, K.M. The psychophysiology of emotion across the lifespan. *Annu. Rev. Gerontol. Geriatr.* **1998**, *17*, 27–65.
55. Gross, J.J. Antecedent- and Response-Focused Emotion Regulation: Divergent Consequences for Experience, Expression, and Physiology. *J. Personal. Soc. Psychol.* **1998**, *74*, 224–237. [CrossRef]
56. Singh, V.; Padmanabhan, B.; de Vreede, T.; de Vreede, G.-J.; Andel, S.; Spector, P.E.; Benfield, S.; Aslami, A. A content engagement score for online learning platforms. In Proceedings of the Fifth Annual ACM Conference Learning Scale—L@S '18, London, UK, 26–28 June 2018; pp. 1–4. [CrossRef]
57. Consedine, N.S.; Moskowitz, J.T. The role of discrete emotions in health outcomes: A critical review. *Appl. Prev. Psychol.* **2007**, *12*, 59–75. [CrossRef]
58. Baños, R.M.; Castilla, D.; Etchemendy, E.; Garcia-Palacios, A. Positive mood induction procedures for virtual environments designed for elderly people. *Interact. Comput.* **2012**, *24*, 131–138. [CrossRef]
59. Choi, N.G.; DiNitto, D.M. Internet Use Among Older Adults: Association with Health Needs, Psychological Capital, and Social Capital. *J. Med. Internet Res.* **2013**, *15*, e97. [CrossRef]

60. Winstead, V.; Yost, E.A.; Cotten, S.R.; Berkowsky, R.W.; Anderson, W.A. The Impact of Activity Interventions on the Well-Being of Older Adults in Continuing Care Com. *J. Appl. Gerontol.* **2014**, *33*, 888–911. [CrossRef]
61. Sander, D.; Grandjean, D.; Scherer, K.R. A systems approach to appraisal mechanisms in emotion. *Neural Netw.* **2005**, *18*, 317–352. [CrossRef]
62. Scherer, K.R.; Schorr, A.; Johnstone, T. Appraisal Processes in Emotion: Theory, Methods, Research. In *Handbook of Affective Sciences*; Oxford University Press: Oxford, UK, 2003; pp. 92–120.
63. Frank, D.L.; Khorshid, L.; Kiffer, J.; Moravec, C.S.; McKee Michael, G. Biofeedback in medicine: Who, when, why and how? *Mental Health in Family Medicine.* **2010**, *7*, 85–91.
64. Wheat, A.L.; Larkin, K.T. Biofeedback of heart rate variability and related physiology: A critical review. *Appl. Psychophysiol. Biofeedback* **2010**, *35*, 229–242. [CrossRef]
65. Gevirtz, R. The Promise of Heart Rate Variability Biofeedback: Evidence-Based Applications. *Biofeedback* **2013**, *41*, 110–120. [CrossRef]
66. Gilbert, C.; Moss, D. Biofeedback and Biological Monitoring. In *Handbook of Mind-Body Medicine for Primary Care: Behavioral and Physiological Tools*; Sage Publications: Thousand Oaks, CA, USA, 2003; pp. 109–122.
67. La Vaque, T.J. Neurofeedback, Neurotherapy, and Quantitative EEG. In *Handbook of Mind-Body Medicine for Primary Care*; Sage Publications: Thousand Oaks, CA, USA, 2003; pp. 123–136.
68. Yucha, C.B.; Montgomery, D. *Evidence-Based Practice in Biofeedback and Neurofeedback*; Association for Applied Psychophysiology and Biofeedback: Wheat Ridge, CO, USA, 2008.
69. Serino, S.; Cipresso, P.; Gaggioli, A.; Riva, G. The potential of pervasive sensors and computing for positive technology. In *Pervasive and Mobile Sensing and Computing for Healthcare: Smart Sensors, Measurement and Instrumentation*; Mukhopadhyay, S.C., Postolache, O.A., Eds.; Springer: New York, NY, USA, 2013.
70. Realdon, O.; Rossetto, F.; Nalin, M.; Baroni, I.; Cabinio, M.; Fioravanti, R.; Saibene, F.L.; Alberoni, M.; Mantovani, F.; Romano, M.; et al. Technology-enhanced multi-domain at home continuum of care program with respect to usual care for people with cognitive impairment: The Ability- TelerehABILITation study protocol for a randomized controlled trial. *BMC Psychiatry* **2016**, 1–9. [CrossRef] [PubMed]
71. Realdon, O.; Rossetto, F.; Nalin, M.; Baroni, I.; Romano, M.; Catania, F.; Frontini, D.; Mancastroppa, S.; Alberoni, M.; Zurloni, V.; et al. The Technology-Enhanced Ability Continuum-of-Care Home Program. for People with Cognitive Disorders: Concept Design and Scenario of Use. In Proceedings of the International Symposium on Pervasive Computing Paradigms for Mental Health, Buenos Aires, Argentina, 23–24 April 2018.
72. Matamala-Gomez, M.; Donegan, T.; Bottiroli, S.; Sandrini, G.; Sanchez-Vives, M.V.; Tassorelli, C. Immersive virtual reality and virtual embodiment for pain relief. *Front. Hum. Neurosci.* **2019**, *13*, 279. [CrossRef] [PubMed]
73. Matamala-Gomez, M.; Gonzalez, A.M.D.; Slater, M.; Sanchez-Vives, M.V. Decreasing Pain Ratings in Chronic Arm Pain Through Changing a Virtual Body: Different Strategies for Different Pain Types. *J. Pain* **2019**, *20*. [CrossRef] [PubMed]
74. Hoffman, H.G.; Patterson, D.R.; Carrougher, G.J.; Sharar, S.R. Effectiveness of virtual reality-based pain control with multiple treatments. *Clin. J. Pain* **2001**, *17*, 229–235. [CrossRef] [PubMed]
75. Baer, R.A. Mindfulness training as a clinical intervention: A conceptual and empirical review. *Clin. Psychol. Pract.* **2003**, *10*, 125–143. [CrossRef]
76. Bingham, P.; Bates, J.H.T.; Thompson-Figueroa, T.; Lahiri, J. A breath biofeedback computer game for children with cystic fibrosis. *Clin. Paediatr.* **2010**, *49*, 337–342. [CrossRef]
77. Fernández-Aranda, F.; Jiménez-Murcia, S.; Penelo, E. Video games as a complementary therapy tool in mental disorders: PlayMancer, a European multicentre study. *J. Ment. Health* **2012**, *21*, 364–374. [CrossRef]
78. Lobel, A.; Gotsis, M.; Reynolds, E.; Annetta, M.; Engels, I.; Granic, R.C.M.E. Designing and utilizing biofeedback games for emotion regulation: The case of nevermind. In Proceedings of the 2016 CHI Conference Extended Abst, San Jose, CA, USA, 7–12 May 2016.
79. Schwartz, M.S. *Biofeedback: A Practitioner's Guide*, 2nd ed.; The Guilford Press: New York, NY, USA, 1995.
80. Peper, E.; Harvey, R.; Takebayashi, N. Biofeedback an evidence based approach inclinical practice. *Jpn. J. Biofeedback Res.* **2009**, *36*, 3–10.
81. Pham, Q.; Khatib, Y.; Fox, S.; Green, T. Feasibility and efficacy of an mHealth game for managing anxiety: 'Flowy' randomized controlled pilot trial and design evaluation. *Games Health J.* **2016**, *5*, 50–67. [CrossRef]
82. Tyson, S.; Selley, A. A content analysis of physiotherapy for postural control in people with stroke: An observational study. *Disabil. Rehabil.* **2006**, *28*, 865–872. [CrossRef] [PubMed]

83. Ryan, R.M.; Deci, E.L. On happiness and human potentials: A review of research on hedonic and eudaimonic well-being. *Annu. Rev. Psychol.* **2001**, *52*, 141–166. [CrossRef] [PubMed]
84. Thibaud, M.; Bloch, F.; Tournoux-Facon, C.; Brèque, C.; Rigaud, A.S.; Dugué, B.; Kemoun, G. Impact of physical activity and sedentary behaviour on fall risks in older people: A systematic review and meta-analysis of observational studies. *Eur. Rev. Aging Phys. Act.* **2012**, *9*, 5–15. [CrossRef]
85. Stuart, M.; Chard, S.; Benvenuti, F.; Steinwachs, S. Community Exercise: A Vital Component to Healthy Aging. *Healthcarepapers* **2009**, *10*, 23–28. [CrossRef] [PubMed]
86. El Khoury, F. The effect of fall prevention exercise programmes on fall induced injuries in community dwelling older adults: Systematic review and meta-analysis of randomised controlled trials. *BMJ Res.* **2013**. [CrossRef]
87. Mohr, D.C.; Cheung, K.; Schueller, S.M.; Brown, H.; Duan, N. Continuous Evaluation of Evolving Behavioral Intervention Technologies. *Am. J. Prev. Med.* **2013**, *45*, 1–11. [CrossRef] [PubMed]
88. Clore, G. Why emotions vary in intensity. In *The Nature of Emotion: Fundamental Questions*; Ekman, P., Davidson, R.J., Eds.; Oxford University Press: Oxford, UK, 1994; pp. 386–393.
89. Richards, J.M.; Gross, J.J. Emotion regulation and memory: The cognitive costs of keeping one's cool. *J. Personal. Soc. Psychol.* **2000**, *79*, 410–424. [CrossRef]
90. Granic, I.; Lobel, A.; Engels, R.C.M.E. The Benefits of Playing Video Games. *Am. Psychol.* **2014**, *69*, 66–78. [CrossRef]
91. Sherry, J.L. Flow and Media Enjoyment. *Commun. Theory* **2004**, *14*, 328–347. [CrossRef]
92. Nakamura, J.; Csikszentmihalyi, M. The Concept of Flow. In *Oxford Handbook of Positive Psychology*; Snyder, U., Ed.; Oxford University Press: Oxford, UK, 2009; pp. 89–105.
93. Riva, G.; Castelnuovo, G.; Mantovani, F. Transformation of flow in rehabilitation: The role of advanced communication technologies. *Behav. Res. Methods* **2006**, *38*, 237–244. [CrossRef]
94. Riva, G.; Waterworth, J.A.; Waterworth, E.L. The layers of presence: A bio-cultural approach to understanding presence in natural and mediated environments. *Cyberpsychol. Behav. Soc. Netw.* **2004**, *7*, 405–419. [CrossRef] [PubMed]
95. Riva, G. From Virtual to Real Body. *J. Cyberther. Rehabil.* **2008**, *1*, 7–22.
96. Steuer, J. Defining Virtual Reality: Characteristics Determining Telepresence. *J. Commun.* **1992**, *42*, 73–94. [CrossRef]
97. Valmaggia, L.R.; Latifa, L.; Kempton, M.J.; Rus-Calafell, M. Virtual reality in the psychological treatment for mental health problems: An systematic review of recent evidence. *Psychiatry Res.* **2016**, *236*, 189–195. [CrossRef] [PubMed]
98. Slater, M.; Steed, A. Depth of Presence in Virtual Environments. *Presence Teleoper. Virtual Environ.* **1994**. [CrossRef]
99. Parsons, T.D. Virtual Reality for Enhanced Ecological Validity and Experimental Control in the Clinical, Affective and Social Neurosciences. *Front. Hum. Neurosci.* **2015**, *9*, 1–19. [CrossRef]
100. Gross, J.J. Emotion regulation: Conceptual and empirical foundations. In *Handbook of emotion regulation*; Gross, J.J., Ed.; Guilford Press: New York, NY, USA, 2014; pp. 3–20.
101. Realdon, O.; Serino, S.; Savazzi, F.; Rossetto, F.; Cipresso, P.; Parsons, T.D.; Cappellini, G.; Mantovani, F.; Mendozzi, L.; Nemni, R.; et al. An ecological measure to screen executive functioning in MS: The Picture Interpretation Test (PIT). *Sci. Rep.* **2019**, 1–8. [CrossRef]
102. Ochsner, K.N.; Gross, J.J. The Neural Architecture of Emotion Regulation. In *Handbook of Emotion Regulation*; Guilford: New York, NY, USA, 2007; pp. 87–109.
103. Linehan, M.M.; Bohus, M.; Lynch, T.R. Dialectical Behavior Therapy for Pervasive Emotion Dysregulation: Theoretical and Practical Underpinnings. In *Handbook of Emotion Regulation*; Guilford: New York, NY, USA, 2007; pp. 581–606.
104. Boals, A.; Klein, K. Word Use in Emotional Narratives about Failed Romantic Relationships and Subsequent Mental Health. *J. Lang. Soc. Psychol.* **2005**, *24*, 252–268. [CrossRef]
105. Petrie, K.J.; Booth, R.J.; Pennebaker, J.W. The Immunological Effects of Thought Suppression. *J. Personal. Soc. Psychol.* **1998**, *75*, 1264–1272. [CrossRef]

106. Ryff, C.D.; Singer, B.H.; Love, G.D. Positive health: Connecting well-being with biology. *Philos. Trans. R. Soc. B Biol. Sci.* **2004**, *359*, 1383–1394. [CrossRef]
107. Ryff, C.D. Psychological Well-Being in Adult Life. *Curr. Dir. Psychol. Sci.* **1995**, *4*, 99–104. [CrossRef]
108. Kroll, C.; Kroll, C.; Delhey, J. A Happy Nation? Opportunities and Challenges of Using Subjective Indicators in Policymaking. *Soc. Indic. Res.* **2013**, *114*, 13–28. [CrossRef]

9

Profiling Dating Apps Users: Sociodemographic and Personality Characteristics

Ángel Castro [1], Juan Ramón Barrada [1,*], Pedro J. Ramos-Villagrasa [2] and Elena Fernández-del-Río [2]

1 Facultad de Ciencias Sociales y Humanas. Universidad de Zaragoza. Calle Atarazanas, 4. 44003 Teruel, Spain; castroa@unizar.es

2 Facultad de Ciencias Sociales y del Trabajo. Universidad de Zaragoza. Calle Violante de Hungría, 23. 50009 Zaragoza, Spain; pjramos@unizar.es (P.J.R.-V.); elenario@unizar.es (E.F.-d.-R.)

* Correspondence: barrada@unizar.es

Abstract: The development of new technologies, the expansion of the Internet, and the emergence of dating apps (e.g., Tinder, Grindr) in recent years have changed the way to meet and approach potential romantic and/or sexual partners. The recent phenomenon has led to some gaps in the literature on individual differences (sociodemographic variables and personality traits) between users (previous and current users) and non-users of dating apps. Thus, the aim of this study was to analyze the relationship between using dating apps, sociodemographics (gender, age, sexual orientation, and relationship status), and bright and dark personality traits. Participants were 1705 university students (70% women, 30% men), aged between 18 and 26 ($M = 20.60$, $SD = 2.09$), who completed several online questionnaires. Through multinomial logistic regression analyses, it was found that men, older youth, and members of sexual minorities were more likely to be current and previous dating apps users. Being single and higher scores in open-mindedness were associated with higher probability to be current dating apps user. The dark personality showed no predictive ability. The discussion highlights the usefulness of knowing and considering the sociodemographic background and the characteristics of personality patterns in the design and implementation of preventive and promotion programs of healthy romantic and sexual relationships to improve people's better health and well-being.

Keywords: dating apps; Tinder; Grindr; Big Five; Dark Core; university students

---

1. Introduction

The development of new technologies has changed people's lives, affecting both their intimacy and how they relate to others. Over the past two decades, the successive popularization of the Internet and smartphone use has changed the way potential couples approach each other for millions of people worldwide. More recently, the use of location-based real-time dating apps has been extended (e.g., Tinder, Grindr), designed to maximize social, romantic, and sexual connections between strangers who are geographically nearby [1–4].

The emergence and development of dating apps have attracted considerable research interest over the past five years. Usage patterns and user profiles have both been studied, as well as the advantages and disadvantages they may have for the mental and relational health of those who use them [5,6]. Among the advantages, their portability, availability, locatability, and multimediality [2] have been highlighted, aspects that facilitate the immediate interaction with possible partners. However, there have also been risks associated with the use of apps, which can affect both mental (e.g., problematic use, related to dark personality patterns) [7] and relational health (e.g., infidelity, performance of risky behaviors, sexual victimization) [5,8].

Previous literature has confirmed that the use of dating apps is associated with different sociodemographic and personality factors. Concerning sex, it has traditionally been considered that men used dating apps more [9]. Currently, it is considered that, although men use them more and more intensely, women use them more selectively and effectively, achieving a greater number of encounters with other users [3,4]. Regarding age, previous studies have mostly evaluated the use of dating apps in college youth aged 18 to 24 [3]. For instance, Shapiro et al. [10] found that 40% of undergraduate students, aged 18–26, used Tinder. However, various investigations suggest that the average age of users could be somewhat older, even up to 31 [1,2,9]. Thus, we expected to find a direct relationship between the age of college students and the use of dating apps.

Sexual orientation also influences the use of these applications. Several studies have found greater use in people of sexual minorities than among heterosexuals [11,12]. Further, it has been emphasized that being able to contact and communicate online can be particularly useful for people of these minorities who have trouble expressing their sexuality and/or finding a partner [13]. Finally, and although there is a stereotype that dating apps are used by singles, several studies have found that a remarkable percentage of users, between 18% and 25%, had a stable partner [4,14]. Nevertheless, it seems that these people use dating apps for different purposes than singles' reasons (e.g., infidelity) [15].

Personality traits play a key role in understanding sexuality and have been essential in the design of sexual health preventive and promotion programs [16]. In the psychosocial area, the personality model that has shown a stronger relationship to a variety of important life outcomes is the five-factor model or the Big Five [17], a taxonomy of five personality traits whose labels can differ according to the authors' denomination (Neuroticism or Negative Emotionality, Extraversion, Openness to Experience or Open-Mindedness, Agreeableness, and Conscientiousness). Thus, for example, the relationship between the Big Five and certain areas of sexuality such as the performance of risky behaviors, sexual functioning, or sexual assault has been studied [16]. However, there is hardly any research to analyze the phenomenon of dating apps in relation to the Big Five traits. The only reference is the study of Timmermans and De Caluwé [18], who found that young single dating apps users scored higher in Extraversion and Open-Mindedness than non-users and obtained lower scores in Conscientiousness.

In recent years, in parallel with the traditional Big Five paradigm, other proposals have emerged focused on the malevolent side of personality, which may be of special interest for the understanding of sexual phenomena [7]. Although some authors defend a multidimensional approach of these socially aversive personality traits (narcissism, Machiavellianism, psychopathy, and sadism), recent evidence about a single common factor, the so-called "Dark Core" [19], based on theoretical and methodological reasons, has gained momentum [19–23]. All of these traits share callousness [24] and the tendency to interpersonal exploitativeness [25]. Previous research found that this dark side of personality was associated with poor quality relationships [26]. Regarding mating behavior, it has been found that people with higher scores in dark personality traits had a less restrictive sociosexuality, more sexual partners, and a greater orientation to short-term mating and casual sexual relationships [27,28]. Concerning the use of dating apps and dark personality, the main conclusions of the few available studies can be summarized in [7,15]: (1) the role of the Dark Core as a single dimension has not been evaluated, but instead, the relationships with the different dark personality traits have been explored; (2) the associations are mediated by the reasons for using the applications, which leads to different relationships depending on the different nature of the personality traits; (3) despite having found partial associations with some patterns (i.e., Machiavellianism), the role of psychopathy has been highlighted, finding higher scores in this personality trait among dating app users than among non-users.

Perhaps due to the recent expansion of the dating apps phenomenon, the existing literature has some gaps. When analyzing the uses and users of dating apps, people who used them at some point and no longer use them have not been included in the same study, nor have they been compared to current users (at the time of study or for a previous short period) [4,8,9,15,18]. To detect possible differences between the two user profiles and to determine their correlates, it would be interesting if research consider both perspectives. In the case of the relationship between the use of dating apps and personality traits, some partial studies either analyze the relationship taking into account only the traits of the Big Five [18] or only the traits of the Dark Tetrad [7]. Only one study has simultaneously contemplated both sides of personality [15]. However, this study is aimed at determining the use of dating apps based on the relational status of the participants and the patterns of infidelity and not so much to explore the differences in individual tendencies between users and non-users.

To fill these gaps, the objective of this study was to analyze the relationship between the previous use and current use (the last three months) of dating apps and the personality traits (Big Five and Dark Core) in a sample of young college students. In this way, we aim to examine the relationships between the use of these applications and personality traits, as well as to know which of those traits can predict the use of dating apps. Further, the predictive role of different sociodemographic variables, such as gender, age, sexual orientation, and relational status, is explored. Knowing the individual tendencies of users of this type of apps can be useful for the design and implementation of preventive and promotion programs for mental health and healthy relationships, both romantic and sexual, in this group.

2. Materials and Methods

2.1. Participants and Procedure

The initial sample comprised 1996 participants. Four inclusion criteria were used: (1) studying a university degree at the time of data collection (76 participants excluded); (2) aged between 18 to 26 years, according to criteria from previous studies with university samples [29–31] (128 participants excluded); (3) labeling themselves as woman or man (13 participants excluded; the small sample size of this group prevented us from incorporating these participants to our analyses); and (4) correctly answering a control question (74 participants excluded; see below).

Considering all these criteria, the final sample included 1705 university students (70% women, 30% men), aged between 18 and 26 (M = 20.60, SD = 2.09). Of the participants, 70.1% described themselves as heterosexual, 22.5% as bisexual, 5.8% as homosexual, and 1.6% as other orientations. Due to the small sample sizes of non-heterosexual groups, those participants were combined into a sexual minority category (29.9%). Concerning relationship status, 52.9% of the participants had a partner, with an average relationship duration of 26.1 months (SD = 22.6), and 47.1% had no partner.

Regarding the procedure, data were collected in December 2019 using a Google Forms survey. To reach participants, a link to the survey was distributed through the e-mail distribution lists of the students of the authors' university. Participants provided informed consent after reading the description of the study, where the anonymity of the responses was clearly stated. The survey remained open for 14 days. This procedure was approved by the Ethics Review Board for Clinical Research of the region (PI18/058).

2.2. Measures

2.2.1. Sociodemographic and Dating App Use Questionnaire

We asked participants about their gender (woman, men, other), age, sexual orientation (heterosexual, homosexual, bisexual, other), and whether they were in a relationship (if they were, for how long). We also asked them whether they had ever used any dating app (Tinder, Grindr or similar) and whether they had used any in the past three months before the study. People who answered "No" to both questions were identified as "nonusers", those who only answered "Yes" to the second one were labeled as "current user", and the rest of the sample were identified as "previous users".

2.2.2. Short Form of the Big Five Inventory–2

This instrument [32] (the short form the original BFI-2) [33] has 30 items that assess the Big Five domains: Negative Emotionality (e.g., "[I am someone who...] is moody, has up and down mood swings"; α = 0.75—all reported alpha values correspond to those observed in the current sample); Extraversion (e.g., "is outgoing, sociable"; $\alpha = 0.71$); Open-Mindedness (e.g., "is curious about many different things"; $\alpha = 0.73$); Agreeableness (e.g., "is compassionate, has a soft heart"; $\alpha = 0.68$); and Conscientiousness (e.g., "is systematic, likes to keep things in order"; $\alpha = 0.75$). These items are rated on a five-point scale, ranging from 1 = *disagree strongly* to 5 = *agree strongly*. The Spanish translation was provided by the first author of the original version of the BFI-2.

2.2.3. Dark Factor of Personality–16

This instrument [20] (a short form of the full 70-item version) has 16 items that assess the dark factor of personality with a single component (e.g., "People who mess with me always regret it"; $\alpha = 0.75$). These items are rated on a five-point scale, ranging from 1 = *strongly disagree* to 5 = *strongly agree*. Following the original instructions, items were presented in random order for each participant [20]. The translation into Spanish was performed for the present research. In our case, three of the co-authors, all native Spanish speakers, translated the scale from English to Spanish, reviewed the translation together, and agreed on a single version of the scale. Finally, a native professional translator reviewed the correspondence between the English and Spanish versions, which agreed with the translated version. The Spanish version can be seen in Appendix A.

2.2.4. Control Question

Embedded in the questionnaire and to check whether the participants paid enough attention to the wording of the items, we introduced an item asking the participants to respond to it with *strongly disagree*. Those participants responding with an option different from the one requested could be considered distracted.

2.3. Data Analyses

Firstly, we computed descriptives and associations between the different variables. The correlations between dichotomous variables (gender, relationship status, and sexual orientation) with age and the six personality scores were transformed to Cohen's *d* [34]. The effect size measure for the associations between the dating apps use groups (never, previous, current) and age and the six personality scores was the *R* statistic from the ANOVA model of means comparison. The association between the dating apps use groups and dichotomous variables was quantified with Cramer's *V*. We chose the effect measure which we considered to allow a potentially easier interpreation of the results [35].

Secondly, we computed a multinomial logistic regression models, with the dating apps use groups as the criteria—nonusers as the reference group—and gender, relationship status, sexual orientation, age, and personality scores as the predictors. As the metric of the personality scores is not easy to interpret, we standardized them before the regression. By doing so, the odds ratio coefficients of personality variables indicate the change in the odds ratio for increments in units of one standard deviation.

The analyses were performed with R 4.0.0 (R Foundation for Statistical Computing, Vienna, Austria) [36]. No missing data were present in our database. The open database and code files for these analyses are available at the Open Science Framework repository (https://osf.io/wjuh6/).

3. Results

The associations among the different variables, with the descriptives, can be seen in Tables 1 and 2. We will focus our attention on the relationship between dating apps use and sociodemographic characteristics and personality scores.

Table 1. Bivariate relations of the different variables and descriptive statistics.

	1	2	3	4	5	6	7	8	9	10	11
				Pearson *r*							
1. Negative Emotionality											
2. Extraversion	**−0.28**										
3. Open-Mindedness	0.01	**0.23**									
4. Agreeableness	**−0.18**	**0.17**	**0.17**								
5. Conscientiousness	**−0.20**	**0.24**	0.02	**0.19**							
6. Dark Core	0.03	**−0.06**	**−0.15**	**−0.59**	**−0.11**						
7. Age	**−0.05**	0.00	0.03	0.02	0.02	−0.02					
				Cohen's *d*							
8. Men	**−0.38**	**−0.17**	−0.01	**−0.42**	**−0.31**	**0.59**	0.02	**Pearson *r***			
9. Single	0.04	−0.08	0.03	**−0.20**	**−0.10**	**0.13**	**−0.27**	**0.15**			
10. Sexual minority	**0.37**	**−0.15**	**0.38**	**−0.12**	**−0.24**	−0.06	**−0.11**	−0.03	0.04		
				ANOVA *R*					**Cramer's *V***		
11. Apps use group	**0.07**	0.00	**0.10**	**0.08**	**0.10**	**0.08**	**0.24**	**0.12**	**0.24**	**0.25**	
Mean	19.02	19.49	22.94	23.16	19.83	27.61	20.60	0.30	0.53	0.30	——
Standard Deviation	4.91	4.54	4.31	3.84	4.75	6.74	2.09	0.46	0.50	0.46	——

Age, measured in years. Men: dummy variable where *women* = 0 and *men* = 1. Single: dummy variable where *in a relationship* = 0 and *single* = 1. Sexual minority: dummy variable where *heterosexual* = 0 and *sexual minority* = 1. —— = Mean and standard deviation for apps use groups are not reported as this variable was nominal with three levels. Bold values correspond to statistically significant associations ($p < 0.05$).

Table 2. Means and standard deviations (for numerical variables), proportions (for categorical variables), and significance testing according to dating app use.

	Nonusers	Previous Users	Current Users		
		Mean (Standard Deviation)		F	p
Negative Emotionality	18.81 (4.95)	19.52 (4.82)	19.61 (4.71)	4.07	0.017
Extraversion	19.49 (4.49)	19.47 (4.73)	19.48 (4.61)	0.00	0.998
Open-Mindedness	22.74 (4.29)	22.97 (4.52)	24.01 (4.00)	8.04	<0.001
Agreeableness	23.34 (3.80)	22.91 (3.83)	22.49 (3.95)	5.20	0.006
Conscientiousness	20.11 (4.77)	19.25 (4.72)	18.94 (4.56)	7.94	<0.001
Dark Core	27.39 (6.62)	27.59 (6.08)	28.93 (7.94)	4.84	0.008
Age	20.31 (1.98)	21.70 (2.16)	20.86 (2.11)	53.85	<0.001
		Proportion		χ^2	p
Women	0.75	0.15	0.10	23.25	<0.001
Men	0.65	0.17	0.18		
In a relationship	0.79	0.17	0.04	100.51	<0.001
Single	0.65	0.15	0.20		
Heterosexual	0.79	0.13	0.08	108.64	<0.001
Sexual minority	0.55	0.23	0.23		

Nonusers: participants reported having never used dating apps. Previous users: participants reported having used dating apps, but not in the last three months. Current users: Participants reported having used dating apps in the last three months. Age, measured in years. Proportions by row.

Of the participants, 71.5% ($n = 1219$) were nonusers, 15.8% ($n = 270$) were previous dating apps users, and 12.7% ($n = 216$) were current users. All sociodemographic variables were associated with the dating apps users groups. With respect to gender, for women, the distributions by group was $p_{\text{nonuser}} = 0.75$, $p_{\text{previous}} = 0.15$, and $p_{\text{current}} = 0.10$; for men, $p_{\text{nonuser}} = 0.65$, $p_{\text{previous}} = 0.17$, and $p_{\text{current}} = 0.18$; $\chi^2(2) = 23.25$, $p < 0.001$, $V = 0.12$. For those in a relationship, $p_{\text{nonuser}} = 0.79$, $p_{\text{previous}} = 0.17$, and $p_{\text{current}} = 0.04$; for single participants, $p_{\text{nonuser}} = 0.65$, $p_{\text{previous}} = 0.15$, and $p_{\text{current}} = 0.20$; $\chi^2(2) = 100.51$, $p < 0.001$, $V = 0.24$. For heterosexual participants, $p_{\text{nonuser}} = 0.79$, $p_{\text{previous}} = 0.13$, and $p_{\text{current}} = 0.08$; for sexual minority participants, $p_{\text{nonuser}} = 0.55$, $p_{\text{previous}} = 0.23$, and $p_{\text{current}} = 0.23$; $\chi^2(2) = 108.64$, $p < 0.001$, $V = 0.25$. Age was associated with the dating apps users groups, with previous users being the older ones ($M = 21.70$, $SD = 2.16$) and nonusers the youngers ($M = 20.31$, $SD = 1.98$), $F(2, 1702) = 53.85$, $p < 0.001$, $R = 0.24$.

Personality means differed by dating apps users group for all considered variables (all $ps \leq 0.017$), except for Extraversion, $F(2, 1702) = 0.00$, $p = 0.998$. All effect sizes could be considered as rather small ($M_R = 0.07$, range [.00, 0.10]). The higher associations were with respect to Open-Mindedness (higher mean for current users) and Conscientiousness (higher mean for nonusers). We note that Conscientiousness and Dark Core showed a high negative correlation ($r = -0.59$, $p < 0.001$).

Results of the multinomial logistic regression models are shown in Table 3. The explanatory capacity of the model was moderate (Nagelkerke's pseudo-$R^2 = 0.25$, McFadden's pseudo-$R^2 = 0.14$). The explanatory ability was basically provided by the sociodemographic information. Being a member of a sexual minority greatly increased the probability of dating apps use ($OR_{previous} = 3.08$, $p < 0.001$; $OR_{current} = 4.11$, $p < 0.001$). Men had a higher probability of use ($OR_{previous} = 1.44$, $p = 0.029$; $OR_{current} = 1.71$, $p = 0.002$). Increments in age were associated with increments in the probability of use ($OR_{previous} = 1.42$, $p < 0.001$; $OR_{current} = 1.27$, $p < 0.001$). Being single showed a very interesting result, as it had an an important impact on the probability of being a current user ($OR_{current} = 6.48$, $p < 0.001$), but not with being a previous user ($OR_{previous} = 1.22$, $p < 0.177$). To better understand the relevance of these variables, we computed the probability of belonging to each group for an 18-year-old heterosexual woman in a relationship and for a 26-year-old single non-heterosexual man (both with mean scores in all personality variables). For that woman, $p_{nonuser} = 0.95$, $p_{previous} = 0.04$, and $p_{current} = 0.01$; for that man, $p_{nonuser} = 0.12$, $p_{previous} = 0.45$, and $p_{current} = 0.44$. All of the personality scores showed statistically non-significant coefficients (*OR*s in the range [0.86, 1.19], $ps \geq 0.058$), except for Open-Mindedness with current use ($OR_{previous} = 1.22$, $p = 0.026$).

Table 3. Multinomial logistic regression analyses of use of dating apps.

	Apps Previous Users					Apps Current Users				
	b	*SE*	*OR*	95% CI	*p*	*b*	*SE*	*OR*	95% CI	*p*
Intercept	**–9.44**	**0.76**	**0.00**	**[0.00, 0.00]**	**<0.001**	**–8.66**	**0.88**	**0.00**	**[0.00, 0.00]**	**<0.001**
Negative Emotionality	0.15	0.08	1.16	[0.99, 1.36]	0.058	0.13	0.09	1.13	[0.95, 1.35]	0.159
Extraversion	0.15	0.08	1.16	[0.99, 1.35]	0.059	0.15	0.09	1.16	[0.98, 1.38]	0.087
Open-Mindedness	–0.07	0.08	0.93	[0.80, 1.08]	0.340	**0.20**	**0.09**	**1.22**	**[1.02, 1.45]**	**0.026**
Agreeableness	–0.05	0.09	0.95	[0.79, 1.13]	0.555	0.00	0.10	1.00	[0.82, 1.22]	0.989
Conscientiousness	–0.13	0.08	0.88	[0.76, 1.02]	0.085	–0.16	0.09	0.86	[0.72, 1.01]	0.067
Dark Core	–0.02	0.09	0.98	[0.82, 1.17]	0.816	0.17	0.10	1.19	[0.99, 1.44]	0.071
Age	**0.35**	**0.03**	**1.42**	**[1.33, 1.52]**	**<0.001**	**0.24**	**0.04**	**1.27**	**[1.17, 1.37]**	**<0.001**
Men	**0.36**	**0.17**	**1.44**	**[1.04, 1.99]**	**0.029**	**0.53**	**0.18**	**1.71**	**[1.21, 2.41]**	**0.002**
Single	0.20	0.15	1.22	[0.91, 1.62]	0.177	**1.87**	**0.21**	**6.48**	**[4.31, 9.73]**	**<0.001**
Sexual minority	**1.12**	**0.16**	**3.08**	**[2.27, 4.17]**	**<0.001**	**1.41**	**0.17**	**4.11**	**[2.95, 5.75]**	**<0.001**

SE = standard error; *OR* = odds ratio; CI = odds ratio confidence interval. All personality variables were standarized. Age, measured in years. Men: dummy variable where *women* = 0 and *men* = 1. Single: dummy variable where *in a relationship* = 0 and *single* = 1. Sexual minority: dummy variable where *heterosexual* = 0 and *sexual minority* = 1. Bold values correspond to statistically significant coefficients ($p < 0.05$). Nonusers was the reference group.

Given the relevant correlation between Agreeableness and Dark Core, which could lead to some problems of multicollinearity, we tested a model without dark personality scores. If multicollinearity was a concern, the pattern of results would be changed for this reduced model, but that was not the case. For the full model, the results for Agreeableness were as follows: $OR_{previous} = 0.95$, $p = 0.555$; $OR_{current} = 1.00$, $p = 0.989$; and for the reduced model: $OR_{previous} = 0.96$, $p = 0.589$; $OR_{current} = 0.90$, $p = 0.215$. We did not test a model without Agreeableness as we considered that, theoretically, it made no sense to exclude one of the dimensions of the Big Five.

4. Discussion

The emergence and popularization of dating apps in recent years have changed the way potential romantic and/or sexual partners meet and interact. Due to the recency and relevance of this phenomenon, it is necessary to deepen our knowledge about the profile of dating apps users. Although some studies have pointed out that the use of these applications varies depending on certain sociodemographic variables and personality traits, such studies are still few, and they present partial analyses, significant limitations in sampling, and their results are inconclusive. Therefore, the objective of this study was to analyze the relationship between the use of dating apps—previous and current—and the personality traits (bright and dark), also taking into account the role of sociodemographic variables such as gender, age, sexual orientation, and relational status, in a sample of young university students.

Of the participants, 71.5% were nonusers of dating apps, 15.8% were previous users, and 12.7% were current users (in the last three months). This is a prevalence of medium use, compared with that found in other studies [2,3,18], although it should be noted that, in these studies, sampling was aimed at finding people who used dating apps or it excluded those who had a partner, even with convenience samples. Therefore, although there are different reasons for the lower prevalence of dating app use in this study compared with those in previous works (e.g., participants' age, proportion of people with partners, cultural differences), we consider that our sampling allows us to better estimate the actual percentage of users of these applications.

From the data obtained, a sociodemographic profile of dating app users can be drawn among young Spanish university students. Individuals who are members of sexual minorities, men, and older youths are more likely to use dating apps. Although the results were expected in accordance with the previous literature, it can be stated that these characteristics are consistent for both groups of users (previous and current use) and both in the bivariate and the regression analyses performed.

The past and current likelihood of using dating apps in people from sexual minorities was more than three times greater than that of heterosexual people, in line with existing evidence. As has already been shown, dating apps are a resource widely used by people from sexual minorities, especially those who have more difficulty expressing their sexuality and/or finding a partner [11–13].

Our data support that men use dating apps more than women, as appears in most studies collected in the review of Anzani et al. [1]. As for age, the data revealed that the older the person is, the more likely they are to have used or to use dating apps currently. In the same vein, previous studies found a higher current use in older college students, noting that the phenomenon of dating apps is more prevalent among slightly older youths [1,2,9]. Concerning previous use, it seems logical to think that older youths, due simply to their lifetime, have been more likely to have used a dating app.

Concerning relational status, the results are especially interesting. Being single greatly increased the likelihood of being a current user of dating apps, but not of being a previous user. There exists a stereotype that considers that these apps are used only for casual sex [9] and that dating app users are not interested in long-term relationships. If that was the case, previous users should still be single to a larger extent. These results indicate that dating apps can be used to find long-term relationships or that looking for casual sex is not incompatible with seeking a romantic relationship [37].

We found that 4% of current users were in a relationship. This could be due to the fact that we considered as "current" those who had used in the last three months, so those participants could be single while using the apps, but not when responding to the questionnaires. Other options are people cheating on their partners [15] or in a consensually non-monogamous relationship. Other studies have found that about 20% of dating app users are in a committed relationship [4,38]. Further research is needed to clarify that important difference.

The relationships found between personality traits and the use of dating apps allow us to draw two relevant and surprising conclusions concerning the previous literature, which we will discuss below. First, although all dimensions—but Extraversion—showed statistically significant, although small, associations with dating app use group, those effects disappeared in the regression model. This lack of effect was found for the Big Five domains and for dark personality. The only exception was Open-Mindedness, which emerged as the only personality trait associated with the current use of dating apps, in line with previous studies [18].

Some explanations are plausible to justify why the Open-Mindedness effect was not the same for previous and current use. First, it could be simply interpreted as statistical noise. Second, we cannot discard that some features of Open-Mindedness (i.e., better tolerance of change) have a higher predictive capacity when the criteria refer to more recent behaviors (i.e., use of dating apps in the last three months). To clarify the predictive value of personality traits, future research should examine in greater depth the role of the Big Five in explaining different types of dating apps use (never users vs. experimental users vs. regular users).

The Dark Core of personality was not a significant predictor of previous and current use of dating apps, contrary to previous research [7,15]. This disparity may be due to the conception of dark personality and, consequently, the way of assessing it. Preceding studies addressed the dark personality from a multidimensional approach, using scales that assess four different dark personality traits (i.e., narcissism, Machiavellianism, psychopathy, and sadism). As we mentioned, we conceived the dark personality as a single latent factor called Dark Core, according to the most recent evidence about the theoretical and empirical overlap among the dark traits [19–23]. Further, previous studies [7,15] used the Short Dark Triad-3 (SD-3) [39]. This instrument includes an item that, while measuring psychopathy, clearly overlaps with high sociosexual orientation ("I enjoy having sex with people I hardly know"). Therefore, higher scores for apps users may be indicative of higher dark personality or higher sociosexuality.

We cannot rule out the influence of cultural differences in the relationship between personality and the use of dating apps. Young Spaniards may conceive of intimate relationships through this type of application differently from young people from other contexts where this phenomenon has been studied (Belgium [15]; United Kingdom, United States, and Canada [7]). In the absence of references in a young population similar to the Spanish one, we would need more studies, preferably cross-cultural, to test this hypothesis. Finally, dating app users may not actually differ from non-users in these antagonistic personality traits. If future research corroborated these results, we would have to banish the negative stereotype that is still associated with dating apps and their users [40].

The study has several limitations that need to be taken into account when interpreting the results. The use of dating apps has been evaluated without delving into the variety of uses, from those who used it on a single afternoon as a joke among friends to those who used it for months looking for a romantic relationship. Our estimation of current use is not a punctual prevalence, but with a timeframe of three months. The sample was mostly female, aged between 18 and 26, and coming from a single university. For this reason, it is difficult to generalize the results to the global population of university students and to young people of these ages who do not study at a university. Further, by grouping all the participating members of sexual minorities, we have lost information about the peculiarities of the use of dating apps and the personality patterns of these people depending on whether they are gay/lesbian, bisexual, or of other orientations. As for the instruments used to evaluate the Big Five and the Dark Core, lower levels of reliability were found than those of the original instrument validation studies [20,32]. For Agreeableness, Cronbach's alpha was only 0.68. Reductions in reliability may have led to reductions in the estimated effect sizes and loss of statistical power. For the BFI-2 Short Form, in the German version [41], an even smaller value of Cronbach's alpha was reported for this dimension ($\alpha = 0.65$), so, apparently, these potential problems in reliability cannot be attributed to undetected problems with our sample. Moreover, our study shares with previous studies based on self-selected samples and self-reported measures the limitation due to the response and recall bias. In this sense, it would be interesting to carry out longitudinal studies that would allow evaluating evolution in personality traits, and their influence on the use of dating apps.

Some readers may consider as a problem the inclusion of instruments that have not been validated in Spanish samples, as we did with the BFI-2 or the Dark Factor of Personality–16. We do not share this concern. We cannot take for granted that an instrument that has shown adequate psychometric properties for specific use with a specific sample will show the same results with other samples. For example, if a validation effort is done for the development or adaptation of a Big Five questionnaire with a sample of university students from the north of Spain in 2018, we cannot guarantee that this instrument will be valid for a sample of nurses from the south of Spain in 2020. We have changed occupation, location, and time and we do not know if any of those changes may be relevant.

The essential point is if there are any theoretical or empirical reasons to expect that the validity will be compromised with the intended sample. We consider that this is not the case for our Big Five measure with our sample. As Costa and McCrae have noted, "the [Big Five] factors are found in different age, sex, race, and language groups" [42]. From the same source, "they may be somewhat differently expressed in different cultures". There are strong reasons to not expect this in our case. First, other measures of the Big Five have shown adequate properties in Spanish samples [43,44]. Second, the previous version of the BFI has also shown that "the Spanish BFI may serve as an efficient, reliable, and factorially valid measure of the Big Five for research on Spanish-speaking individuals" [45]. Third, the BFI-2 has shown adequate psychometric properties in different adaptations: German [41] or Russian [46]. In the case of dark personality, other measures of this construct have been previously validated into Spanish without any problem [47]. In any case, all our data are fully available for further research about the psychometric properties of those instruments (https://osf.io/wjuh6/).

Despite the above limitations, the study is considered to make some relevant contributions. First, information on the prevalence of dating apps use among Spanish university students has been provided, and this is one of the first studies to evaluate this phenomenon in Spanish-speaking youth. Second, both previous and current use have been taken into account, a novel aspect with respect to previous research that only evaluated the most recent use. In addition, this has been done in an unbiased sample, in which no attempt was made to overrepresent dating app users, as was the case in previous studies [2,3,18]. Thirdly, a profile of the dating apps user has been developed based on individual differences, with special relevance of sociodemographic variables (gender, age, sexual orientation, and relationship status), as all of them allowed for predicting use. Fourth, the traditional personality traits of the Big Five and dark personality have been simultaneously evaluated. Fifth, it has been found that, among personality dimensions, only Open-Mindedness can help to explain current use, although the contribution is of low magnitude.

5. Conclusions

The findings of this study have allowed us to plot a profile of the dating apps user based on some sociodemographic and personality characteristics. Men, older individuals, without a stable relationship (for current use), and belonging to a sexual minority are more likely to have used and/or to use such applications to relate with others and establish romantic relationships. However, the Big Five personality traits are not associated with past or recent use of dating apps, except for recent use being related to higher Open-Mindedness. Having dark or socially aversive personality traits does not help to explain the use of dating apps. The profile of previous and current users is largely equivalent.

In any case, the results obtained have revealed that the predictive power of personality for past and recent use of dating apps is very small compared to other individual features. In this sense, perhaps it would be appropriate to explore in more detail the influence of cognitive, motivational, and affective elements, more linked to situational and sociocultural influences, and therefore more changeable and adaptable to the characteristics of the environment, rather than focusing on more stable elements (i.e., traits). Although the individual's behavior will depend on the continuous interrelationship of both elements, those who are more easily modifiable will be key aspects of mental and sexual health promotion programs in young people (e.g., negative emotions, low perception of risk of certain behaviors, etc.).

Dating apps, due to their huge use among adolescents and early adults, could be taken into account in the design of mental health protocols, including sexual and reproductive health strategies. For instance, as we found, people from sexual minorities are frequent users of dating apps. Meta-analytic evidence reported elevated risks for different mental health problems for sexual minority individuals [48]. Although dating apps can be useful to express their sexual identity and initiate a romantic relationship, these apps have also some characteristics (e.g., over-exposure) that could increase even more the risk for several mental health problems in vulnerable users (e.g., youth with low self-esteem). However, the popularity of dating apps could be used to promote sexual health among diverse and at-risk populations.

Author Contributions: Conceptualization, Á.C. and J.R.B.; methodology, J.R.B. and P.J.R.-V.; validation, J.R.B.; formal analysis, J.R.B. and P.J.R.-V.; investigation, Á.C. and E.F.-d.-R.; resources, Á.C., J.R.B., P.J.R.-V. and E.F.-d.-R.; data curation, J.R.B.; writing—original draft preparation, Á.C., P.J.R.-V. and E.F.-d.-R.; writing—review and editing, J.R.B., E.F.-d.-R., P.J.R.-V. and Á.C.; project administration, Á.C.; funding acquisition, Á.C. and J.R.B. All authors have read and agreed to the published version of the manuscript.

Appendix A

Table A1. Spanish version of the Dark Core Scale [20].

Please read each statement and decide how much you agree or disagree with that statement. Note that there are no "correct" or "incorrect" answers to the statements. Please answer every statement, even if you are not completely sure of your response. If not specified otherwise, the items refer to your behavior (towards others) in general.	Por favor, lee cada oración y decide en qué grado estás de acuerdo o en desacuerdo con la misma. Recuerda que no hay respuestas correctas o incorrectas. Por favor, responde a cada afirmación, aunque no estés completamente seguro/a de tu respuesta. Las preguntas se refieren a tu comportamiento en general con los demás, a menos que se especifique lo contrario.
It is hard for me to see someone suffering.	Me resulta duro ver sufrir a alguien.
Payback needs to be quick and nasty.	La venganza debe ser rápida y cruel.
All in all, it is better to be humble and honest than important and dishonest.	En general, es mejor ser humilde y honesto que ser importante y deshonesto.
My own pleasure is all that matters.	Mi propio placer es lo único que importa.
I cannot imagine how being mean to others could ever be exciting.	NO puedo imaginar cómo ser desagradable con los demás puede ser excitante.
People who get mistreated have usually done something to bring it on themselves.	Las personas que son maltratadas generalmente han hecho algo para provocarlo.
Hurting people would make me very uncomfortable.	Hacer daño a alguien me haría sentir muy incómodo.
It's wise to keep track of information that you can use against people later.	Es inteligente guardar información que puedas utilizar más adelante contra otras personas.
I feel sorry if things I do upset people.	Me siento mal/triste si las cosas que hago molestan a la gente.
People who mess with me always regret it.	La gente que se mete conmigo siempre se arrepiente.
Why should I care about other people, when no one cares about me?	¿Por qué debería preocuparme por otras personas cuando nadie se preocupa por mí?
I would like to make some people suffer, even if it meant that I would go to hell with them.	Me gustaría hacer sufrir a algunas personas, aunque eso significara hundirme con ellas.
Most people deserve respect.	La mayoría de la gente merece respeto.
I make a point of trying not to hurt others in pursuit of my goals.	Procuro NO hacer daño a otras personas mientras persigo mis objetivos.
I would be willing to take a punch if it meant that someone I did not like would receive two punches.	Estaría dispuesto a recibir un puñetazo si eso significara que alguien que NO me gusta recibiera dos puñetazos.
I avoid humiliating others.	Evito humillar a otros.

1 = Totalmente en desacuerdo / 2 = En desacuerdo / 3 = Neutral/Ni de acuerdo ni en desacuerdo / 4 = De acuerdo / 5 = Totalmente de acuerdo.

References

1. Anzani, A.; Di Sarno, M.; Prunas, A. L'utilisation des applis de smartphones pour trouver des partenaires sexuels. *Sexologies* **2018**, *27*, 144–149. [CrossRef]
2. Ranzini, G.; Lutz, C. Love at first swipe? Explaining Tinder self-presentation and motives. *Mob. Media Commun.* **2016**, *5*, 80–101. [CrossRef]

3. Sumter, S.; VandenBosch, L. Dating gone mobile: Demographic and personality-based correlates of using smartphone-based dating applications among emerging adults. *New Media Soc.* **2018**, *21*, 655–673. [CrossRef]
4. Timmermans, E.; Courtois, C. From swiping to casual sex and/or committed relationships: Exploring the experiences of Tinder users. *Inf. Soc.* **2018**, *34*, 59–70. [CrossRef]
5. Albury, K.; Byron, P. Safe on My Phone? Same-Sex Attracted Young People's Negotiations of Intimacy, Visibility, and Risk on Digital Hook-Up Apps. *Soc. Media Soc.* **2016**, *2*, 205630511667288. [CrossRef]
6. Aretz, W.; Gansen-Ammann, D.-N.; Mierke, K.; Musiol, A. Date me if you can: Ein systematischer Überblick über den aktuellen Forschungsstand von Online-Dating. *Z. Sex.* **2017**, *30*, 7–34. [CrossRef]
7. Lyons, M.; Messenger, A.; Perry, R.; Brewer, G. The Dark Tetrad in Tinder: Hook-up app for high psychopathy individuals, and a diverse utilitarian tool for Machiavellians? *Curr. Psychol.* **2020**, 1–8. [CrossRef]
8. Alexopoulos, C.; Timmermans, E.; McNallie, J. Swiping more, committing less: Unraveling the links among dating app use, dating app success, and intention to commit infidelity. *Comput. Hum. Behav.* **2020**, *102*, 172–180. [CrossRef]
9. Lefebvre, L. Swiping me off my feet. *J. Soc. Pers. Relatsh.* **2017**, *35*, 1205–1229. [CrossRef]
10. Shapiro, G.; Tatar, O.; Sutton, A.; Fisher, W.; Naz, A.; Perez, S.; Rosberger, Z. Correlates of Tinder Use and Risky Sexual Behaviors in Young Adults. *Cyberpsychology Behav. Soc. Netw.* **2017**, *20*, 727–734. [CrossRef]
11. Badal, H.J.; Stryker, J.E.; DeLuca, N.; Purcell, D.W. Swipe Right: Dating Website and App Use Among Men Who Have Sex With Men. *AIDS Behav.* **2017**, *22*, 1265–1272. [CrossRef] [PubMed]
12. Ferris, L.; Duguay, S. Tinder's lesbian digital imaginary: Investigating (im)permeable boundaries of sexual identity on a popular dating app. *New Media Soc.* **2019**, *22*, 489–506. [CrossRef]
13. Korchmaros, J.D.; Ybarra, M.L.; Mitchell, K. Adolescent online romantic relationship initiation: Differences by sexual and gender identification. *J. Adolesc.* **2015**, *40*, 54–64. [CrossRef] [PubMed]
14. Orosz, G.; Tóth-Király, I.; Bőthe, B.; Melher, D. Too many swipes for today: The development of the Problematic Tinder Use Scale (PTUS). *J. Behav. Addict.* **2016**, *5*, 518–523. [CrossRef]
15. Timmermans, E.; De Caluwé, E.; Alexopoulos, C. Why are you cheating on tinder? Exploring users' motives and (dark) personality traits. *Comput. Hum. Behav.* **2018**, *89*, 129–139. [CrossRef]
16. Allen, M.S.; Walter, E.E. Linking big five personality traits to sexuality and sexual health: A meta-analytic review. *Psychol. Bull.* **2018**, *144*, 1081–1110. [CrossRef]
17. Ozer, D.; Benet-Martinez, V. Personality and the Prediction of Consequential Outcomes. *Annu. Rev. Psychol.* **2006**, *57*, 401–421. [CrossRef]
18. Timmermans, E.; de Caluwé, E. To Tinder or not to Tinder, that's the question: An individual differences perspective to Tinder use and motives. *Personal. Individ. Differ.* **2017**, *110*, 74–79. [CrossRef]
19. Bertl, B.; Pietschnig, J.; Tran, U.S.; Stieger, S.; Voracek, M. More or less than the sum of its parts? Mapping the Dark Triad of personality onto a single Dark Core. *Personal. Individ. Differ.* **2017**, *114*, 140–144. [CrossRef]
20. Moshagen, M.; Zettler, I.; Hilbig, B.E. Measuring the dark core of personality. *Psychol. Assess.* **2020**, *32*, 182–196. [CrossRef]
21. Muris, P.; Merckelbach, H.; Otgaar, H.; Meijer, E. The Malevolent Side of Human Nature. *Perspect. Psychol. Sci.* **2017**, *12*, 183–204. [CrossRef] [PubMed]
22. O'Boyle, E.H.; Forsyth, D.R.; Banks, G.C.; Story, P.A.; White, C. A Meta-Analytic Test of Redundancy and Relative Importance of the Dark Triad and Five-Factor Model of Personality. *J. Personal.* **2014**, *83*, 644–664. [CrossRef] [PubMed]
23. Volmer, J.; Koch, I.K.; Wolff, C. Illuminating the 'dark core': Mapping global versus specific sources of variance across multiple measures of the dark triad. *Personal. Individ. Differ.* **2019**, *145*, 97–102. [CrossRef]
24. Paulhus, D.L. Toward a Taxonomy of Dark Personalities. *Curr. Dir. Psychol. Sci.* **2014**, *23*, 421–426. [CrossRef]
25. Book, A.; Visser, B.; Blais, J.; Hosker-Field, A.; Methot-Jones, T.; Gauthier, N.Y.; Volk, A.; Holden, R.R.; D'Agata, M.T. Unpacking more "evil": What is at the core of the dark tetrad? *Personal. Individ. Differ.* **2016**, *90*, 269–272. [CrossRef]
26. Ali, F.; Chamorro-Premuzic, T. The dark side of love and life satisfaction: Associations with intimate relationships, psychopathy and Machiavellianism. *Personal. Individ. Differ.* **2010**, *48*, 228–233. [CrossRef]
27. Fernández-Del-Río, E.; Ramos-Villagrasa, P.J.; Castro, Á.; Barrada, J.R. Sociosexuality and Bright and Dark Personality: The Prediction of Behavior, Attitude, and Desire to Engage in Casual Sex. *Int. J. Environ. Res. Public Health* **2019**, *16*, 2731. [CrossRef]

28. Jonason, P.K.; Luevano, V.; Adams, H.M. How the Dark Triad traits predict relationship choices. *Personal. Individ. Differ.* **2012**, *53*, 180–184. [CrossRef]
29. Barthels, F.; Barrada, J.R.; Roncero, M. Orthorexia nervosa and healthy orthorexia as new eating styles. *PLoS ONE* **2019**, *14*, e0219609. [CrossRef]
30. Barrada, J.R.; Castro, Á.; Correa, A.B.; Ruiz-Gómez, P. The Tridimensional Structure of Sociosexuality: Spanish Validation of the Revised Sociosexual Orientation Inventory. *J. Sex Marital. Ther.* **2017**, *44*, 149–158. [CrossRef]
31. Barrada, J.R.; Ruiz-Gómez, P.; Correa, A.B.; Castro, Á. Not all Online Sexual Activities Are the Same. *Front. Psychol.* **2019**, *10*, 339. [CrossRef] [PubMed]
32. Soto, C.J.; John, O.P. Short and extra-short forms of the Big Five Inventory–2: The BFI-2-S and BFI-2-XS. *J. Res. Personal.* **2017**, *68*, 69–81. [CrossRef]
33. Soto, C.J.; John, O.P. The Next Big Five Inventory (BFI-2): Developing and Assessing a Hierarchical Model With 15 Facets to Enhance Bandwidth, Fidelity, and Predictive Power. *J. Personal. Soc. Psychol.* **2017**, *113*, 117–143. [CrossRef] [PubMed]
34. McGrath, R.E.; Meyer, G.J. When effect sizes disagree: The case of r and d. *Psychol. Methods* **2006**, *11*, 386–401. [CrossRef] [PubMed]
35. Wilkinson, L. Statistical methods in psychology journals: Guidelines and explanations. *Am. Psychol.* **1999**, *54*, 594–604. [CrossRef]
36. R Core Team. *R: A Language and Environment for Statistical Computing*; R Foundation for Statistical Computing: Vienna, Austria, 2020.
37. Jackson, J.J.; Kirkpatrick, L.A. The structure and measurement of human mating strategies: Toward a multidimensional model of sociosexuality. *Evol. Hum. Behav.* **2007**, *28*, 382–391. [CrossRef]
38. Orosz, G.; Benyó, M.; Berkes, B.; Nikoletti, E.; Gal, E.; Tóth-Király, I.; Bőthe, B. The personality, motivational, and need-based background of problematic Tinder use. *J. Behav. Addict.* **2018**, *7*, 301–316. [CrossRef]
39. Jones, D.N.; Paulhus, D.L. Introducing the Short Dark Triad (SD3). *Assessment* **2013**, *21*, 28–41. [CrossRef]
40. Choi, E.P.H.; Wong, J.Y.H.; Lo, H.H.M.; Wong, W.; Chio, J.H.M.; Fong, D.-T.; Lo, H.H. Association Between Using Smartphone Dating Applications and Alcohol and Recreational Drug Use in Conjunction With Sexual Activities in College Students. *Subst. Use Misuse* **2016**, *52*, 1–7. [CrossRef]
41. Rammstedt, B.; Danner, D.; Soto, C.J.; John, O.P. Validation of the Short and Extra-Short Forms of the Big Five Inventory-2 (BFI-2) and Their German Adaptations. *Eur. J. Psychol. Assess.* **2020**, *36*, 149–161. [CrossRef]
42. Costa, P.T.; McCrae, R.R. Four ways five factors are basic. *Personal. Individ. Differ.* **1992**, *13*, 653–665. [CrossRef]
43. Ortet, G.; Martínez, T.; Mezquita, L.; Morizot, J.; I Ibáñez, M. Big Five Personality Trait Short Questionnaire: Preliminary Validation with Spanish Adults. *Span. J. Psychol.* **2017**, *20*. [CrossRef] [PubMed]
44. Costa, P.T., Jr.; McCrae, R.R. *Inventario De Personalidad NEO Revisado (NEO PI-R). Inventario NEO Reducido De Cinco Factores (NEO-FFI). Manual 3a Edición [NEO PI-R Revised Neo Personality Inventory and NEO Five-Factor Inventory (NEO-FFI)]*; TEA: Madrid, Spain, 2008.
45. Benet-Martinez, V.; John, O.P. Los Cinco Grandes across cultures and ethnic groups: Multitrait-multimethod analyses of the Big Five in Spanish and English. *J. Personal. Soc. Psychol.* **1998**, *75*, 729–750. [CrossRef]
46. Shchebetenko, S.; Kalugin, A.Y.; Mishkevich, A.M.; Soto, C.J.; John, O.P. Measurement Invariance and Sex and Age Differences of the Big Five Inventory–2: Evidence From the Russian Version. *Assessment* **2019**, *27*, 472–486. [CrossRef] [PubMed]
47. Pineda, D.; Sandín, B.; Muris, P. Psychometrics properties of the Spanish version of two Dark Triad scales: The Dirty Dozen and the Short Dark Triad. *Curr. Psychol.* **2018**, 1–9. [CrossRef]
48. Plöderl, M.; Tremblay, P. Mental health of sexual minorities. A systematic review. *Int. Rev. Psychiatry* **2015**, *27*, 367–385. [CrossRef]

10

Current State and Future Directions of Technology-Based Ecological Momentary Assessment and Intervention for Major Depressive Disorder

Desirée Colombo [1,*], Javier Fernández-Álvarez [2], Andrea Patané [3], Michelle Semonella [4], Marta Kwiatkowska [3], Azucena García-Palacios [1,5], Pietro Cipresso [2,4], Giuseppe Riva [2,4] and Cristina Botella [1,5]

1 Department of Basic Psychology, Clinic and Psychobiology, Universitat Jaume I, Av. Sos Baynat, s/n, 12071 Castellón, Spain; azucena@uji.es (A.G.-P.); botella@uji.es (C.B.)

2 Department of Psychology, Università Cattolica del Sacro Cuore, Largo Gemelli, 1, 20100 Milan, Italy; javier.fernandezkirszman@unicatt.it (J.F.-Á.); pietro.cipresso@unicatt.it (P.C.); giuseppe.riva@unicatt.it (G.R.)

3 Department of Computer Science, University of Oxford, Wolfson Building, Parks Rd, Oxford OX1 3QD, UK; andrea.patane@cs.ox.ac.uk (A.P.); marta.kwiatkowska@cs.ox.ac.uk (M.K.)

4 Applied Technology for Neuro-Psychology Lab, IRCCS Istituto Auxologico Italiano, 20149 Milan, Italy; semonellamichelle@gmail.com

5 CIBER Fisiopatología Obesidad y Nutrición (CIBERobn), Instituto Salud Carlos III, 28029 Madrid, Spain

* Correspondence: dcolombo@uji.es

Abstract: Ecological momentary assessment (EMA) and ecological momentary intervention (EMI) are alternative approaches to retrospective self-reports and face-to-face treatments, and they make it possible to repeatedly assess patients in naturalistic settings and extend psychological support into real life. The increase in smartphone applications and the availability of low-cost wearable biosensors have further improved the potential of EMA and EMI, which, however, have not yet been applied in clinical practice. Here, we conducted a systematic review, using the Preferred Reporting Items for Systematic Reviews and Meta-Analyses (PRISMA) guidelines, to explore the state of the art of technology-based EMA and EMI for major depressive disorder (MDD). A total of 33 articles were included (EMA = 26; EMI = 7). First, we provide a detailed analysis of the included studies from technical (sampling methods, duration, prompts), clinical (fields of application, adherence rates, dropouts, intervention effectiveness), and technological (adopted devices) perspectives. Then, we identify the advantages of using information and communications technologies (ICTs) to extend the potential of these approaches to the understanding, assessment, and intervention in depression. Furthermore, we point out the relevant issues that still need to be addressed within this field, and we discuss how EMA and EMI could benefit from the use of sensors and biosensors, along with recent advances in machine learning for affective modelling.

Keywords: major depressive disorder; ecological momentary assessment; ecological momentary intervention

---

1. Introduction

Major depressive disorder (MDD) is a common debilitating psychiatric disease characterized by mood disturbances, loss of interest and pleasure in daily activities, disturbed appetite and sleep, loss of energy, and psychomotor retardation or agitation. According to the World Health Organization, depression is one of the leading causes of disease and disability in the world, annually affecting 4.4%

of the general adult population [1]. In addition to producing high costs for the public health system, depression seriously impairs patients' functioning, leading to increased mortality, high suicide rates, exacerbated medical conditions, and high consumption of alcohol and illegal drugs [2–5].

As a result of the increased availability of smartphones and portable and wearable devices, a growing body of research has begun to explore new digital technologies as potential tools to foster assessments and interventions in clinical practice. More specifically, technology-based ecological momentary assessment (EMA) and ecological momentary intervention (EMI) have been proposed as alternative strategies to assess patients ecologically in naturalistic settings and deliver psychological support in daily life.

1.1. Ecological Momentary Assessment

Traditional clinical assessments are based on retrospective self-reports in which patients are asked to summarize their symptoms and affective experiences over the past few weeks. Nevertheless, increasing evidence shows that these tools are not able to capture MDD dynamics, such as symptom fluctuations or mood shifts over time [6,7]. Likewise, self-reports are affected by recall bias. In other words, depressed patients have been found to alter the content of past experiences when asked to retrieve them retrospectively [8,9], judging symptoms as more severe [10] or increasing the elaboration of negative information [11].

EMA emerged as an alternative assessment strategy to better grasp affective and behavioural dynamics in daily life [12–14]. Not surprisingly, a growing body of research has applied this approach to exploring mood disorders [15,16]. On the one hand, the term "ecological" refers to the environment where the data are collected. Behaviours, thoughts, and affect are repeatedly written down in real-world contexts. On the other hand, the term "momentary" refers to the focus of the assessment, i.e., close in time to the experience. The first studies to use this approach adopted paper-and-pencil daily diaries, but the discomfort, low compliance, and low experimental control over backfilling made them not very efficacious [14]. The exponential progress of information and communication technologies (ICTs) and the increasing availability of smartphones offered novel opportunities to ecologically assess patients. On the one hand, mobile technologies allow the shortcomings of traditional diaries to be overcome by eliminating the need for manual data entry and by increasing control on backfilling, thus obtaining more accurate data. On the other hand, all the necessary processes can be integrated in one tool, for instance, a smartphone, thus decreasing intrusiveness and increasing users' comfort, and providing a more engaging and dynamic experience. During the day, indeed, patients are automatically prompted by the device to fill in self-reports that are subsequently stored and safely sent to clinicians and/or researchers. More recently, the potential of EMA was extended due to the integration of self-reports with data gathered from embedded sensors and wearable biosensors, hence allowing for a multimodal approach. Unobtrusive wearable biosensors can continuously monitor physiological parameters throughout the day with high precision [17], whereas smartphone embedded sensors make it possible to indirectly collect data about patients' behaviours and habits, such as their social media use, physical activity, or social interactions [18,19]. Overall, the integration of these tools has the potential to revolutionize traditional assessments, leading to the exploration of new facets of MDD obtained in daily life contexts that are often difficult to capture in laboratory settings.

1.2. Ecological Momentary Intervention

According to statistics, 70% of people suffering from mental disorders do not receive adequate psychological treatment or reach complete clinical remission [20]. Affordances of technological developments, as Kazdin and Blase suggested, may facilitate new solutions for disseminating evidence-based psychotherapy [21].

The same "ecological" and "momentary" principles have been applied to the development of innovative interventions (EMI) [22] that go beyond traditional clinical settings and extend the delivery of psychological support into real life [23]. EMI has the advantage of providing psychological support directly on hand-held mobile technologies during the flow of daily experiences, in real-time settings, and at specific time points in the day, without the need for face-to-face meetings with a clinician [24]. EMIs can be delivered both as stand-alone treatments or in combination with other treatments. Moreover, similarly to EMAs, the use of data gathered from biosensors and embedded sensors along with machine learning techniques can increase the customization of the proposed interventions [16,25].

1.3. Objectives

Recent studies have confirmed the feasibility of mobile health (mHealth) applications and patients' interest in and adherence to these technologies, suggesting the great potential of this approach in the clinical field [23,26]. Nevertheless, no systematic review has explored technology-based EMA and EMI for MDD to date. Although two reviews focused on EMAs for mood disorders [15,16], most of the included studies were based on paper-and-pencil daily diaries, and the target population included adults and adolescents with bipolar disorder (BD) and borderline personality disorder (BPD).

Coinciding with our field of interest, the aim of this systematic review is to provide an overview of the state of the art of technology-based EMA and EMI for MDD from both a clinical and technological point of view. Our final objective is to show how and why clinical practice could benefit from the use of these approaches. In doing so, we will describe the potential of new technologies in this field, and we will discuss how EMAs and EMIs could be performed with sensors and biosensors along with recent advances in machine learning for affective modelling.

2. Methods

Preferred Reporting Items for Systematic Reviews and Meta-Analyses (PRISMA) criteria [27] were followed. For the systematic review protocol, see [28].

2.1. Search Strategy

To collect relevant publications, a computer-based search was performed (March 2019). We searched in two high-order databases, PubMed and Web of Science (Web of Knowledge), using the following string: ((EMA) OR ("ecological momentary assessment") OR (EMI) OR ("mobile health") OR (mhealth) OR (smartphone) OR ("ecological momentary intervention") OR (ESM) OR ("experience sampling method") OR ("ambulatory assessment") OR ("personal digital assistant") OR ("ambulatory monitoring") OR ("real time data capture") OR ("real time monitoring") OR ("real time interventions") OR ("electronic diary") OR ("repeated observations") OR ("diary data") OR ("time series")) AND (("affective disorder") OR ("mood disorder") OR (depress*) OR (depression) OR (MDD) OR ("major depressive disorder") OR ("major depression") OR ("unipolar depression") OR ("affective symptoms").

This search produced a total of 4993 articles. After eliminating duplicate papers, we made a first selection by reading titles and abstracts, and 401 articles were retrieved. We finally selected publications by applying the selection criteria described in the following paragraph, obtaining 40 papers.

Three individual researchers (D.C., J.F.-Á., and M.S.) performed the search for publications in the English language. More details are provided in Table 1 and in the flow diagram (Figure 1), in order to make this search replicable in the future.

Table 1. Detailed search strategy.

Process	Results
PubMed/Medline	2758
Web of Science	2235
Total	4993
Not duplicated	3613
Excluded (after reading title and abstract)	3212
Retrieved	401
Excluded (after applying inclusion criteria)	361
Excluded (missing experimental data)	0
Final included articles	40

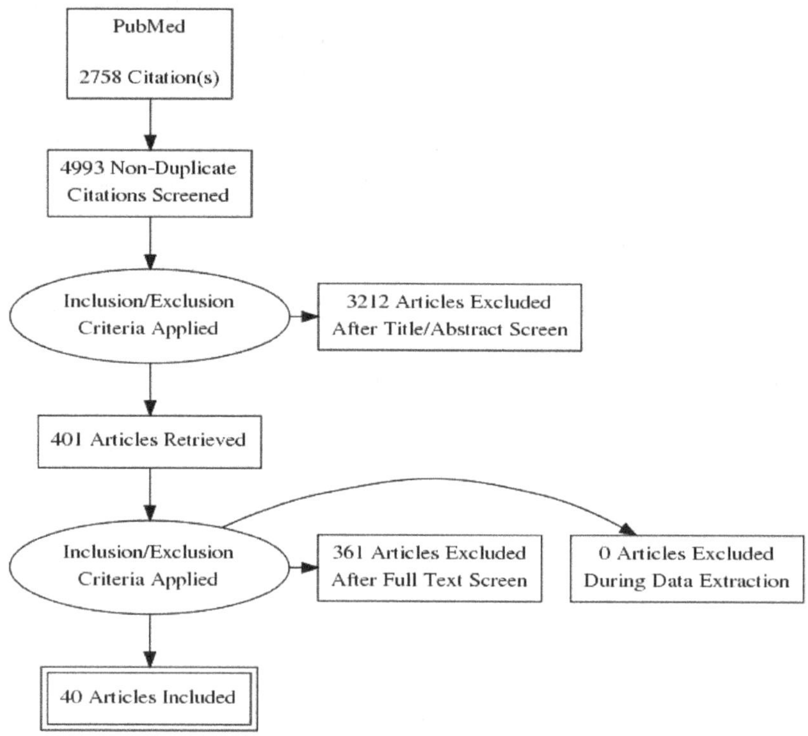

Figure 1. PRISMA (Preferred Reporting Items for Systematic Reviews and Meta-Analyses) flow diagram.

2.2. Selection Criteria

We included all studies involving a sample of adults with a primary (both current or past) diagnosis of MDD, using recognised diagnostic criteria (Diagnostic and Statistical Manual of Mental Disorders—DSM; International Classification of Disease—ICD). We excluded non-English papers and studies that did not meet the inclusion criteria. We also excluded articles that did not have full-text available, and the following types of manuscripts: Conference papers, reviews and systematic reviews, metanalyses, meeting abstracts, notes, case reports, letters to the editor, editor's notes, extended abstracts, proceedings, patents, editorials, and other editorial materials. We tried to contact the corresponding authors, when necessary, to obtain missing or supplementary data.

Ecological momentary assessment: We included studies that adopted an ecological momentary assessment by means of hand-held technologies (such as smartphones, personal digital assistants, or hand-held computers) for the collection of daily self-reports, thus excluding studies that used paper-and-pencil diaries. Additionally, we included studies that integrated daily self-reports with data supplied by sensors and biosensors.

Ecological momentary interventions: We included EMIs that were provided to patients through hand-held technologies. We selected studies in which the proposed EMI was either a stand-alone intervention or combined with other types of treatment. We also included EMI that collected data from wearable biosensors or device-embedded sensors. Because providing continuous feedback to patients has been shown to be a valuable therapeutic procedure [29], we also included studies that adopted EMA-based feedback as a therapeutic tool for clinically depressed patients.

2.3. *Quality Assessment and Data Abstraction*

To control for the risk of bias, PRISMA recommendations for systematic literature analysis were followed. Studies were independently selected by three different authors (D.C., M.S., and J.F.-Á.), who first analysed titles and abstracts and subsequently selected the full papers that met the inclusion criteria, resolving disagreements through consensus. For what concerns the EMA included studies, the main aim was to provide a perspective of clinical, technical, and technological issues related to this approach: In other words, we were interested in EMA as a clinical and experimental tool to be used in the psychological field, regardless of the study design or variables of outcome (Colombo et al., 2018). No risk of bias assessment was therefore performed. Differently, risk of bias of EMI studies was assessed by two independent reviewers (D.C and J.F.-Á.). As both randomized and non-randomized controlled trials were included, quality assessment was assessed with the Downs and Black quality index [30].

The data extracted from each study were as follows: Author(s), sample(s), variable(s), device(s), sensor(s), duration, prompt(s) per day, sampling schema, primary outcome(s) for the selected studies on EMA (Table 2); and author(s), name of the intervention, sample(s), content of the intervention, duration, device(s), sensor(s), and primary outcome(s) for the studies proposing an EMI (Table 3).

3. Results

3.1. *Ecological Momentary Assessment in MDD*

After applying the inclusion criteria, 32 studies were retrieved that investigated and assessed MDD through a technology-based EMA.

A synthesis of the results is provided in Table 2.

3.1.1. Electronic Devices and Use of Sensors

Most of the selected studies administered daily self-reports either through a personal digital assistant (PDA) or a smartphone. Only three studies adopted different technological solutions that allowed them to collect both self-reports and data gathered from sensors and biosensors. Conrad et al. [31] used the LifeShirt System (Vivometrics, Inc., Ventura, CA, USA), a comfortable garment with integrated biosensors that can continuously monitor various cardiopulmonary parameters, including heart rate (HR), respiration, and posture. With an embedded hand-held computer, patients can also complete self-reports following daily beep signals. In another study, Kim and colleagues adopted ECOLOG [32], a watch-type computer characterized by an 8-direction joystick and an integrated actimetry sensor. Via a beep signal, the wristwatch prompts patients to complete momentary assessments directly on the watch screen. Similarly, a compact wrist–worn electronic diary was used by Littlewood et al. to collect both self-reports and sleep/wake cycles with an embedded actimetry sensor [33].

Although a growing number of studies analyse data from embedded-sensors and biosensors in research on mental health disorders [34], their use in association with EMA has been low in the field of MDD. Among our selected studies, only seven of the 32 studies collected physiological measures in addition to self-reports. Conrad and colleagues collected cardiac and respiratory measures as indices of vagal activity, along with physical activity measured through an embedded actimetry sensor [31], whereas Ottaviani and colleagues collected ambulatory HR [35]. The remaining five articles investigated the association of depressive symptoms with sleep/wake cycles [32,33,36] and physical activity [37,38] using actimetry sensors.

Table 2. More detailed information about the selected Ecological Momentary Assessment studies.

	Authors	Sample	Variables	Device(s)	Duration	Prompts Per Day	Sampling Schema	Compliance	Sensor(s)	Primary Outcome(s)
Recall bias	[8]	MDD (n = 26), and HCG (n = 25)	Affect	Palm Tungsten E2	7 days	8	Semi-randomized	89%	No	Both depressed and non-depressed participants overestimate the retrospective recall of PA and NA. Depressed patients are more inaccurate in recalling NA.
	[26]	MDD (n = 13)	Randomized items from PHQ-9 questionnaire	"Mindful Moods" mobile application	29/30 days	3	Randomized	78%	No	Even if strongly correlated, the PHQ-9 scores collected through the mobile application are significantly higher than those obtained though the retrospective paper-and-pencil PHQ-9.
Symptoms monitoring	[39]	MDD (n = 20), and BD (n = 21)	Affect; stressors; behaviours; environment; social context	PDA	3 days	5	Fixed sampling scheme	85.7%	No	High rates of acceptance and compliance are observed among both samples. Participants show a practice effect, i.e., faster responses over the course of the study.
	[40]	MDD (n = 26)	Depressive and anxiety symptoms	Palm Treo 650 Smartphone (Mental Health Telemetry mobile application)	14 days	1	Selected by the patient	Not specified	No	Self-reported ratings of improvement at day 7 predict response to the treatment.
	[41]	MDD (n = 59)	Symptoms, sleep patterns, cognitive functioning	iHOPE smartphone application	8 weeks	2 (symptoms) 1 (sleep duration and quality)	Not specified	Not specified	No	Baseline depression scores evaluated with HAM-D are associated with scores of PHQ-9, VAS for depression and anxiety symptoms collected with the application.
Cortisol	[42]	MDD (n = 32), mD (n = 18), and HCG (n = 50)	Daily activities (frequency, social contacts); cortisol	Palm Pilot M100	4 days (over a maximum period of 7 days)	4 (saliva samples) 1 (self-report)	Fixed sampling scheme	Not specified	No	In the control sample, daily activities are negatively associated with cortisol levels. This association is not observed in depressed patients.
	[43]	MDD (n = 37), and HCG (n = 36)	Sleep patterns; social contacts; cortisol	Palm Pilot M100	3 non-consecutive days (over a maximum period of 7 days)	3 (saliva samples) 1 (self-report)	Fixed sampling scheme	93%	No	Depressed patients show lower cortisol awakening response, lower sleep quality, and more negative social interactions.
	[31]	MDD (n = 46) and HCG (n = 19)	Physiological indices (HR, respiration, accelerometer, cortisol); mood	LifeShirt System, with an integrated hand-held computer	1 day	6 (self-reports) 5 (saliva samples)	Fixed sampling scheme	91%	LifeShirt System (HR, respiration, actigraphy)	Cortisol level and HRV do not differ between the two groups. Interestingly, NA is negatively correlated with HRV only in the control sample.
	[44]	Remitted MDD (n = 31) and HCG (n = 32)	Mood; ruminative self-focus; stressful events; cortisol	Palm Tungsten E2	2 consecutive days	10	Semi-randomized	94%	No	Rumination and low mood are associated with increased activation of the HPAA. In remitted patients, HPAA is less responsive to subtle emotional events.
	[36]	MDD (n = 15), and HCG (n = 15)	Affect; cognition; daily activities; cortisol	PsyMate	30 days	3	Fixed sampling scheme	92.5%	ActiCal (Respironics, Bend, OR, USA)	Compared to healthy participants, depressed patients report higher cortisol levels, higher α-amylase levels, and a greater ratio of α-amylase over cortisol. This latter association, however, disappears when correction for lifestyle factors is applied.
	[45]	MDD (n = 15), and HCG (n = 15)	Affect; cortisol	PsyMate	30 days	3	Fixed sampling scheme	92.5%	No	PA and NA are bidirectionally associated with cortisol levels. Nevertheless, the direction, sign, and timing of this association show great variability among subjects.

Table 2. *Cont.*

	Authors	Sample	Variables	Device(s)	Duration	Prompts Per Day	Sampling Schema	Compliance	Sensor(s)	Primary Outcome(s)
Sleep patterns	[46]	MDD (n = 35), mD (n = 25), and HCG (n = 36)	Positive and negative affects	PDA	3 days	10	Semi-randomized	65%	No	Sleep quality predicts lower PA, but not NA. Low PA is associated with poor subjective sleep quality and self-reported daily dysfunction.
	[47]	MDD and mD (n = 60), and HCG (n = 35)	Positive and negative affects; events appraisal	Palm Pilot Zire 22	3 days	10	Semi-randomized	65%	No	In the non-clinical sample, sleep disturbances are associated with enhanced NA in response to negative events. Considering depressed patients, sleep disturbances negatively influence the emotional reactivity to both neutral and negative events.
	[48]	MDD (n = 27), and HCG (n = 27)	PA and NA, sleep quality; tiredness; rumination	PsyMate	30 days	3	Fixed sampling scheme	96%	No	Sleep quality directly influences PA and NA experienced during the following day, but not vice versa. Tiredness is a mediator.
	[49]	MDD (n = 14) and HCG (n = 15)	PA; NA; fatigue; sleep; activities; cognition; melatonin	PsyMate	30 days	3	Fixed sampling scheme	93%	No	Melatonin is associated with changes in affect and fatigue. However, changes in affect and fatigue are also predictors of melatonin levels. Individuals that do not show this association report higher depression severity and worse sleep quality.
	[38]	MDD (n = 27), and HCG (n = 27)	Sleep patterns	PsyMate	30 days	3	Fixed sampling scheme	96%	ActiCal (Respironics, Bend, OR, USA)	Sleep duration affects next-day physical activity. Depression does not moderate this association.
	[33]	MDD (n = 51)	Sleep patterns and quality; suicide ideation; entrapment perception	PRO-Diary actigraph watch (CamNtech)	7 days	6	Semi-randomized	89%	Accelerometer	Poor sleep quality, both objectively and subjectively evaluated, is associated with higher next-day suicide ideations. Suicide ideation does not influence sleep patterns and quality.
Physical activity	[50]	MDD (n = 53), and HCG (n = 53)	Physical activity; positive and negative affects	Palm Pilot Zire 22	7 days	8	Randomized	75%	No	Both samples show higher PA following physical activity. More specifically, depressed patients show a significantly higher increase in experienced PA levels after physical activity.
	[32]	MDD (n = 14) and HCG (n = 43)	Mood; physical symptoms; physical activity	Ruputer ECOLOG	Average: 37.43 days (range:18–67 days)	4	Semi-randomized	93%	Ambulatory Monitors Inc.—actigraph	Depressive mood is associated with increased intermittency of locomotor activity.
	[37]	MDD (n = 10), and HCG (n = 10)	Mood; cognition; daily activities; physical activity	PsyMate	30 days	3	Fixed sampling scheme	91%	ActiCal Respironics—actigraph	Despite the observation of large interindividual differences, results show a positive effect of physical activity on PA in all participants.
Rumination	[51]	MDD (n = 6) and HCG (n = 7)	Context; mood; depressive symptoms; EEG (at baseline)	Palm Pilot and EEG (at baseline)	7 days	5	Not specified	Not specified	No	Lower activation of bilateral PFC predicts higher rates of rumination, whereas higher levels of self-esteem are associated with lower right PFC activity.
	[35]	MDD (n = 18) and HCG (n = 18)	Thoughts; disturbing events; feelings; possible influencing factors; feelings; HR	Electronic diary implemented on a smartphone	1 day	Not reported	Semi-randomized	Not specified	RS 800CX; Bodyguard2 (HR and HRV)	Depressed participants show higher rates of perseverative cognition, which are associated with lower HRV.
	[52]	MDD (n = 38), GAD (n = 36), MDD with GAD comorbidity (n = 38), and HCG (n = 33)	Events stressfulness; rumination	Palm Pilot Zire 22	7 days	8	Randomized	72%	No	MDD and GAD participants show the same level of rumination, which is even more severe in comorbid cases. Higher rates of rumination are predictive of worse affect, more maladaptive behaviours, and more severe symptoms.
	[53]	MDD (n = 16), GAD (n = 15), MDD with GAD comorbidity (n = 20), and HCG (n = 19)	Rumination; worry; PA and NA; significant events	Palm Pilot Zire 22	6 to7 days	8	Semi-randomized	65%	No	Levels of rumination among all the clinical samples are higher in response to significant events. Decreased PA and increased NA are associated with higher momentary rumination.

Table 2. *Cont.*

	Authors	Sample	Variables	Device(s)	Duration	Prompts Per Day	Sampling Schema	Compliance	Sensor(s)	Primary Outcome(s)
Emotional reaction	[54]	Remitted MDD (n = 55) and HCG (n = 55)	Perceived stress; mood	Hand held Psion "Revo" computer	7 days	5	Randomized	90%	No	Past episodes of depression are likely to increase the vulnerability to stressful events, especially in male participants.
	[55]	MDD (n = 35), mD (n = 26), and HCG (n = 38)	Context; mood; events (nature of the event; location; people involved; affective rating)	Palm Pilot Zire 22	3 non-consecutive days (over a period of 5 days)	10	Semi-randomized	65%	No	Both MDD and mD patients show lower levels of positive affect and rate events as more stressful and unpleasant than the control group. Furthermore, they show a higher reduction in negative feelings after positive events.
	[50]	MDD (n = 53), and HCG (n = 53)	Affect; significant events	Palm Pilot Zire 22	7/8 days	8	Randomized	78%	No	Results point out greater emotional instability with respect to NA in depressed patients. No differences are observed in terms of reactivity, inertia, and instability in PA.
	[56]	MDD (n = 21) and MDD with BPD comorbidity (n = 20)	Affect and mood; events; subjective affective reactivity	Smartphone to access a web platform	7 days	5	Randomized	94%	No	Comorbidity with BPD does not imply major affective instability, but it is associated with lower subjective perception of affective reactivity.
	[57]	Remitted MDD (n = 10) and HCG (n = 11)	Mood; PA and NA; visual mental imagery	"Imagine your Mood", smartphone application	3 days a week, for 8 weeks	10	Semi-randomized	Not specified	No	In both samples, higher levels of visual imagery-based processing are associated with higher levels of PA and better mood, regardless of the valence of the imagery content. Elevated levels of visual imagery-based processing are not associated with daily affective reactivity.
	[58]	MDD (n = 51), and BPD (n = 80)	PA, NA, fear; hostility; sadness; interpersonal events	Palm Pilot Zire 31	28 days	6	Semi-randomized	86%	No	Rejection and disagreement increase NA (especially hostility and sadness) both at a momentary and daily level, regardless of the diagnosis. The association between rejection/disagreement and hostility is stronger in BPD patients.
	[59]	MDD (n = 12), DD (n = 3), BD (n = 15)	Affect; location; social context; gambling desire/motivation/activities	Palm Pilot Zire 22	30 days	3	Randomized	73%	No	High levels of sadness and arousal are predictive of gambling desire, regardless of the diagnosis. Depressed individuals are likely to gamble to increase PA or for social reasons.
	[60]	MDD (n = 15), GAD (n = 25)	Symptoms, PA, NA, rumination, behavioural avoidance, reassurance seeking	Web-based survey	30 days	4	Not specified	Not specified	No	Using a person-by-person approach, results show that moment-to-moment symptomatology is mainly driven by positive mood, hopelessness, anger, and irritability, but not depressed mood, anhedonia, or worry.

MDD: major depressive disorder; mD: minor depression; HCG: healthy control group; BDP: borderline personality disorder; GAD: generalized anxiety disorders; PDA: personal digital assistant; DD: dysthymic disorder; PFC: prefrontal cortex; PA: positive affect; NA: negative affect; HRV: heart rate variability; PHQ-9: Patient Health Questionnaire-9; QUID-SR: Quick Inventory of Depressive Symptomatology—Self Report; HADS-A: Hospital Anxiety and Depression Scale; PANAS: Positive and Negative Affect Schedule; HPAA: hypothalamic-pituitary-adrenal axis.

Table 3. More detailed information about the selected Ecological Momentary Intervention studies.

Authors	Name	Sample	Intervention	Duration	Prompts	Sampling Schema	Sensor(s)	Primary Outcome(s)
[61]	Mobylize!	MDD ($n = 7$), with different comorbidities	Mobylize! is a context-aware system, composed of three main elements: (1) A mobile application for the collection of self-reports; (2) a website with feedback and theoretical lessons; (3) periodic contacts with trained coaches	8 weeks	5/day	Randomized	38 concurrent sensors integrated in the phone	Mobylize! significantly reduced depressive symptoms. Predictive models did not reach high levels of accuracy, especially for mood.
[62]	PsyMate	MDD ($n = 102$): Experimental condition ($n = 33$), pseudo-experimental condition ($n = 36$), control condition ($n = 33$)	Daily assessment of self-reports and weekly EMA-derived feedback through face-to-face sessions	3 days per week, for 6 weeks	10/day	Semi-randomized	No	The use of EMA-derived feedback as a complementary intervention to pharmacological treatment significantly decreased depressive symptoms. These improvements were also maintained over time.
[63]	PsyMate	MDD ($n = 102$): Experimental condition ($n = 33$), pseudo-experimental condition ($n = 36$), control condition ($n = 33$)	Daily assessment of self-reports and weekly EMA-derived feedback through face-to-face sessions	3 days per week, for 6 weeks	10/day	Semi-randomized	No	The use of Psymate as a technique of self-monitoring could improve patients' feelings of empowerment.
[64]	PsyMate	MDD ($n = 102$): Experimental condition ($n = 33$), pseudo-experimental condition ($n = 36$), control condition ($n = 33$)	Daily assessment of self-reports and weekly EMA-derived feedback through face-to-face sessions	3 days per week, for 6 weeks	10/day	Semi-randomized	No	Face-to-face EMA-derived feedback sessions did not increase the rate of PA experienced during or shortly after the intervention.
[65]	Medlink	MDD ($n = 8$)	Medlink is a mobile application delivering psychological support to MDD patients. The application provides users with: (1) psychoeducation; (2) weekly symptom assessment; (3) medication adherence monitoring; (4) monthly communication with a professional based on the previous points	4 weeks	1/week	Not specified	No	Medlink was positively evaluated by participants, especially regarding the weekly psychoeducation lessons. Depression severity of participants significantly decreased over the course of the experiment.

Table 3. *Cont.*

Authors	Name	Sample	Intervention	Duration	Prompts	Sampling Schema	Sensor(s)	Primary Outcome(s)
[66]	Help4Mood	MDD (n = 28): Experimental condition (n = 14) and control condition (n = 14)	Web platform providing daily assessment of symptoms, self-monitoring, and tailored activities. The delivered content is created in response to the user's actions through a virtual agent	About 5 weeks	CESD-VAS-VA: 1/day PHQ-9: 1/week	Not specified	Accelerometer and acoustic speech analysis	Only half of the participants used Help4Mood regularly. Significant changes in depressive symptoms were observed only among regular users.
[67]	PsyMate	MDD (n = 102): Experimental condition (n = 33), pseudo-experimental condition (n = 36), control condition (n = 33)	Daily assessment of self-reports and weekly EMA-derived feedback through face-to-face sessions	3 days per week, for 6 weeks	10/day	Semi-randomized	No	The use of EMA-derived feedback decreased depressive symptoms and improved maladaptive behaviours.
[68]	PsyMate	MDD (n = 79): Experimental condition (n = 25), pseudo-experimental condition (n = 30), control condition (n = 24)	Daily assessment of self-reports and weekly EMA-derived feedback through face-to-face sessions	3 days per week, for 6 weeks	10/day	Semi-randomized	No	The use of a self-monitoring EMA improves negative emotion differentiation.

MDD: major depressive disorder; PA: positive affect; CESD-VAS-VA: brief visual analogue scale version of the Center of Epidemiological Studies Depression. Scale; PHQ-9: Patient Health Questionnaire.

3.1.2. Sampling Methods

Currently, different EMA designs can be used to define prompt scheduling, depending on the main purpose of the study. It is possible to prompt participants using fixed time periods or randomized/semi-randomized samplings (time-based sampling). Alternatively, participants can be asked to personally fill in the assessment after the occurrence of a specific behaviour or event (event-based sampling). Whereas time-based samplings depend on a signal emitted by the device (signal-contingent), event-based samplings are not preceded by a prompt (event-contingent). Signal-contingent schemas are useful when repeated measures are needed to obtain a representative value of a variable or when the objective is to capture dynamic variables (e.g., mood), whereas event-contingent schemas are more likely to be adopted when the main focus is on a specific behaviour that occurs randomly or less frequently during the day (e.g., smoking a cigarette). Regarding our selected studies, none of them adopted event-based sampling. Most of the studies collected data using randomized or semi-randomized schemas, whereas nine studies prompted participants to note information at fixed time points during the day. This latter approach was adopted especially by the studies that investigated the association between cortisol or melatonin and depression, i.e., when the assessed variable required greater temporal precision and accuracy.

The duration of the data collection showed great variability. Some studies collected self-reports for a brief time period (less than 3 days); this choice was especially observed in the field of cortisol and sleep pattern research. Other studies required longer periods of assessment, where participants were involved for one or two months. This was especially true for studies investigating physical activity and its association with depressive symptoms. The same high variability was observed in the number of prompts, which varied from 1 to 20 prompts per day.

3.1.3. Compliance and Dropout Rates

With the term "compliance", we refer to the percentage of answered prompts. A few studies did not report this information [35,40–42,51,57,60]. However, the majority clearly addressed this issue. Sixteen studies reported compliance rates higher than 85%, five studies showed rates between 84% and 70%, and four studies collected 65% of the total possible answers. Patient dropout was related to diagnosis change, subjective burden, technical problems, incomplete data, retrospective completion of the electronic diary, missed prompts, worsening of symptoms, or non-attendance at follow-up sessions.

To prevent backfilling, different solutions were adopted. In most of the studies, participants could complete self-reports for a fixed time period after the prompt, ranging from a few minutes to a maximum of one hour. To increase compliance, two studies also gave participants the possibility of postponing prompts.

3.1.4. Contribution of EMA to the Study of MDD

As Table 4 shows, so far EMA has been applied to seven different fields. In the following paragraph, we will provide an overview of EMA's contribution to the understanding and assessment of MDD.

Table 4. Fields of application of EMAs for Major Depressive Disorder.

Field of Application	Retrieved Articles	Aim	Advantages
Recall bias	[8,26]	Experimental	No retrospective bias; control over backfilling; repeated momentary measurements.
Symptoms monitoring	[39–41]	Clinical	Continuous monitoring (symptoms assessment, treatment progress); real-time feedback to clinicians (e.g., crisis plan) and users (e.g., patterns visualization).

Table 4. *Cont.*

Field of Application	Retrieved Articles	Aim	Advantages
Cortisol dysregulation	[31,36,42–45]	Experimental	Role of contextual variables; temporal relationship between physiological measures and self-reports.
Sleep patterns	[33,38,46–49]	Experimental	Control over backfilling; no retrospective bias; integration of self-reports with passive data supplied by sensors and biosensors.
Physical activity	[32,37,50]	Experimental	Role of contextual variables; integration of self-reports with passive data supplied by sensors; temporal relationship between physiological measures and self-reports.
Rumination	[35,51–53]	Experimental	Role of contextual variables; rumination deployment across time.
Affect and emotional reactivity	[50,54–60],	Experimental	Role of contextual variables; temporal deployment of affect and emotional reactivity.

Recall Bias

Increasing evidence shows that memories often have inaccurate and imprecise content due to recall bias. In the case of EMAs, two studies were carried out to investigate this bias, comparing EMA daily data to retrospective assessments. Ben-Zeev and colleagues compared positive (PA) and negative (NA) affect collected through an EMA to scores obtained by means of traditional paper-and-pencil retrospective questionnaires [8]. When retrospectively recalled, both PA and NA were overestimated, regardless of the diagnosis. Interestingly, the control group was more likely to exaggerate the retrieval of PA rather than NA, but this trend was not observed in depressed patients. By contrast, Torous and colleagues developed a smartphone application to administer randomized subsets of items taken from the Patient Health Questionnaire (PHQ-9) [69], compared to the traditional paper-based PHQ-9. Symptoms were evaluated as more severe in daily EMA evaluations, compared to the retrospective PHQ-9 assessment. According to the authors, this discrepancy could be due to different factors, such as recall bias or stigma.

Symptom Monitoring

Unexpectedly, we could only retrieve three studies within this research field, i.e., studies that actually applied EMA to monitor clinically depressed patients. Husky and colleagues investigated the acceptability of a three-days computerized ambulatory monitoring on MDD and BD patients, showing encouraging compliance and acceptance rates among both samples. Practice effects were observed (faster response time over the course of the study), thus suggesting the importance of considering the potential effects of EMA duration on self-reports [39]. Schaffer et al. developed a system called "Mental Health Telemetry" to monitor symptoms of patients receiving pharmacological treatment [40]. According to the results, a reduction in depressive symptoms was already observable one day after beginning the treatment, and symptoms on day 7 were predictive of treatment outcome. Similarly, iHOPE is a smartphone application for the daily monitoring of depressive symptoms and sleep patterns [41]. EMA assessments of depression, sleep quality, and anxiety were highly associated with the Hamilton Depression Rating Scale (HAM-D), administered at baseline. Nevertheless, application use decreased significantly over the weeks, from 3.4 days per week to 0.4 days per week after 8 weeks, highlighting the important issue of compliance in EMA assessments.

Cortisol Secretion

Stetler and colleagues investigated the associations among cortisol and sleep patterns, social interactions [43], and daily activities [42]. Not only were cortisol levels after awakening different in depressed and healthy participants, but the impact of psychosocial variables on cortisol secretion was also dissimilar. Consistently, the Hypothalamic–pituitary–adrenal (HPA) axis of depressed patients was no longer able to respond to the timing of the sleep-wake cycle, daily routines, and external social experiences. One study explored the impact of cortisol on affect, showing a bidirectional association between PA and NA and daily cortisol levels [45]. Nevertheless, high variability was observed among participants regarding the timing, direction, and sign of this association. For instance, NA was positively associated with cortisol 50% of the time, while the association between cortisol and PA was almost always negative. Booij et al. identified higher cortisol and α-amylase levels among depressed individuals [36]. Similarly, when applying individual correction for lifestyle factors, the association of depression to cortisol and the ratio of α-amylase over cortisol was no longer significant, suggesting that generalization from groups does not always reflect the single individual. Nevertheless, Conrad and colleagues could not find cortisol differences between depressed and non-depressed participants. Interestingly, a negative correlation between NA and heart rate variability (HRV) was observed only in the control group, suggesting that constant NA may alter the normal interaction between affectivity and the autonomic nervous system [31].

Finally, interesting outcomes were also observed among remitted MDD patients [44]. Despite remission, patients showed reduced cortisol levels throughout the day and a different interaction between affect and cortisol, thus suggesting a reduction in the HPA axis' responsiveness as a potential marker of recurrent depression.

Sleep Patterns

According to our search, six studies adopted an EMA to explore sleep disturbances in depression. Through the daily administration of morning self-reports about sleep patterns, O'Leary et al. found that depression was associated with lower perceived sleep quality, which in turn affected negative emotional reactivity to both neutral and unpleasant events during the day [47]. However, in healthy participants, sleep disturbances only affected emotional reactivity to unpleasant events. In other words, depression could be a factor affecting the relationship between sleep quality and emotional reactivity. Similarly, two studies analysed the influence of sleep quality on daily affect [46,48]. As expected, higher sleep quality was associated with higher PA in both healthy and depressed participants. Surprisingly, there was no evidence of the moderating role of depression in the association between sleep and affect. Nevertheless, sleep quality affected daily mood, but not vice versa, because higher sleep quality was associated with increased PA and decreased NA the following day. This association did not differ between depressed and healthy participants. Similarly, sleep duration was found to affect next-day physical activity, but again, no difference between depressed and non-depressed individuals was observed [38]. An EMA was finally adopted to investigate the association between sleep patterns and suicide ideation in a sample of depressed patients [33]. Poor sleep quality, both at subjective and objective levels, was associated with increased suicide ideations the following day. However, suicidal thoughts did not predict sleep patterns the following night.

Bouwmans and colleagues also collected repeated saliva samples to analyse the association of depression with melatonin, an important hormone related to sleep onset [49]. A bidirectional relationship between affect and fatigue, and melatonin was pointed out: Melatonin is associated with changes in affect and fatigue; however, affect and fatigue are also predictors of melatonin levels. Participants that did not show this association were likely to report higher rates of depression, worse sleep quality, and lower energy expenditure.

Physical Activity

In order to analyse the effect of self-initiated physical activity on mood, clinically depressed patients were asked to report their daily physical activity [50]. Both healthy and depressed participants showed higher levels of PA following physical activity, but no decrease in NA. Notably, the increase in PA after physical exercise was greater in depressed patients, which is consistent with the ample evidence supporting behavioural activation in general, and physical activity in particular, for the treatment of depression. Confirming these results, another study found that physical activity was associated with subsequent increased PA, regardless of the diagnosis [37]. However, the analysis also revealed high subjective variability in the association between physical activity and mood in terms of strength, direction, and temporal aspects. Finally, Kim and colleagues developed a statistical model with cross validity that identified a significant association between higher intermittency of locomotor activity and worse mood ratings [32], suggesting the possibility of predicting patients' moods through the analysis of momentary locomotor patterns. According to their model, a worsening of depressive mood was associated with increased intermittency of locomotor activity.

Rumination

Ruscio and colleagues investigated the relationship between stressful events and rumination in MDD and GAD patients [52]. Both clinical samples showed higher levels of rumination in response to stressful situations, which were further worsened by symptom severity and extensive comorbidity. In addition, rumination significantly mediated the impact of stress on symptoms and affect; that is, higher rumination after a stressful event predicted greater NA and more maladaptive behaviours. Putman and colleagues investigated rumination and self-esteem through the assessment of resting baseline PFC alpha activity, along with the momentary assessment of affect and depressive symptoms, in a sample of clinically depressed individuals [51]. Rumination was found to be associated with an increased alpha signal in the bilateral prefrontal cortex (i.e., decreased neural activation), whereas an increased alpha signal in the right prefrontal cortex was positively correlated with higher self-esteem ratings. One study investigated perseverative thoughts (i.e., depressive rumination, worry, and reactive rumination) in relation to mind wandering [35]. Participants were instructed to complete a smartphone diary every 30 min for one day, and these self-reports were integrated with continuous HR monitoring. Confirming the hypothesis that mind wandering is not a maladaptive behaviour per se, only perseverative cognition was associated with health risk factors, such as lower HRV, worse mood, and higher interference in daily functioning. Finally, one study examined the dynamics of worry and rumination in daily life [53]. Contrary to the hypothesis, levels of worry were not significantly associated with the occurrence of significant events, whereas rumination was significantly higher in response to these circumstances. Compared to the control group, clinically depressed individuals showed decreased PA and increased NA as a consequence of high rumination levels.

Affect and Emotional Reactivity

Thompson and colleagues investigated emotional reactivity, emotional inertia, and emotional instability in depressed patients [50]. Compared to healthy participants, clinically depressed patients showed higher NA instability, whereas no differences in PA instability were observed. Both samples reported increased NA after a negative event; however, depressed patients showed a greater decrease in NA and increase in PA after a positive event. These results were confirmed by another study that showed a greater reduction in NA following positive events in depressed individuals [55]. When considering BPD comorbidity, depressed patients were found to be less emotionally influenced by events, and to perceive themselves as less emotionally reactive [56]. Other factors that affect emotional reactivity are gender and past depression [54]. In one study, women and remitted patients evaluated daily events as more negative than men, and they showed worse mood and higher emotional reactivity in response to daily stressors. Finally, a smartphone application was developed to assess visual mental imagery and its impact on mood and affective reactivity in healthy people and remitted MDD patients [57]. Participants were asked to focus on their mental representations, i.e., what they had in mind, eight times per day. Imagery-based processing was associated with better mood, regardless of the valence of the mental representation. This pattern was similar in healthy and depressed participants. However, no association between mental imagery and affective reactivity was observed.

Regarding daily affect, one study explored the impact of gambling desire on mood in a sample of depressed individuals [59]. Higher levels of sadness and arousal were associated with higher rates of gambling desire. Consistently, depressed participants were also likely to perform gambling behaviours to increase their current PA levels. However, momentary affect did not predict actual gambling behaviours. An EMA was also used to investigate the influence of social rejection and disagreement on daily affect in MDD and BPD patients [58]. As expected, momentary and daily negative interpersonal events triggered higher NA (fear, hostility, and sadness) in both groups. High levels of hostility predicted rejection and disagreements, whereas sadness was only a predictor of social rejection. The aforementioned relationships were stronger in BPD patients than in depressed participants.

Finally, one study investigated the topology and temporal dynamics of depression and anxiety symptoms using contemporaneous and temporal network models [60]. Positive (positive, content, enthusiastic, energetic) and negative (down) mood were the most representative variables of patients' core symptoms. While "worried" and "down" did not show temporal influence, "positive mood", "hopelessness", "anger", and "irritability" were the strongest drivers of moment-to-moment symptomatology.

3.2. Ecological Momentary Intervention in MDD

The selection process resulted in eight studies that administered an EMI to clinically depressed patients. In all, four different interventions were identified: Psymate, Mobylize, Hel4Mood, and Medlink.

3.2.1. General Overview of the Interventions

Psymate is a PDA-based EMA for symptom monitoring that aims to increase awareness about depression and the dynamics that characterize this disorder [62–64,67,68]. Psymate allows patients to record daily symptoms and affect. Based on these daily assessments, patients meet a clinician weekly and receive graphical feedback on the association between PA levels and daily life activities, events, or social interactions, as well as on the association between PA changes and the number of depressive complaints. In this way, patients have the chance to reflect on their affective state and the relationship between symptoms and contextual variables with a professional. According to Heron's definition, "the key feature of all EMIs is that the treatment is provided to people during their everyday lives (i.e., in real time) and settings (i.e., real world)" [22]. Therefore, Psymate does not meet all the criteria for an EMI, as EMA-feedbacks are provided during weekly face-to-face sessions. However, we decided to include this intervention because we think it provides important insights about the potential of self-monitoring EMA as a therapeutic tool.

Likewise, Mobylize! constitutes an ecological intervention composed of a mobile application, an interactive website, and a system for email/telephone support [61]. The most innovative aspect of this application is the integration of self-reports with data from smartphone sensors. Mobylize! is provided with a context-aware system. Thanks to a machine learning algorithm, the application can predict the state of the patient (mood, emotions, cognitive/motivational states, activities, environmental context, and social context). Specifically, the system works in three different phases: (1) Data collection, during which 38 sensors collect sensor information; (2) learners, during which prompted self-reports are matched and paired with simultaneously labelled state data to develop predictive models; and (3) action components, a continuous process that analyses sensor data in order to update previous predictive models without the direct input of the user. Mobylize! is designed to prompt patients to assess mood, intensity of emotions, fatigue, pleasure, accomplishment, concentration, engagement, perceived control, location, and interactions five or more times a day. To accommodate new data, every new self-report is subsequently associated with the generation and modification of previous models. Thanks to this complex system, the mobile application sends tailored feedback to participants. Through the website, users can graphically visualize self-report patterns, read theoretical lessons, and use interactive tools, such as tailored plans and calendars, for monitoring daily activities. Lastly, a trained clinician contacts users periodically by phone or email to provide technical support, reinforce adherence, and enhance motivation.

Help4Mood is a web-platform to self-monitor daily symptoms, mood, activities, and thoughts [66]. Based on a Cognitive Behavioural Therapy (CBT) approach, Help4Mood helps patients to reflect on the emotional and cognitive patterns related to depression. In addition to collecting daily self-reports, the application receives data from an actimetry sensor and acoustic analysis of speech. The innovative aspect of Help4Mood is the use of a virtual agent, completely customizable in terms of voice, clothing style, sex, and language, that communicates with users to provide tailored exercises and activities and guide them through the daily questionnaires. The application also has an emergency section called the "crisis plan": As soon as symptom worsening is detected, the application prompts users to contact a professional or a relative.

Finally, Medlink is a mobile application to support and monitor MDD patients taking antidepressant medication [65]. The main purpose of the app is to address the failure points that usually occur between professionals and newly diagnosed patients. On the one hand, the application provides users with weekly psychoeducation material and sends suggestions about medication management and how to deal with depressive symptoms. On the other hand, it monitors patients' treatment and depressive symptoms. Every four weeks, personal communication with a professional is scheduled to give patients monthly feedback about disease progression.

3.2.2. Effectiveness of the Intervention

Psymate was tested in a sample of 102 clinically depressed patients in a three-arm randomized controlled trial [62–64,67] with an experimental condition (treatment as usual – TAU - and six-week Psymate treatment, with weekly face-to-face feedback sessions), a pseudo-experimental condition (TAU and Psymate without EMA face-to-face feedbacks), and a control condition (TAU). Three different categories of weekly feedback were provided: (1) Positive affect, (2) positive affect in relation to events appraised with an internal versus external locus of control, and (3) positive affect in relation to social interactions. Results showed a significant reduction in depressive symptoms in the experimental group that was maintained in the follow-up assessment. Participants in the pseudo-experimental condition reported decreased depressive symptoms in the first weeks of the treatment, but this gain was not maintained across the weeks. Notably, the use of Psymate was associated with increased levels of perceived empowerment, regardless of the presence of weekly feedback, and with increased experienced PA throughout the treatment. Decreased depressive symptoms were also associated with increased positive daily behaviours. Finally, Widdershoven and colleagues observed a significant improvement in negative emotions' differentiation and a close-to-significance improvement in positive emotions' differentiation after 6-weeks of self-monitoring, regardless of EMA-derived feedbacks [68].

Mobylize! was tested in a small pilot study with a sample of 7 MMD patients [61]. According to the results, the use of Mobylize! significantly reduced depressive symptoms, both on a self-rated measure (PHQ-9) and a clinician-based evaluation (Quick Inventory of Depressive Symptomatology-Clinician Rating, QUIDS-C), as well as anxiety symptoms, measured with the Generalized Anxiety Disorder Scale (GAD-7). At the end of the treatment, participants were also less likely to meet MDD diagnostic criteria. Nevertheless, the accuracy of the predictive model was low, especially for mood; higher accuracy was achieved by models that predicted location, conversational state, and social interactions (accuracy between 60% and 90%).

A randomized controlled trial was conducted to evaluate Help4Mood [66]. Twenty-eight depressed patients were recruited and randomized into two treatment groups: Help4Mood and TAU. Outcome measures, which included the Beck Depression Inventory (BDI) and Quick Inventory of Depressive Symptomatology—Self Report (QIDS-SR), indicated reduced symptoms in both samples. Nevertheless, patients in the TAU group achieved greater clinical improvement compared to patients who used the application. Notably, regular users were more likely to obtain greater clinical improvement compared to users with low compliance.

Finally, a preliminary study tested the efficacy of Medlink with 8 MDD patients [65]. On the one hand, medication monitoring showed promising outcomes. Patients reported taking 84% of their medication, which is significantly higher than medication adherence rates reported in the literature. On the other hand, depressive symptoms significantly decreased over the course of 4 weeks.

3.2.3. Compliance and Dropout Rates

Regarding Psymate, the number of answered prompts in both the experimental and pseudo-experimental groups was 135.5 out of 180 (75.3%); participants completed 39.7 out of 50 pre-assessments (79.4%) and 23.7 out of 30 (79%) post-assessment observations. Moreover, 27 of the 33 participants (81.9%) allocated to the experimental group completed the intervention, whereas 32 out of 36 participants (88.89%) allocated to the pseudo-experimental group completed it.

Throughout the 8-week treatment with Mobylize, the mean number of log-ins to the mobile application was 7.9 (approximately one per week), whereas the number of completed lessons on the website was 4.8 out of 9 (53.3%). The number of answered prompts drastically decreased throughout the treatment, from 15.3 in the first week to 4.8 in the last week, due to technical difficulties and connectivity problems. Seven out of eight participants (87.5%) completed the intervention: The only dropout was caused by technical problems with the smartphone.

Regarding Help4Mood, the authors indicated great variability in terms of time of use. Two participants used the application for one or two days, whereas three participants used it between 3 and 7 days. The remaining six participants used it more than 10 times, approximately twice a week. The mean use was 134 min. Eleven out of 13 (84.6%) participants completed the protocol and were assessed for the follow-up. One participant withdrew due to worsening mood.

Finally, participants entered the Medlink application approximately 17.4 times during the 4 weeks of data collection and answered 96% of the prompts. Seven out of nine users read the psychoeducation lessons from the first and second week, whereas only half of them read the third and fourth lessons. No dropouts were reported.

3.2.4. Participants' Feedback and Satisfaction

Using Likert scales ranging from 1 to 7, participants found that Psymate was very simple to use and provided clear instructions (verbal instructions = 6.6 ± 0.7; written instructions = 6.5 ± 1.0; Psymate answers = 2.6 ± 1.5). The number of daily prompts and the time needed to complete assessments was not stressful (number of beeps per day = 3.1 ± 1.6; time to answer = 2.5 ± 1.5). Finally, satisfaction with its most important feature, i.e., receiving EMA-derived feedback, indicated that the feedback was highly appreciated (usefulness of feedback = 6.2 ± 0.7) and considered valuable (feedback to improve daily skills = 5.4 ± 1.1). However, participants would have appreciated receiving more specific and practical advice related to the EMA-based feedback (3.2 ± 2.0).

Regarding Mobylize, satisfaction with the application was rated as 5.71 on a scale from 1 to 7. Criticism was related to technical problems, such as loss of connectivity and subsequent failure to receive prompts. Interestingly, 86% of the participants reported that the intervention was particularly helpful for identifying NA triggers and avoiding distressing and maladaptive behaviours. Participants also suggested lengthening the intervention and adding more activities, such as a blog to talk with other users or a message service between patients and coaches.

Participants involved in the Help4Mood study were quite satisfied with the application. Most of them would use it in everyday life and suggest it to other patients. The idea of a virtual agent to guide participants in completing the assessments was appreciated; however, some participants perceived the agent as too cold, repetitive, and not sufficiently realistic. Among the limitations, patients reported sometimes being bored by excessively long sessions. They would have appreciated receiving more psychoeducational material and a more tailored experience, allowing them to access their preferred materials and activities without restrictions.

Medlink's usability was assessed using 4 items from the Usefulness, Satisfaction, and Ease of Use Questionnaire (USE). On a scale from 1 to 7, participants reported encouraging scores for ease of use (mean = 5.7 ± 1.1) and learnability (mean = 6.1 ± 1.5), but low scores for perceived usefulness (mean = 4.6 ± 1.0) and satisfaction (mean = 4.8 ± 0.8). Furthermore, encouraging ratings were observed for the weekly psychoeducation lessons (liking = 6.0 ± 1.1; ease of use = 6.6 ± 0.5; learnability = 6.6 ± 0.5; and usefulness = 5.8 ± 1.7), which were also reported to be the most interesting and useful parts of the application. Finally, feedback interviews showed neutral comments regarding daily self-reports, that were perceived as not very useful; contrasting opinions were collected regarding feedback graphs.

4. Discussion

To date, the scientific literature has mostly been based on studies conducted in laboratory settings, thus understudying the daily dynamics of psychopathology [70]. Therefore, unobtrusively monitoring behavioural (i.e., sensors), physiological (i.e., biosensors), and cognitive/emotional (i.e., self-reports) factors in ecological settings collected through portable and wearable devices can provide new information about elusive psychological constructs that are usually defined by the complex dynamics of contexts and variability. Accordingly, the research field could benefit from the use of novel technologies to better explore MDD mechanisms and delineate new theoretical models based on ecological observations.

Compared to paper and pencil daily diaries, the use of electronic devices, and especially smartphones, could further increase the six EMA advantages identified by Ebner-Premier (Table 5) [16]: (a) The automation of the entire process directly on a mobile device, such as a smartphone, can provide greater control over backfilling and higher temporal precision in the administration, planning, and randomization of prompts; (b) the use of ICTs can offer additional possibilities for multimodal assessments, with data supplied by embedded sensors and wearable unobstructed biosensors that can automatically be coordinated with the collection of self-reports; (c) the use of mobile devices reduces the effort required of users in completing daily assessments and prevents errors by researchers and clinicians due to manual data entry; (d) smartphones offer the possibility of providing real-time EMA-derived feedback that can be an important therapeutic tool for patients' self-monitoring, in addition to the possibility of sending real-time alerts to clinicians in case of need. In this regard, smartphones have the potential of becoming global low-cost tools that can also be adopted in the clinical field. Currently, 2.32 billion people in the world use smartphones, and it has been estimated that, by 2020, 70% of the world's population will own one [71]. The potential of these devices is also supported by the evidence showing that people with serious mental and physical illnesses own and regularly use smartphones [72] and are interested in using applications for their health [26].

As pointed out in this review, the widespread adoption of EMA for the investigation of depression has led to novel insights into different aspects of the disease, including emotion reactivity, cortisol patterns, or daily rumination. We discussed different sampling methods that can be used in EMA protocols, showing that the signal-contingent design with prompt randomization or semi-randomization is the most widely adopted option when dealing with variables, such as affect and symptom monitoring. We also reported compliance and dropout rates, which showed encouraging results, with most of the studies reporting more than 70% adherence. Nevertheless, the gap between clinical practice and research is still quite wide, as revealed by the low number of studies that adopt this approach to assess and monitor patients for clinical purposes or implement EMA in clinical settings. Accordingly, many issues still need to be addressed. To date, no standard and validated sets of items have been developed for EMA protocols, raising the problem of context validity. Moreover, further research should be conducted to improve patients' compliance and reduce dropout. Due to the intrinsic nature of the disease, depressed patients could be less likely to consistently complete daily assessments. In a previous study, we observed that compliance was higher in EMA administered through a smartphone and when patients were prompted less than 8 times a day [73]. However, a meta-analysis should be conducted to more precisely identify the factors that improve adherence (see, for example, [74]), thus providing some sort of guideline for the design of EMA. Indeed, we strongly believe that clinical practice could benefit from the use of EMAs for several reasons. First, EMAs can be useful for diagnostic purposes. Traditional diagnostic procedures usually involve a static moment in time, including semi-structured interviews (e.g., Mini-International Neuropsychiatric Interview) complemented by self-report measures. However, ample evidence shows the dynamic nature of affective states and mood [75]. Furthermore, these dynamics greatly vary from person to person, reasons for which ideographic approaches may shed light upon the structure of individual symptom dynamics [60]. Consequently, by means of EMAs, a more accurate diagnostic process could be pursued. Likewise, the continuous monitoring of patients' symptoms would allow clinicians to monitor the efficacy of a treatment over time [76], predict short-term mood changes [77], detect symptoms' worsening in an early stage [78], and create continuous communication between clinicians and patients. On the other hand, the use of daily mood and symptom self-ratings could provide more ecological assessments, overcoming recall bias and capturing the dynamics of human functioning in daily life that cannot be detected with traditional tools.

Table 5. Benefits of using EMA for mood dysregulation and mood disorders as described by Ebner-Premier [16].

	Advantages	Implications
1	Real-time assessments	Reduction in retrospective bias and increase in accuracy.
2	Repeated measurements	Better comprehension of time-dependent processes and dynamic changes in symptoms.
3	Multimodal assessments	Contemporary analysis of behaviours, physiological signals, and subjective experiences.
4	Context-specific information	Assessment of symptoms as context-dependent.
5	Interactive assessments	Real-time customizable and interactive feedback.
6	Generalizability	Higher ecological validity and collection of more representative data.

Our results also highlight the existence of a small number of EMIs for depression. In the current literature, only four ecological interventions have been developed, and only two of them were tested in a randomized-controlled trial (RCT). Our review showed promising results in terms of patient satisfaction and clinical efficacy, further supporting the need for more efforts in this direction. However, compliance rates were sometimes not encouraging, and a major challenge is to encourage regular use of these technologies throughout the entire treatment process [79]. Accordingly, future research should focus on the concept of users' motivation and engagement, taking into consideration the adoption of focus groups with patients during treatments, using mixed quantitative and qualitative designs to obtain as much information as possible to guide future developments, and extending the effects of gamification features on adherence and compliance [80]. In other words, greater attention should be paid to the needs and characteristics of the target population. Considering feedback from users, here, we were able to identify three EMI features that were highly appreciated: The possibility of receiving visual feedback about daily assessments and, therefore, self-monitoring of daily patterns;

the availability of psychoeducational material on depression and its mechanisms; and the opportunity to have continuous or periodic communication with a trained clinician.

In this review, we found that most of the EMAs were based only on self-reports, whereas more attempts to integrate this information with data gathered from sensors and biosensors were observed for EMIs. Recent advances in sensor technologies have had an impact on applications for remote health [81], such as postoperative recovery [82], treatment for chronic patients [83], and monitoring of elderly individuals [84]. Consistently, the hierarchical sensing model proposed by Mohr highlights the great revolution that new sensors and biosensors can bring to the field of mental health [85], making it possible to collect raw sensor data (i.e., the lower level of the hierarchy) that can be converted into "behavioural markers" through machine learning and data mining methods [18].

Smartphone sensors further increase the potentially collectable information, allowing the reconstruction of people's habits, sleep patterns, or social life by using embedded sensors, such as accelerometers, calls, short message service (SMS), social network data, or geolocation. In other words, it is now possible to infer and collect behavioural information without necessarily asking the person to report it.

Even though they were not investigated in the studies targeted at MDD patients discussed here, several opportunities can be found in the integration of EMA and EMI platforms with behavioural and physiological signal processing, further mediated by machine learning algorithms. On the one hand, several behavioural signals are readily collectable with the use of smartphone sensors, even though they may lack the required specificity for mood recognition and prediction, as found by the Mobylize! study [61]. On the other hand, due to recent advancements in sensor technologies, physiological signals can be nowadays recorded unobtrusively by means of, for example, smartwatches and chest bands. These could provide an EMA and/or EMI platform with additional markers that more closely correlate to a person's affective state, and that can be used as input to the analysis performed [61]. Consistently, models can be automatically learned that continuously estimate the patient's affective state by extracting and analysing salient features of physiological signals [86]. For instance, electrodermal activity (EDA) and heart rate variability (HRV) have been extensively investigated as correlates of users' affective state, and they are considered non-invasive. They do not involve recording sensitive information (as opposed to, for example, cameras and acoustic signals), and associated sensors do not interfere with users' daily routines. Consistently, patient-specific models can be automatically learned that continuously estimate the patient's affective state by extracting and analysing salient features of physiological signals [86].

Unfortunately, the relation between physiological signals and affective states is not trivial and mixed results are discussed in the literature [87]. Building on recent advances of machine learning, recent studies obtained promising results by means of model personalisation for stress recognition [88] and deep learning for mood prediction [89] using a combination of behavioural and physiological markers in non-clinical populations. If thoroughly tested and consolidated through experimental validations in EMA settings, a model of this type could provide a finer-grained description of the evolution of the patient's disorder throughout a long-term study, compared to surveys that are usually filled in just a few times a day. It can be considered less obstructive to the patient's life because physiological data are recorded passively and do not require extra effort from the patient. Furthermore, in EMI settings, if the recognition algorithm detects that the patient is in a critical state, it can automatically trigger an intervention module associated with the platform or open a communication channel between the patient and his/her therapist. Alternatively, predictive models that combine information from physiological and behavioural signals to estimate the patient's future mood, stress level, and self-reported health (one or a few days in advance) can be automatically inferred [89]. After identifying a risk threshold, these models would make it possible to plan interventions (or involve the therapist) in advance, that is, before the patient's affective state reaches a critical state.

We should, however, recognize that the use of EMAs and EMIs has some limitations. These approaches are time-consuming and may be perceived as invasive by users. Patients are required to complete multiple assessments throughout a day, and protocols often last weeks. Moreover, people might not be willing to share personal information. Finally, in terms of more ecological validity, they may be advantageous for clinical purposes, but disadvantageous for research aims, because they imply less experimental control. Because the data are collected during everyday life and in naturalistic environments, it becomes hard or even impossible to have complete control over the setting, and, therefore, it is not possible to rule out the role of confounding variables. Nevertheless, due to the implementation of novel statistical procedures, a balance between research necessities and clinical utility could be achieved [90]. If this were the case in the near future, EMAs and EMIs would undoubtedly transform the field of mental health, greatly contributing to the bridging of science and practice [91,92].

Overall, this systematic review clearly shows the emergence of ecological assessment and intervention as a promising avenue for clinical psychology. The focus of the review was limited to a specific clinical population. Still, promising results have been already shown also regarding the application of EMA and EMI to anxiety disorders [93,94] and stress-related disorders [95,96], highlighting the potential of these tools to provide psychological support in daily life and to investigate symptom fluctuations across time. However, similar limitations and burning issues were also evidenced, including the need for more high-quality trials, the gap between the clinical and research field, and the importance of making EMAs and EMIs as engaging and tailored as possible. Altogether, there is evidence showing the feasibility and preliminary efficacy of these approaches, but much more research should be conducted before drawing definite conclusions.

Author Contributions: Conceptualization, D.C., J.F.-Á., A.G.P. and C.B.; methodology: D.C., J.F.-Á., M.S. and C.B.; writing—original draft preparation: D.C., J.F.-Á. and A.P.; writing—review and editing: C.B., A.G.P., P.C., M.K. and G.R.

References

1. World Health Organization. *Depression and Other Common Mental Disorders: Global Health Estimates*; World Health Organization: Geneva, Switzerland, 2017; pp. 1–24.
2. Katon, W.; Ciechanowski, P. Impact of major depression on chronic medical illness. *J. Psychosom. Res.* **2002**, *53*, 859–863. [CrossRef]
3. Simon, G.E. Social and economic burden of mood disorders. *Biol. Psychiatry* **2003**, *54*, 208–215. [CrossRef]
4. Sullivan, L.E.; Fiellin, D.A.; O'Connor, P.G. The prevalence and impact of alcohol problems in major depression: A systematic review. *Am. J. Med.* **2005**, *118*, 330–341. [CrossRef] [PubMed]
5. Swendsen, J.D.; Merikangas, K.R. The comorbidity of depression and substance use disorders. *Clin. Psychol. Rev.* **2000**, *20*, 173–189. [CrossRef]
6. McConville, C.; Cooper, C. Mood variability and the intensity of depressive states. *Curr. Psychol.* **1996**, *14*, 329–338. [CrossRef]
7. Peeters, F.; Berkhof, J.; Delespaul, P.; Rottenberg, J.; Nicolson, N.A. Diurnal mood variation in major depressive disorder. *Emotion* **2006**, *6*, 383–391. [CrossRef] [PubMed]
8. Ben-Zeev, D.; Young, M.A.; Madsen, J.W. Retrospective recall of affect in clinically depressed individuals and controls. *Cogn. Emot.* **2009**. [CrossRef]
9. Chamberlain, S.R.; Sakakian, B.J. The neuropsychology of mood disorders. *Curr. Psychiatry Rep.* **2006**, *8*, 458–463. [CrossRef] [PubMed]
10. Möller, H.J.; von Zerssen, D. Self-rating procedures in the evaluation of antidepressants: Review of the literature and results of our studies. *Psychopathology* **1995**, *28*, 291–306. [CrossRef]
11. Gotlib, I.H.; Joormann, J. Cognition and Depression: Current Status and Future Directions. *Annu. Rev. Clin. Psychol.* **2010**, *6*, 285–312. [CrossRef]
12. Csikszentmihalyi, M.; Larson, R. Validity and Reliability of the Experience- Sampling Method. *J. Nerv. Ment. Dis.* **1987**, *175*, 526–536. [CrossRef] [PubMed]
13. Shiffman, S.; Stone, A.A.; Hufford, M.R. Ecological Momentary Assessment. *Annu. Rev. Clin. Psychol.* **2008**, *4*, 1–32. [CrossRef] [PubMed]

14. Stone, A.A.; Shiffman, S.; Atienza, A.A.; Nebeling, A. Historical roots and rationale of ecological momentary assessment (EMA). In *The Science of Real-Time Data Capture: Self-Reports in Health Research*; Oxford University Press: Oxford, MI, USA, 2007; pp. 3–10.
15. Aan het Rot, M.; Hogenelst, K.; Schoevers, R.A. Mood disorders in everyday life: A systematic review of experience sampling and ecological momentary assessment studies. *Clin. Psychol. Rev.* **2012**, *32*, 510–523. [CrossRef] [PubMed]
16. Ebner-Priemer, U.W.; Trull, T.J. Ecological momentary assessment of mood disorders and mood dysregulation. *Psychol. Assess.* **2009**, *21*, 463–475. [CrossRef] [PubMed]
17. Marzano, L.; Bardill, A.; Fields, B.; Herd, K.; Veale, D.; Grey, N.; Moran, P. The application of mHealth to mental health: Opportunities and challenges. *Lancet Psychiatry* **2015**, *2*, 942–948. [CrossRef]
18. Mohr, D.C.; Zhang, M.; Schueller, S.M. Personal Sensing: Understanding Mental Health Using Ubiquitous Sensors and Machine Learning. *Annu. Rev. Clin. Psychol.* **2017**, *13*, 23–47. [CrossRef] [PubMed]
19. van de Ven, P.; O'Brien, H.; Henriques, R.; Klein, M.; Msetfi, R.; Nelson, J.; Rocha, A.; Ruwaard, J.; O'Sullivan, D.; Riper, H. ULTEMAT: A mobile framework for smart ecological momentary assessments and interventions. *Internet Interv.* **2017**, *9*, 74–81. [CrossRef] [PubMed]
20. Henderson, C.; Evans-Lacko, S.; Thornicroft, G. Mental illness stigma, help seeking, and public health programs. *Am. J. Public Health* **2013**, *103*, 777–780. [CrossRef] [PubMed]
21. Kazdin, A.E.; Blase, S.L. Rebooting Psychotherapy Research and Practice to Reduce the Burden of Mental Illness. *Perspect. Psychol. Sci.* **2011**, *6*, 21–37. [CrossRef] [PubMed]
22. Heron, K.E.; Smyth, J.M. Ecological momentary interventions: Incorporating mobile technology into psychosocial and health behaviour treatments. *Br. J. Health Psychol.* **2010**, *15*, 1–39. [CrossRef] [PubMed]
23. Donker, T.; Petrie, K.; Proudfoot, J.; Clarke, J.; Birch, M.R.; Christensen, H. Smartphones for smarter delivery of mental health programs: A systematic review. *J. Med. Internet Res.* **2013**, *15*, e247. [CrossRef]
24. Cuijpers, P.; Donker, T.; Van Straten, A.; Li, J.; Andersson, G. Is guided self-help as effective as face-to-face psychotherapy for depression and anxiety disorders? A systematic review and meta-analysis of comparative outcome studies. *Psychol. Med.* **2010**, *40*, 1943–1957. [CrossRef] [PubMed]
25. Asada, H.H.; Shaltis, P.; Reisner, A.; Rhee, S.; Hutchinson, R.C. Mobile Monitoring with Wearable Photoplethysmographic Biosensors. *IEEE Eng. Med. Biol. Mag.* **2003**, *22*, 28–40. [CrossRef] [PubMed]
26. Torous, J.; Friedman, R.; Keshvan, M. Smartphone ownership and interest in mobile applications to monitor symptoms of mental health conditions. *J. Med. Internet Res.* **2014**, *16*. [CrossRef]
27. Moher, D.; Liberati, A.; Tetzlaff, J.; Altman, D.G.; PRISMA Group. Preferred reporting items for systematic reviews and meta analyses: The Prisma Statement. *PLoS Med.* **2009**, *6*, 1–15. [CrossRef] [PubMed]
28. Colombo, D.; Palacios, A.G.; Alvarez, J.F.; Patané, A.; Semonella, M.; Cipresso, P.; Kwiatkowska, M.; Riva, G.; Botella, C. Current state and future directions of technology-based ecological momentary assessments and interventions for major depressive disorder: Protocol for a systematic review. *Syst. Rev.* **2018**, *7*, 233. [CrossRef] [PubMed]
29. Delgadillo, J.; de Jong, K.; Lucock, M.; Lutz, W.; Rubel, J.; Gilbody, S.; Ali, S.; Aguirre, E.; Appleton, M.; Nevin, J.; et al. Feedback-informed treatment versus usual psychological treatment for depression and anxiety: A multisite, open-label, cluster randomised controlled trial. *Lancet Psychiatry* **2018**. [CrossRef]
30. Downs, S.H.; Black, N. The feasibility of creating a checklist for the assessment of the methodological quality both of randomised and non-randomised studies of health care interventions. *J. Epidemiol. Community Health* **1998**, *52*, 377–384. [CrossRef] [PubMed]
31. Conrad, A.; Wilhelm, F.H.; Roth, W.T.; Spiegel, D.; Taylor, C.B. Circadian affective, cardiopulmonary, and cortisol variability in depressed and nondepressed individuals at risk for cardiovascular disease. *J. Psychiatr. Res.* **2008**. [CrossRef]
32. Kim, J.; Nakamura, T.; Kikuchi, H.; Yoshiuchi, K.; Sasaki, T.; Yamamoto, Y. Covariation of Depressive Mood and Spontaneous Physical Activity in Major Depressive Disorder: Toward Continuous Monitoring of Depressive Mood. *IEEE J. Biomed. Heal. Inform.* **2015**, *19*, 1347–1355. [CrossRef]
33. Littlewood, D.L.; Kyle, S.D.; Carter, L.-A.; Peters, S.; Pratt, D.; Gooding, P. Short sleep duration and poor sleep quality predict next-day suicidal ideation: An ecological momentary assessment study. *Psychol. Med.* **2018**. [CrossRef] [PubMed]
34. Adams, Z.W.; McClure, E.A.; Gray, K.M.; Danielson, C.K.; Treiber, F.A.; Ruggiero, K.J. Mobile devices

for the remote acquisition of physiological and behavioral biomarkers in psychiatric clinical research. *J. Psychiatr. Res.* **2017**. [CrossRef] [PubMed]
35. Ottaviani, C.; Shahabi, L.; Tarvainen, M.; Cook, I.; Abrams, M.; Shapiro, D. Cognitive, behavioral, and autonomic correlates of mind wandering and perseverative cognition in major depression. *Front. Neurosci.* **2015**. [CrossRef] [PubMed]
36. Booij, S.H.; Bos, E.H.; Bouwmans, M.E.J.; Van Faassen, M.; Kema, I.P.; Oldehinkel, A.J.; De Jonge, P. Cortisol and α-amylase secretion patterns between and within depressed and non-depressed individuals. *PLoS ONE* **2015**. [CrossRef] [PubMed]
37. Stavrakakis, N.; Booij, S.H.; Roest, A.M.; de Jonge, P.; Oldehinkel, A.J.; Bos, E.H. Temporal dynamics of physical activity and affect in depressed and nondepressed individuals. *Health Psychol.* **2015**, *34S*, 1268–1277. [CrossRef] [PubMed]
38. Bouwmans, M.E.J.; Oude Oosterik, N.A.M.; Bos, E.H.; de Groot, I.W.; Oldehinkel, A.J.; de Jonge, P. The Temporal Order of Changes in Physical Activity and Subjective Sleep in Depressed Versus Nondepressed Individuals: Findings From the MOOVD Study. *Behav. Sleep Med.* **2018**. [CrossRef] [PubMed]
39. Husky, M.M.; Gindre, C.; Mazure, C.M.; Brebant, C.; Nolen-Hoeksema, S.; Sanacora, G.; Swendsen, J. Computerized ambulatory monitoring in mood disorders: Feasibility, compliance, and reactivity. *Psychiatry Res.* **2010**. [CrossRef]
40. Schaffer, A.; Kreindler, D.; Reis, C.; Levitt, A.J. Use of Mental Health Telemetry to Enhance Identification and Predictive Value of Early Changes During Augmentation Treatment of Major Depression. *J. Clin. Psychopharmacol.* **2013**. [CrossRef] [PubMed]
41. Hung, S.; Li, M.-S.; Chen, Y.-L.; Chiang, J.-H.; Chen, Y.-Y.; Hung, G.C.-L. Smartphone-based ecological momentary assessment for Chinese patients with depression: An exploratory study in Taiwan. *Asian J. Psychiatr.* **2016**, *23*, 131–136. [CrossRef] [PubMed]
42. Stetler, C.; Dickerson, S.S.; Miller, G.E. Uncoupling of social zeitgebers and diurnal cortisol secretion in clinical depression. *Psychoneuroendocrinology* **2004**, *29*, 1250–1259. [CrossRef]
43. Stetler, C.; Miller, G.E. Blunted cortisol response to awakening in mild to moderate depression: Regulatory influences of sleep patterns and social contacts. *J. Abnorm. Psychol.* **2005**, *114*, 697–705. [CrossRef] [PubMed]
44. Huffziger, S.; Ebner-Priemer, U.; Zamoscik, V.; Reinhard, I.; Kirsch, P.; Kuehner, C. Effects of mood and rumination on cortisol levels in daily life: An ambulatory assessment study in remitted depressed patients and healthy controls. *Psychoneuroendocrinology* **2013**, *38*, 2258–2267. [CrossRef] [PubMed]
45. Booij, S.H.; Bos, E.H.; de Jonge, P.; Oldehinkel, A.J. The temporal dynamics of cortisol and affective states in depressed and non-depressed individuals. *Psychoneuroendocrinology* **2016**. [CrossRef] [PubMed]
46. Bower, B.; Bylsma, L.M.; Morris, B.H.; Rottenberg, J. Poor reported sleep quality predicts low positive affect in daily life among healthy and mood-disordered persons: Sleep quality and positive affect. *J. Sleep Res.* **2010**, *19*, 323–332. [CrossRef] [PubMed]
47. O'Leary, K.; Small, B.J.; Panaite, V.; Bylsma, L.M.; Rottenberg, J. Sleep quality in healthy and mood-disordered persons predicts daily life emotional reactivity. *Cogn. Emot.* **2017**, *31*, 435–443. [CrossRef] [PubMed]
48. Bouwmans, M.E.J.; Bos, E.H.; Hoenders, H.J.R.; Oldehinkel, A.J.; de Jonge, P. Sleep quality predicts positive and negative affect but not vice versa. An electronic diary study in depressed and healthy individuals. *J. Affect. Disord.* **2017**, *207*, 260–267. [CrossRef] [PubMed]
49. Bouwmans, M.E.J.; Beltz, A.M.; Bos, E.H.; Oldehinkel, A.J.; de Jonge, P.; Molenaar, P.C.M. The person-specific interplay of melatonin, affect, and fatigue in the context of sleep and depression. *Personal. Individ. Differ.* **2018**. [CrossRef]
50. Thompson, R.J.; Mata, J.; Jaeggi, S.M.; Buschkuehl, M.; Jonides, J.; Gotlib, I.H. The everyday emotional experience of adults with major depressive disorder: Examining emotional instability, inertia, and reactivity. *J. Abnorm. Psychol.* **2012**, *121*, 819–829. [CrossRef] [PubMed]
51. Putnam, K.M.; McSweeney, L.B. Depressive symptoms and baseline prefrontal EEG alpha activity: A study utilizing Ecological Momentary Assessment. *Biol. Psychol.* **2008**. [CrossRef]
52. Ruscio, A.M.; Gentes, E.L.; Jones, J.D.; Hallion, L.S.; Coleman, E.S.; Swendsen, J. Rumination Predicts Heightened Responding to Stressful Life Events in Major Depressive Disorder and Generalized Anxiety Disorder. *J. Abnorm. Psychol.* **2015**, *124*, 17–26. [CrossRef]
53. Kircanski, K.; Thompson, R.J.; Sorenson, J.; Sherdell, L.; Gotlib, I.H. The everyday dynamics of rumination

and worry: Precipitant events and affective consequences. *Cogn. Emot.* **2018**, *32*, 1424–1436. [CrossRef] [PubMed]

54. Husky, M.M.; Mazure, C.M.; MacIejewski, P.K.; Swendsen, J.D. Past depression and gender interact to influence emotional reactivity to daily life stress. *Cognit. Ther. Res.* **2009**, *33*, 264–271. [CrossRef]
55. Bylsma, L.M.; Taylor-Clift, A.; Rottenberg, J. Emotional reactivity to daily events in major and minor depression. *J. Abnorm. Psychol.* **2011**. [CrossRef]
56. Kohling, J.; Moessner, M.; Ehrenthal, J.C.; Bauer, S.; Cierpka, M.; Kammerer, A.; Schauenburg, H.; Dinger, U.; Köhling, J.; Moessner, M.; et al. Affective Instability and Reactivity in Depressed Patients With and Without Borderline Pathology. *J. Personal. Disord.* **2015**, *30*, 1–20. [CrossRef] [PubMed]
57. Slofstra, C.; Nauta, M.H.; Holmes, E.A.; Bos, E.H.; Wichers, M.; Batalas, N.; Klein, N.S.; Bockting, C.L.H. Exploring the relation between visual mental imagery and affect in the daily life of previously depressed and never depressed individuals. *Cogn. Emot.* **2018**, *32*, 1131–1138. [CrossRef] [PubMed]
58. Hepp, J.; Lane, S.P.; Carpenter, R.W.; Niedtfeld, I.; Brown, W.C.; Trull, T.J. Interpersonal Problems and Negative Affect in Borderline Personality and Depressive Disorders in Daily Life. *Clin. Psychol. Sci.* **2017**. [CrossRef] [PubMed]
59. Quilty, L.C.; Watson, C.; Toneatto, T.; Bagby, R.M. A Prospective Investigation of Affect, the Desire to Gamble, Gambling Motivations and Gambling Behavior in the Mood Disorders. *J. Gambl. Stud.* **2017**. [CrossRef] [PubMed]
60. Fisher, A.J.; Reeves, J.W.; Lawyer, G.; Medaglia, J.D.; Rubel, J.A. Exploring the idiographic dynamics of mood and anxiety via network analysis. *J. Abnorm. Psychol.* **2017**. [CrossRef] [PubMed]
61. Burns, M.N.; Begale, M.; Duffecy, J.; Gergle, D.; Karr, C.J.; Giangrande, E.; Mohr, D.C. Harnessing context sensing to develop a mobile intervention for depression. *J. Med. Internet Res.* **2011**, *13*. [CrossRef]
62. Kramer, I.; Simons, C.J.P.; Hartmann, J.A.; Menne-Lothmann, C.; Viechtbauer, W.; Peeters, F.; Schruers, K.; van Bemmel, A.L.; Myin-Germeys, I.; Delespaul, P.; et al. A therapeutic application of the experience sampling method in the treatment of depression: A randomized controlled trial. *World Psychiatry* **2014**, *13*, 68–77. [CrossRef]
63. Simons, C.J.P.; Hartmann, J.A.; Kramer, I.; Menne-Lothmann, C.; Höhn, P.; van Bemmel, A.L.; Myin-Germeys, I.; Delespaul, P.; van Os, J.; Wichers, M. Effects of momentary self-monitoring on empowerment in a randomized controlled trial in patients with depression. *Eur. Psychiatry* **2015**. [CrossRef]
64. Hartmann, J.A.; Wichers, M.; Menne-Lothmann, C.; Kramer, I.; Viechtbauer, W.; Peeters, F.; Schruers, K.R.J.; Van Bemmel, A.L.; Myin-Germeys, I.; Delespaul, P.; et al. Experience sampling-based personalized feedback and Positive affect: A randomized controlled trial in depressed patients. *PLoS ONE* **2015**, *10*. [CrossRef] [PubMed]
65. Mohr, D.C.; Stiles-Shields, C.; Brenner, C.; Palac, H.; Montague, E.; Kaiser, S.M.; Carty-Fickes, E.; Duffecy, J. MedLink: A Mobile Intervention to Address Failure Points in the Treatment of Depression in General Medicine. *Int. Conf. Pervasive Comput. Technol. Healthc.* **2015**, *2015*, 100–107. [PubMed]
66. Burton, C.; Szentagotai Tatar, A.; McKinstry, B.; Matheson, C.; Matu, S.; Moldovan, R.; Macnab, M.; Farrow, E.; David, D.; Pagliari, C.; et al. Pilot randomised controlled trial of Help4Mood, an embodied virtual agent-based system to support treatment of depression. *J. Telemed. Telecare* **2016**, *22*, 348–355. [CrossRef]
67. Snippe, E.; Simons, C.J.P.; Hartmann, J.A.; Menne-Lothmann, C.; Kramer, I.; Booij, S.H.; Viechtbauer, W.; Delespaul, P.; Myin-Germeys, I.; Wichers, M. Change in daily life behaviors and depression: Within-person and between-person associations. *Health Psychol.* **2016**, *35*, 433–441. [CrossRef] [PubMed]
68. Widdershoven, R.L.A.; Wichers, M.; Kuppens, P.; Hartmann, J.A.; Menne-Lothmann, C.; Simons, C.J.P.; Bastiaansen, J.A. Effect of self-monitoring through experience sampling on emotion differentiation in depression. *J. Affect. Disord.* **2019**. [CrossRef] [PubMed]
69. Torous, J.; Staples, P.; Shanahan, M.; Lin, C.; Peck, P.; Keshavan, M.; Onnela, J.-P. Utilizing a Personal Smartphone Custom App to Assess the Patient Health Questionnaire-9 (PHQ-9) Depressive Symptoms in Patients With Major Depressive Disorder. *JMIR Ment. Health* **2015**, *2*, e8. [CrossRef]
70. Nilsen, W.J.; Pavel, M. Moving behavioral theories into the 21st century: Technological advancements for improving quality of life. *IEEE Pulse* **2013**, *4*, 25–28. [CrossRef]
71. Ericsson Consumer Lab Eurupe Ericsson Mobility Report Appendix. *Ericsson Mobil. Rep.* **2015**, 1–8. [CrossRef]

72. Ben-Zeev, D.; Davis, K.E.; Kaiser, S.; Krzsos, I.; Drake, R.E. Mobile technologies among people with serious mental illness: Opportunities for future services. *Adm. Policy Ment. Health* **2013**, *40*, 340–343. [CrossRef]
73. Colombo, D.; Cipresso, P.; Fernández Alvarez, J.; Garcia Palacios, A.; Riva, G.; Botella, C. An Overview of Factors Associated with Adherence and Dropout to Ecological Momentary Assessments in Depression. *Annu. Rev. CyberTherapy Telemed.* **2018**, in press.
74. Karyotaki, E.; Kleiboer, A.; Smit, F.; Turner, D.T.; Pastor, A.M.; Andersson, G.; Berger, T.; Botella, C.; Breton, J.M.; Carlbring, P.; et al. Predictors of treatment dropout in self-guided web-based interventions for depression: An "individual patient data" meta-analysis. *Psychol. Med.* **2015**. [CrossRef] [PubMed]
75. Kuppens, P.; Verduyn, P. Emotion dynamics. *Curr. Opin. Psychol.* **2017**, *17*, 22–26. [CrossRef] [PubMed]
76. Boswell, J.F.; Kraus, D.R.; Miller, S.D.; Lambert, M.J. Implementing routine outcome monitoring in clinical practice: Benefits, challenges, and solutions. *Psychother. Res.* **2015**. [CrossRef] [PubMed]
77. Mikus, A.; Hoogendoorn, M.; Rocha, A.; Gama, J.; Ruwaard, J.; Riper, H. Predicting short term mood developments among depressed patients using adherence and ecological momentary assessment data. *Internet Interv.* **2018**, *12*, 105–110. [CrossRef]
78. Nuij, C.; van Ballegooijen, W.; Ruwaard, J.; de Beurs, D.; Mokkenstorm, J.; van Duijn, E.; de Winter, R.F.P.; O'Connor, R.C.; Smit, J.H.; Riper, H.; et al. Smartphone-based safety planning and self-monitoring for suicidal patients: Rationale and study protocol of the CASPAR (Continuous Assessment for Suicide Prevention And Research) study. *Internet Interv.* **2018**. [CrossRef] [PubMed]
79. Saranummi, N.; Spruijt-Metz, D.; Intille, S.S.; Korhonen, I.; Nilsen, W.J.; Pavel, M. Moving the science of behavioral change into the 21st century: Part 2. *IEEE Pulse* **2013**, *4*, 32–33. [CrossRef] [PubMed]
80. Brown, M.; O'Neill, N.; van Woerden, H.; Eslambolchilar, P.; Jones, M.; John, A. Gamification and Adherence to Web-Based Mental Health Interventions: A Systematic Review. *JMIR Ment. Health* **2016**, *3*, e39. [CrossRef] [PubMed]
81. Majumder, S.; Mondal, T.; Deen, M. Wearable Sensors for Remote Health Monitoring. *Sensors* **2017**, *17*, 130. [CrossRef] [PubMed]
82. Aziz, O.; Atallah, L.; Lo, B.; ElHelw, M.; Wang, L.; Yang, G.Z.; Darzi, A. A pervasive body sensor network for measuring postoperative recovery at home. *Surg. Innov.* **2007**. [CrossRef]
83. Patel, S.; Park, H.; Bonato, P.; Chan, L.; Rodgers, M. A review of wearable sensors and systems with application in rehabilitation. *J. Neuroeng. Rehabil.* **2012**, *9*, 21. [CrossRef]
84. Ohta, S.; Nakamoto, H.; Shinagawa, Y.; Tanikawa, T. A health monitoring system for elderly people living alone. *J. Telemed. Telecare* **2002**. [CrossRef]
85. Seppälä, J.; De Vita, I.; Jämsä, T.; Miettunen, J.; Isohanni, M.; Rubinstein, K.; Feldman, Y.; Grasa, E.; Corripio, I.; Berdun, J.; et al. Mobile Phone and Wearable Sensor-Based mHealth Approaches for Psychiatric Disorders and Symptoms: Systematic Review. *JMIR Ment. Health* **2019**, *6*, e9819. [CrossRef]
86. Lisetti, C.L.; Nasoz, F. Using noninvasive wearable computers to recognize human emotions from physiological signals. *EURASIP J. Appl. Signal Process.* **2004**, *2004*, 1672–1687. [CrossRef]
87. Choi, K.H.; Kim, J.; Kwon, O.S.; Kim, M.J.; Ryu, Y.H.; Park, J.E. Is heart rate variability (HRV) an adequate tool for evaluating human emotions? A focus on the use of the International Affective Picture System (IAPS). *Psychiatry Res.* **2017**. [CrossRef]
88. Kocielnik, R.; Sidorova, N.; Maggi, F.M.; Ouwerkerk, M.; Westerink, J.H.D.M. Smart technologies for long-term stress monitoring at work. In Proceedings of the CBMS 2013—26th IEEE International Symposium on Computer-Based Medical Systems, Porto, Portugal, 20–22 June 2013.
89. Shen, N.; Levitan, M.-J.; Johnson, A.; Bender, J.L.; Hamilton-Page, M.; Jadad, A.A.R.; Wiljer, D. Finding a Depression App: A Review and Content Analysis of the Depression App Marketplace. *JMIR Mhealth Uhealth* **2015**, *3*, e16. [CrossRef]
90. Lin, X.; Mermelstein, R.J.; Hedeker, D. A 3-level Bayesian mixed effects location scale model with an application to ecological momentary assessment data. *Stat. Med.* **2018**. [CrossRef]
91. Goldfried, M.R. The future of psychotherapy integration: Closing the gap between research and practice. *J. Psychother. Integr.* **2010**, *20*, 386–396. [CrossRef]
92. Fernández-Álvarez, J.; Fernández-Álvarez, H.; Castonguay, L.G. Summarizing Novel Efforts to Integrate Practice and Research from a Practice Oriented Research Perspective. *Rev. Argent. Clín. Psicol.* **2018**, *27*, 353–362. [CrossRef]
93. Walz, L.C.; Nauta, M.H.; aan het Rot, M. Experience sampling and ecological momentary assessment for

studying the daily lives of patients with anxiety disorders: A systematic review. *J. Anxiety Disord.* **2014**, *28*, 925–937. [CrossRef]

94. Schueller, S.M.; Aguilera, A.; Mohr, D.C. Ecological momentary interventions for depression and anxiety. *Depress. Anxiety* **2017**, *34*, 540–545. [CrossRef] [PubMed]
95. Yoshiuchi, K.; Yamamoto, Y.; Akabayashi, A. Application of ecological momentary assessment in stress-related diseases. *Biopsychosoc. Med.* **2008**, *2*, 13. [CrossRef] [PubMed]
96. Gee, B.L.; Griffiths, K.M.; Gulliver, A. Effectiveness of mobile technologies delivering Ecological Momentary Interventions for stress and anxiety: A systematic review. *J. Am. Med. Inform. Assoc.* **2016**. [CrossRef]

11

Machine Learning and Virtual Reality on Body Movements' Behaviors to Classify Children with Autism Spectrum Disorder

Mariano Alcañiz Raya [1], Javier Marín-Morales [1], Maria Eleonora Minissi [1], Gonzalo Teruel Garcia [1], Luis Abad [2] and Irene Alice Chicchi Giglioli [1,*]

1 Instituto de Investigación e Innovación en Bioingeniería (i3B), Universitat Politécnica de Valencia, 46022 Valencia, Spain; malcaniz@i3b.upv.es (M.A.R.); jamarmo@i3b.upv.es (J.M.-M.); meminiss@upvnet.upv.es (M.E.M.); gonzaloteruelg@gmail.com (G.T.G.)

2 Red Cenit, Centros de Desarrollo Cognitivo, 46020 Valencia, Spain; lam@redcenit.com

* Correspondence: alicechicchi@i3b.upv.es

Abstract: Autism spectrum disorder (ASD) is mostly diagnosed according to behavioral symptoms in sensory, social, and motor domains. Improper motor functioning, during diagnosis, involves the qualitative evaluation of stereotyped and repetitive behaviors, while quantitative methods that classify body movements' frequencies of children with ASD are less addressed. Recent advances in neuroscience, technology, and data analysis techniques are improving the quantitative and ecological validity methods to measure specific functioning in ASD children. On one side, cutting-edge technologies, such as cameras, sensors, and virtual reality can accurately detect and classify behavioral biomarkers, as body movements in real-life simulations. On the other, machine-learning techniques are showing the potential for identifying and classifying patients' subgroups. Starting from these premises, three real-simulated imitation tasks have been implemented in a virtual reality system whose aim is to investigate if machine-learning methods on movement features and frequency could be useful in discriminating ASD children from children with typical neurodevelopment. In this experiment, 24 children with ASD and 25 children with typical neurodevelopment participated in a multimodal virtual reality experience, and changes in their body movements were tracked by a depth sensor camera during the presentation of visual, auditive, and olfactive stimuli. The main results showed that ASD children presented larger body movements than TD children, and that head, trunk, and feet represent the maximum classification with an accuracy of 82.98%. Regarding stimuli, visual condition showed the highest accuracy (89.36%), followed by the visual-auditive stimuli (74.47%), and visual-auditive-olfactory stimuli (70.21%). Finally, the head showed the most consistent performance along with the stimuli, from 80.85% in visual to 89.36% in visual-auditive-olfactory condition. The findings showed the feasibility of applying machine learning and virtual reality to identify body movements' biomarkers that could contribute to improving ASD diagnosis.

Keywords: autism spectrum disorder; body movements; repetitive behaviors; virtual reality; machine learning

---

1. Introduction

1.1. Autism Spectrum Disorder and Repetitive Behaviors

Autism spectrum disorder (ASD) is a neurodevelopmental disorder mainly based on impairments in social communication and interactions' abilities and on the presence of restricted, repetitive patterns of behavior, interests, or activities [1]. It affects 1 in 160 children [2] and its symptomatology tends to appear from two to four years old, although in some cases it is possible to detect in six months old toddlers [3,4]. ASD studies primarily examine the weaknesses in social interaction abilities', and less on the stereotyped and repetitive motor behaviors that also affect educational, social, and daily life [1,5].

Repetitive behaviors (RBs) are defined as heterogeneous observable motor stereotyped or repetitive sequences characterized by rigidity, invariance, inappropriateness, and being purposeless [6,7]. RBs can occur currently with small changes of the routine or in presence of new and unknowns stimuli to reduce subjective arousal and to cope with unfamiliar events, to maintain homeostasis [8–10].

Furthermore, RBs can be classified into two groups: common behaviors and complex behaviors [11]. Common behaviors are for example nail-biting, thumb sucking, and hair twirling and they tend to be also frequent in typical development population (TD), particularly situations that might cause stress or anxiety [12]. On the other hand, complex behaviors include more complex stereotypies, such as flapping hands, fingers wiggling, head spinning and banging, stamping the feet, and high levels of head movement and body rocking. Although complex RBs are possible to find in TDs, complex head spinning and banging, arm flapping, finger wiggling, and body rocking are mostly related to ASD; indeed, ASD individuals tend to exhibit RBs more frequently and severely than age-matched TD controls [13–15].

Several studies have demonstrated the high presence of RBs behaviors in ASD, ranging from 60% to 100% of cases [13–15]. The relevance of this study lies in understanding if movement features and frequency can be used as a diagnostic biomarker to classify children with and without ASD.

1.2. Traditional Assessment in ASD: Advantages and Limitations

Traditional ASD assessment and diagnosis involve qualitative and quantitative measures, such as semi-structured behavioral task observations (Autism Diagnostic Observation Schedule, ADOS) [16] and structured interview (Autism Diagnostic Interview-Revised, ADI-R) [17].

ADOS consists of several structured and semi-structured tasks on communication, use of imagination, social interaction, play, and restrictive and repetitive behavior analysis. The examiner introduces to the child one task at a time, observing whether ASD symptoms are manifested [16]. ADI-R is a semi-structured interview for family caregivers, who answer to questions related to communication, social interaction, and restricted, repetitive, and stereotyped behaviors [17] (see Materials and Methods for a detailed description of both ADOS and ADI-R). Since in ADOS examiner has to judge a child's performance giving scoring and rating, evaluation relies on the examiner's expertise and subjectivity; likewise, in ADI-R ASD diagnosis is based on caregivers' reports rather than on objective evaluation. Although these measures have been always considered as the gold standard for ASD assessment [18], they present some limitations [19,20].

Regarding ADOS and ADI-R, limitations are related to the absence of both objective assessment methods and the ecological validity of the setting. Examiners need to be trained and prepared to avoid inappropriate task presentation and administration, which might cause symptoms over- or under-interpretation, providing misleading outcomes [21,22]. Moreover, traditional assessment methods might not tap and conceal compensatory capabilities that have been already developed by the child [23], and social desirability [24] might affect responses veracity to tests. Because of social desirability bias, individuals might respond to tasks or questions in a manner conceived as favorable by others [25]. Likewise, in semi-structured interviews, such as ADI-R, family caregivers might report differently certain child's behaviors according to their interpretation and will [26].

Furthermore, traditional ASD assessment takes place in settings that lack ecological validity (i.e., laboratory) [27–29], and results do not mirror performance in real life [30,31]. Indeed, in ASD assessment at a laboratory, children might have learned how to behave according to specific rules and scripts [32]. Concerning RB traditional assessment limitations, direct observation consists of watching individual behavioral sequences, and several weaknesses affect measure reliability, such as difficulties in observing high-speed RBs, analyzing two concomitant RBs, detecting RB sequence beginning, ending, and environmental antecedents [18]. Paper-and-pencil rating scales report RBs frequency and intensity from caregivers' general observations and impressions, yielding objective methodological issues related to self-report measures, that, as well as in ADI-R, are not accurate and do not properly tap individual RBs characteristics [33,34]. Finally, video-based RB assessment is an off-line RB coding procedure made by experts. Although a video-based procedure is more reliable than direct observation methods and paper-and-pencil procedures, it is laborious, and it takes a long time [33]; moreover, the examiner's coding ability depends on individual levels of training and expertise [21].

To overcome the lack of ecological validity, and to avoid the use of subjective observational diagnostic methods in ASD, there is a need to automatically quantify and assess RBs, that could be fulfilled using technology [35,36]. Indeed, item-independent methods can grant accurate estimation of RB incidence and co-occurrence [9,35,36], and new technologies, such as virtual reality, can provide more ecological validity and controlled methodologies.

1.3. Implicit Methods: Biomarkers as Supports for ASD Assessment

Recent advances in social cognitive neuroscience (SCN) shed light on how humans analyze and report beliefs, feelings, and behaviors [37]. SCN is a research area that studies biological processes and related cognition-based elements [38], and it is showing that social interactions rely on implicit psychophysiological processes uncontrolled by conscious awareness [39].

Implicit measures tend to assess automatic biological processes outside conscious awareness [38] that ensue from the interaction with environmental external stimuli and their internal processing. Such biomarkers are a valid alternative to explicit measures, which cannot tap implied brain processes on their own [40]. Thus, to overcome explicit measure weaknesses in the ASD diagnosis, more recent research has included biomarkers along with traditional assessment techniques [41,42].

To date, the available utmost biomarkers to study unconscious processes are the electrodermal activity (EDA) [43,44], the functional magnetic resonance imaging (fMRI) [45], the functional near-infrared spectroscopy (fNIRS) [46], the electroencephalography (EEG) [47], the eye tracking [48], and the heart rate variability (HRT) [49]. In ASD assessment, fMRI research showed that ASD is related to hyperactivity in neural activation and alterations in the cingulate posterior cortex and portions of the insula [50]; whereas EEG research suggested that in social context ASD individuals exhibit greater activity in the left hemisphere [51]. Furthermore, recently developed technological tools, such as cameras and/or sensors, allowed the detection and classification of behavioral biomarkers, as body movements [52].

Initial studies on RBs with such devices showed that more automatic and objective assessment is possible, achieving the recognition of RBs [19,33,36,53–58]. For instance, to disentangle RBs from other movements in ASD, three wireless accelerometers placed on six ASD children's wrists and chest in two different settings were able to accurately identify respectively in lab and classroom 86% and 89.5% of spontaneous hand flapping and body rocking cases [33].

Also, RGB color camera equipped with depth sensor and microphones array for simulated-hand flapping discernment was used in a laboratory setting; the application of the dynamic time warping (DTW) algorithm on-camera recorded data showed that it can recognize and isolate all simulated hand flapping instances, leading to claim that RBs detection is possible even involving sensors that not have necessarily to be worn [19].

1.4. Repetitive Behaviors Recognition in ASD

To overcome issues related to traditional RB assessment [18,19], a new research area about movement analysis based on video recordings and automatic tagging has emerged [19,33,36,53–58].

The first attempt has been developing systems that involve video recordings and accelerometers placed on the subject's body to register movements and to transmit data via wireless [35,36,54,59–61].

These measures have yielded promising results in RB classification, although some studies have involved typical population and not ASD individuals [61], and to our knowledge, no studies have assessed RBs involving quantitative methods and have compared them between ASD and other clinical populations. However, accelerometer and video-based methods are expensive in terms of time and effort, and ASD children might feel as uncomfortable wearing accelerometers. For this reason, this work involved an RGB-D camera for real-time analysis. RGB-D camera is a video recording device able to augment the conventional image with depth information, related to how much the recorded moving body is far from the sensor.

Owing to deep learning and big data techniques [62–64], algorithms have been developed that can estimate real-time subjects' posture and categorize automatically their movements. Over the last decades, great progress has been made in posture estimation and modern technologies, allowing classifying postures regardless of the worn clothes and the considered point of view [65–69]. Furthermore, machine-learning methods (ML) are improving the predictive value of motor behavioral biomarkers' measures in ASD, enhancing the development of objective measures in the diagnostic standpoint [70,71]. For example, Crippa et al. (2015) developed a ML to discriminate preschool children with ASD from children with typical development using a simple upper-limb reach-to-drop task. The resulting model showed an accuracy rate of 96.7%, suggesting that ML can be a useful method of classification and discrimination in the diagnosis process [70].

1.5. Use of Virtual Reality in ASD

Virtual reality (VR) is a three-dimensional computer-generated environment that allows users to experience simulated and unreal worlds. VR provides ecological validity to experienced situations and consequent users' reactions, becoming promising in psychological assessment, training, and treatment [72,73].

Over the last two decades, the VR market has deeply grown because of the broad amount of enterprise birth and consequent wide offer of virtual devices. Overall, head-mounted displays (HMDs) are the most important, affordable, and available in the VR market [74]. However, a different VR device has been suggested as more suitable to our target (ASD children): the CAVE-Automatic Virtual Environment (CAVE™) that is a semi-immersive room where 3 to 6 rear-projected surfaces are installed [74–78].

As a semi-immersive system, CAVE™ overcomes users' risk to experience cyber-sickness that is the possible user's discomfort because of sensory-motor incongruence and cognitive dissonance in the virtual world [79]. Furthermore, specifically to ASD children, CAVE system can overcome the significant restrictions of HMDs that, on one hand, are not suitable for small heads, and on the other, can affect and worsen their sensory and cognitive difficulties [80,81]. Previous studies on feasibility, safety of use, and learning skills of CAVE environments in children with ASD have showed no significant negative effect differences between ASD and TD children and improvements in various skills (e.g., pedestrian crossing) [82].

Regardless of the involved technology and the brand, VR systems share three main features: immersion, interaction, and sense of being present in the environment [83–88]. Immersion refers to system capability to isolate the user from reality [86,88]. Interaction allows users to interact with virtual objects in real-time through control sticks or gloves, providing engagement, motivation, and fun [84,89]. Sense of presence is a consequence of immersion and real-time interaction, and it is defined as the psychological feeling related to the sensation of being physically in the virtual environment, even though the awareness of not being there [88,90–94]. Finally, another feature to consider, less addressed in studies and especially in ASD population, concerns the perception and interaction with virtual agents. Virtual agents have been mainly used in social trainings and interventions showing positive results on skills in ASD children [82]. These positive results suggest that virtual agents are perceived not as cartoons or passive objects to watch, but actively as an intentional being that wants to communicate with the child and with mutually directed behaviors. To our knowledge, one study examined the perception of ASD children in the interaction with a virtual agent for performing a task (pick up flowers) [95]. The quantitative data (accuracy and reaction times) showed that ASD children could complete the task and the qualitative data showed that most of the ASD children perceived the virtual agent as an intentional being with mutually directed behavioral intentions, able to engage and motivate the ASD peer.

There is a great involvement of VR in psychological ASD treatment and it taps all important field macro-areas, such as clinical psychology, neuropsychology, and cognitive and motor rehabilitation [75,85,96–105]. Specifically, treatment studies, applying VR to ASD, mainly referred to social competence [101,102,104], emotional recognition [103], and anxiety and phobias [105] showing initial positive effects of this technique. Regarding ASD VR assessment, it has been less addressed and mainly focused on social communication and interaction symptoms. For example, it has been observed that during a virtual interview about personal life, ASD children looked less to social avatars than their TD control peers, identifying correctly 76% of ASD cases [102]. Also, ASD children made atypical social judgments on the kindness of faces photographs in a virtual environment compared to TD controls [103]. Despite VR potential in ASD assessment has already been strengthened [75], to our knowledge, no one has investigated whether it is possible to disentangle ASD in a VR experience using RBs movement analysis.

Starting from these premises, the main aim of this study is to discriminate ASD children from children with typically developing through body movements' data analysis in a multimodal VR experience, characterized by three stimuli: visual, auditory, and olfactory. Applying ML methods to the dataset, we explored: (a) If through movement data it is possible to discriminate between the two populations; (b) which body parameters better discriminate between the two populations; and (c) which virtual stimuli condition better discriminate body parameters between the two populations.

2. Materials and Methods

2.1. Participants

This study included a sample of 49 children between the ages of 4 and 7 years; 24 children with a diagnosis of ASD (age: 5.13 ± 1.35; male = 21, female = 3) and 25 with a typical development (TD) (age: 4.86 ± 0.91; male = 16, female = 9).

The ASD group sample was provided by the Development Neurocognitive Centre, Red Cenit, Valencia, Spain. TD and ASD participants presented an individual assessment report that included the ADOS-2 and ADI-R tests [16,17,21]. TD group was recruited by a management company through mailings to families.

To participate in the study, family caregivers received written information about the study and were required to give their written consent. Ethical Committee of the Polytechnic University of Valencia approved the study. The study procedure was in accordance with the ethical standards of the institutional and national research committee and with the 1964 Helsinki declaration and its later amendments or comparable ethical standards.

2.2. Psychological Assessment

The following test and scales have been administered to participants and their family caregivers.

2.2.1. Autism Diagnostic Observation Schedule (ADOS-2)

The Autism Diagnostic Observation Schedule (ADOS) [16,21] is a semi-structured set of observation tasks that measure autism symptoms in social relatedness, communication, play, and repetitive behaviors. A standardized severity score within these domains can be calculated to compare autism symptoms across the different modules, which differ in age and linguistic level. From the trained psychologist observation of these behaviors, the items are scored between 0 to 3 (from no evidence of abnormality related to autism to definitive evidence) and from the sum of scores are obtained two specific indexes (social affectation and restricted and repetitive behavior) and an ASD's global total index. The ADOS-2 presents excellent test-retest reliability (0.87 for the social affectation index, 0.64 for the repetitive behavior index, and 0.88 for the total global index). In the study, the assessment was performed using module 1.

2.2.2. Autism Diagnostic Interview-Revised (ADI-R)

The ADI-R [17] is a semi-structured interview for family caregivers, designed to provide the developmental history framework for a lifetime to detect the presence of ASD for individuals from early childhood to adult life. It consists of 111 questions with three separate domains: communication, social interaction and restricted, repetitive and stereotyped behaviors. The answers are scored on a 0–3 Likert scale, from the absence of the behavior to a clear presentation of the determined behavior. ADI-R presents a high test-retest reliability ranging from 0.93 to 0.97.

2.3. *The Multimodal Virtual Environment (VE) and the Imitation Tasks*

The multimodal VE consisted of a simulated city street intersection and was divided into three experimental stimuli conditions: visual (V), visual-auditory (VA), and visual-auditory-olfactory (VAO) (Figure 1a).

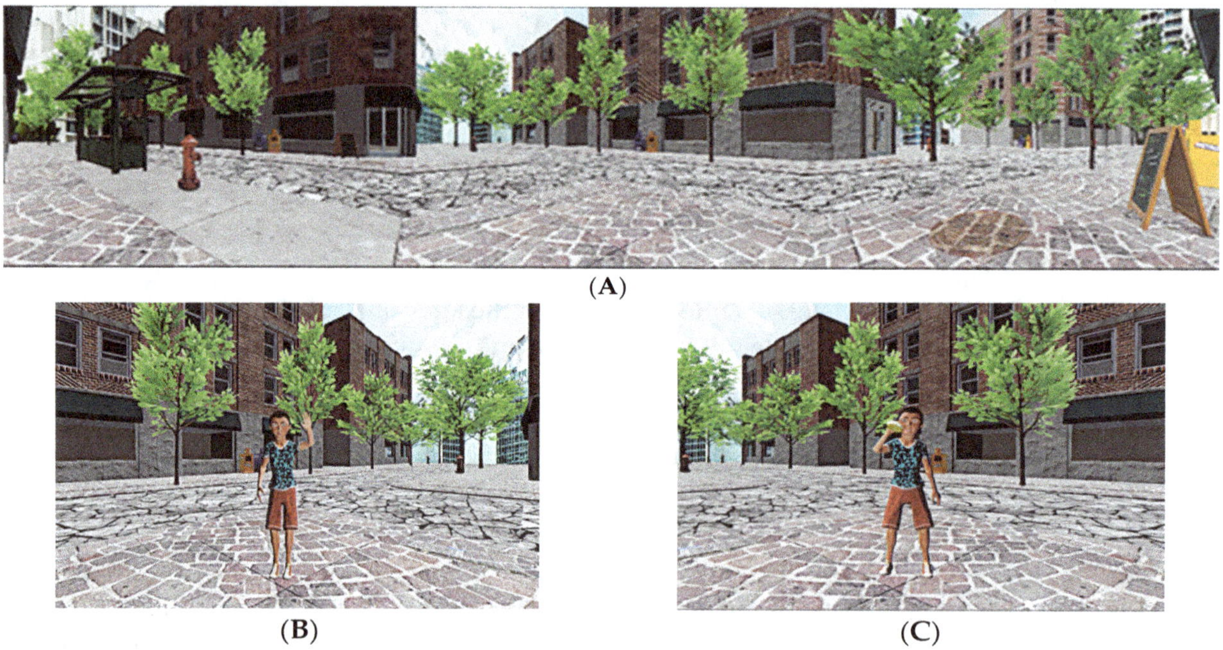

Figure 1. The virtual environment. (**A**) City street intersection; (**B**) visual (V) condition, boy's avatar saying hello; (**C**) visual-auditory-olfactory (VAO) condition, boy's avatar eating a muffin.

First, in the V condition, a boy's avatar appeared from the left side of the surface CAVE™, walking to the middle of the virtual environment, where he stopped and waved to say hello to the participant three times, just before to leave the virtual scene disappearing from behind (Figure 1b).

Next, a girl's avatar appeared in the center of the surface CAVE™, walking to the right of the virtual scene, where she also stopped and repeated the three waves to say hello to the participant, just before leaving the virtual scene disappearing from behind. This sequence was identically repeated three times.

Consecutively, in the second VA stimuli condition, the same avatars appeared in the same first order from the same directions, and they danced over an animated disco song for 10 s three times.

Finally, in the last condition (VAO), the same avatars from the two previous conditions, in the same order and from the same directions, bit a buttered muffin, accompanied with an artificial butter odor (Figure 1c). In the three stimuli conditions, participants were asked to imitate the actions performed by the avatars. Specifically, in the first virtual condition, they should wave three times, dance three times in the second virtual condition, and they should imitate the action of biting a muffing three times.

The selection of the stimuli and the gradual exposition to the three stimuli conditions depended on the hyper-and-hypo sensitivities to sensory stimuli of the ASD population. More in detail, with respect to visual and auditive stimuli (e.g., bright lights or noisy sounds), ASD population presented a hypersensitivity [106,107]; conversely, they present hypo-sensitiveness to olfactive stimuli [108,109]. Sensory hyper-and-hypo sensitivities consequently can affect the information processing in ASD and it has been suggested it may cause RBs [110,111].

The Institute for Research and Innovation in Bioengineering (i3B) of the Polytechnic University of Valencia (UPV) developed the 3D modeling. The environment was projected inside a three surfaces Cave Assisted Virtual Environment (CAVE™) with dimensions of $4 \times 4 \times 3$ mt. It was equipped with three ceiling ultra-short lens projectors, which can project a 100° image from just 55 cm and a Logitech Speaker Z906 500W 5.1 THX sound system (Logitech, Canton of Vaud, Switzerland) (Figure 2).

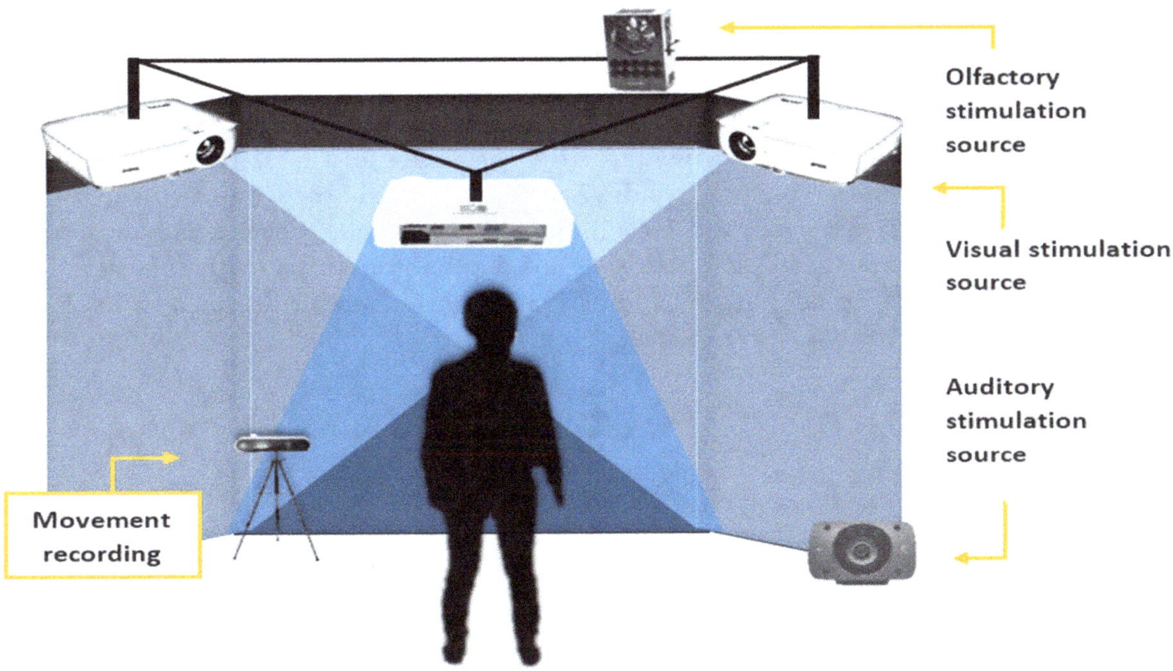

Figure 2. Experimental setting.

2.4. The Olfactory System

Olorama Technology™ (www.olorama.com) a wireless freshener delivered the olfactory stimuli. It can encompass until 12 scents arranged in 12 pre-charged channels, which can be selected and triggered by employing a UDP packet. The device includes a programmable fan time system that controls the duration and intensity of the scent delivery. In the VAO condition, we used a butter scent to evocate the real muffin smell. The scent valve was opened all the time during the last stimuli condition (VAO).

2.5. Experimental Procedure

First, the family caregivers of participants were informed about the general objectives of the research, and, before the experimental session, the setting was also shown and explained to them.

Second, the participant was accompanied in the CAVE™, by the researcher, and by his or her family caregiver according to the child's needs. The participant was placed in the middle of the virtual room, standing in front of the central surface at 1.5 m. The presentation order of VR stimuli conditions for all participants was: visual, visual-auditory, and visual-auditory-olfactory. Before each stimuli VR condition, a two-minute baseline was recorded, and subsequently, the stimuli VR experience condition was presented. The presentation order was maintained the same for all participants to avoid and prevent sensory overload and stress that they could experience.

The total duration of the experiment was of 14 min, and each stimulus condition lasted 2 min and 40 s. Movement recording was turned on during the virtual experience. The researcher monitored the child state during the entire experiment.

2.6. Behavioural Motor Assessment and Data Processing

In the experiment design, it was proposed to use an efficient method to estimate the pose in real-time using an RGB-D camera. The participant's experiment was recorded using an Intel® RealSense™ camera D435 (FRAMOS, Munich, Germany) and Intel RealSense SDK 2.0 (Intel RealSense Technology, Santa Clara, CA, USA) with the cross-platform support. This camera has a depth sensor that uses stereo vision to calculate it. It works like a USB and is equipped with a pair of depth sensors, an RGB sensor, an infrared project a great global image obturator (91.2° × 65.5° × 100.6°).

The detection of the body joints in each frame of the recording was calculated using the deep learning algorithm OpenPose [112], which includes the 2D position related to the video and a confidence level for each joint identification between 0 and 1. The skeleton (Figure 3) includes 25 joints that can be divided into different parts of the body: head (0 nose, 15/16 eyes and 17/18 ears), trunk (1 neck and 8 mid hip), arms (2/5 shoulders, 3/6 elbows and 4/7 wrists), legs (9/12 hips, 10/13 knees, 11/14 ankles), and feet (19/22 big toes, 20/23 small toes and 21/24 heels). After detecting the skeleton, the 3D position of each joint during the experiment was obtained using the depth information of the camera. A computer with an Nvidia GTX1060 graphics card with the NVIDIA Pascal architecture capable of executing neural networks very efficiently in a compact size was used.

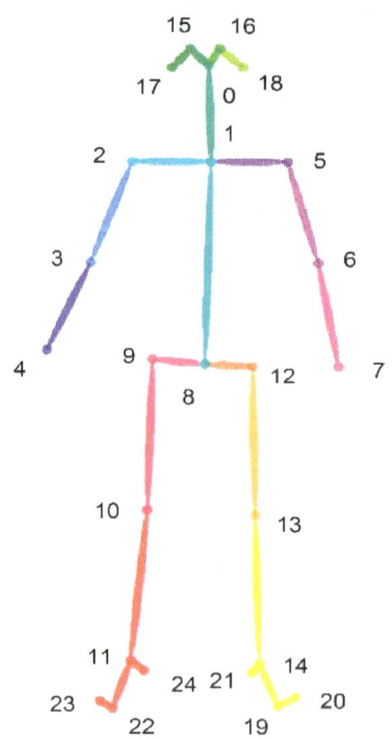

Figure 3. Joint virtual disposition.

After extracting the 3D position of the body's joints from all the experiments, the data recording was segmented for each stimulus condition, excluding the samples of the joints that have a confidence below 0.5. The displacement of the joints was computed using the Euclidean distance between consecutive frames. Finally, the level of movement of a joint during a stimulus was characterized by computing the mean of all displacement.

2.7. Statistical Analysis

First, to characterize behavior differences between ASD and TD children on each stimuli condition, we analyzed the movement frequency of each joint. Since data followed a non-normal distribution (Shapiro-Wilk test: $p < 0.05$), Wilcoxon signed-rank tests were applied.

Second, we applied a set of machine learning models to analyze if the frequency of the movement could discriminate between ASD and TD children. The body was divided into five parts: head (joints 15, 16, 17, and 18), trunk (joints 1 and 8), arms (joints 2, 3, 4, 5, 6, and 7), legs (9, 10, 11, 12, 13, and 14), and feet (19, 20, 21, 22, 23, and 24). The machine learning analysis based on 24 features-based dataset included the five body parts, one related to the whole body, the three stimuli conditions (V, VA, VAO) and one related to the entire experiment. Because of a large number of features, a reduction strategy was adopted to decrease the dimensions in each dataset. Principal component analysis method (PCA) was applied to select features that explain 95% of the variability of the dataset. Finally, a supervised machine-learning model was developed using the PCA features in each dataset.

To implement the models, support vector machine (SVM)-based pattern recognition with a leave-one-subject-out (LOSO) cross-validation procedure has been applied [113]. Within the LOSO scheme, the training set was normalized by subtracting the median value and dividing by the median absolute deviation over each dimension. In each iteration, the validation set consisted of one specific subject and it was normalized using the median and deviation of the training set. We used a C-SVM optimized using a Gaussian Kernel function, changing the parameters of cost and gamma using a vector with seven parameters logarithmically spaced between 0.1 and 1000. Also, a SVM recursive feature elimination (SVM-RFE) procedure was included in a wrapper approach. RFE was performed on the training set of each fold and we computed the median rank for each feature among all folds. In particular, a nonlinear SVM-RFE was implemented, which includes a correlation bias reduction strategy in the feature elimination procedure [114]. To analyze the performance of the models, a set of metrics were considered: accuracy, i.e., percentage of subjects who correctly recognized, true positive rate, i.e., percentage of actual ASD subjects recognized as ASD, true negative rate, i.e., percentage of actual control subjects recognized as controls, and Cohen's kappa, which describes the performance of the model from 0 to 1, 0 being a random class assignation and 1 a perfect classification. The model was optimized to achieve best Cohen's kappa. The algorithms were implemented using Matlab© R2016a and LIBSVM toolbox [115].

3. Results

3.1. Analysis of Total Movement

Figure 4 shows the body joints' significant differences obtained applying Wilcoxon signed-rank. In V stimuli condition, 4 joints of the legs, 2 of the head and 1 of the trunk presented higher movements in ASD population than TD children. In VA stimuli condition, 1 joint of the legs and 2 of the head also presented higher movements in ASD population than TD children. Also in VAO stimuli condition, 3 joints of the head presented the same tendency. Conversely, 1 joint of the head (16) presented lower movement in ASD population in the visual condition baseline (BL_V) and in visual-auditive-olfactive condition baseline (BL_VAO).

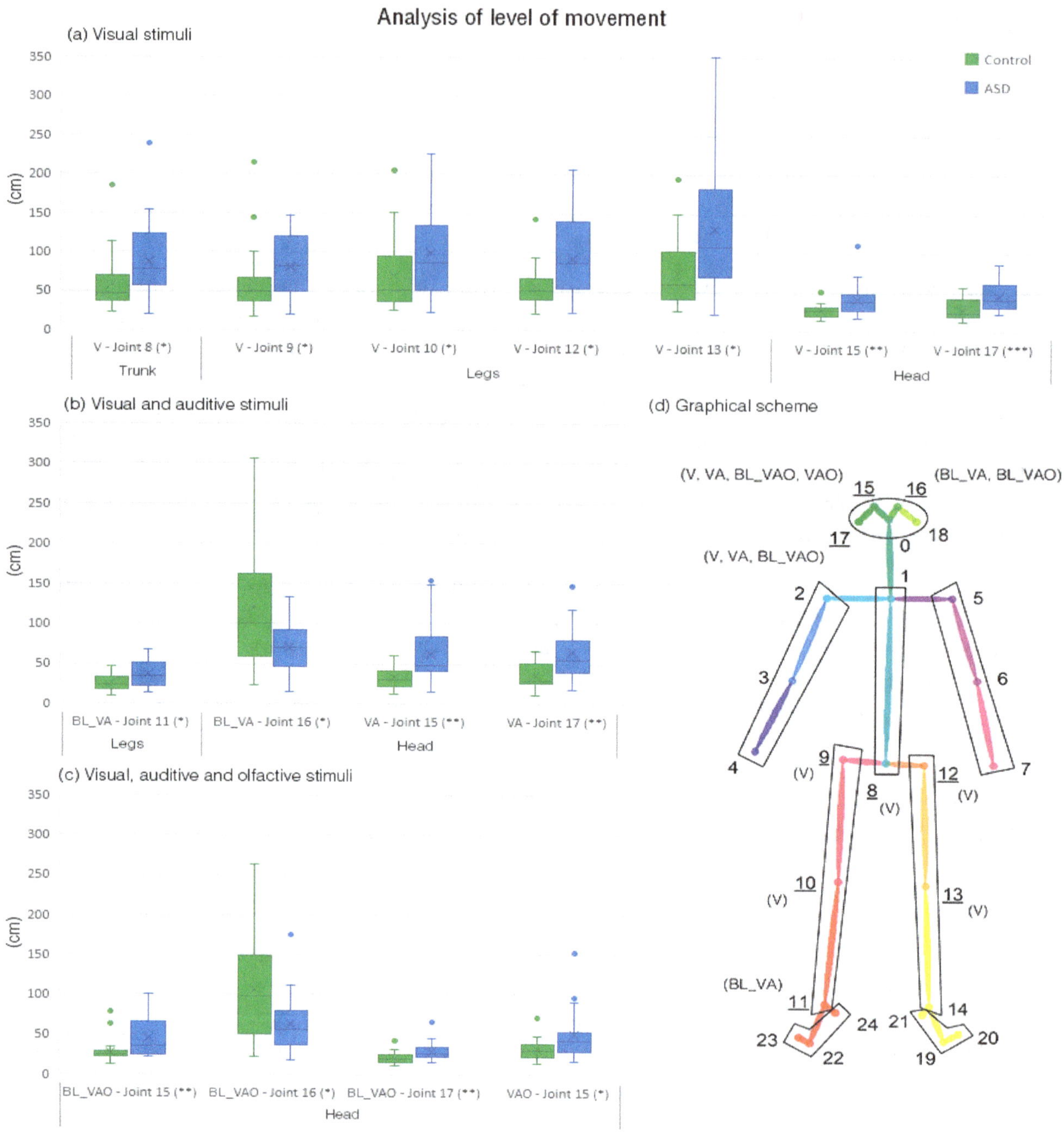

Figure 4. Analysis of the level of movement of joints that presents statistical differences: (**a**) Boxplot of joints in visual stimuli; (**b**) boxplot of joints in visual and auditory stimuli; (**c**) boxplot of joints in visual, auditory, and olfactory stimuli; (**d**) scheme of the joints including the stimuli where differences are found. Note. * $p < 0.05$. ** $p < 0.01$. *** $p < 0.001$.

3.2. ASD Classification Performance

Tables 1 and 2 show the performance of the computed machine learning models, considering the combination of a set of joints and virtual stimuli conditions. Regarding body parameters, the models including the head and trunk joints presented an accuracy of 82.98% and unbalanced confusion matrices. Conversely, the model that uses the feet joints present the same accuracy (82.98%) and a balanced confusion matrix. In addition, the models including arms and legs movements achieved a lower accuracy than the other body joints (74.47% and 72.4% respectively). Finally, the model including all joints and virtual stimuli conditions showed the lowest accuracy (70.21%) and the lower true positives (45.45%).

Table 1. Overview of the accuracy of each model considering the stimuli and set of joints.

		Stimuli			
		V	VA	VAO	All
Set of Joints	Head	80.85%	82.98%	89.36%	82.98%
	Trunk	70.21%	72.34%	76.60%	82.98%
	Arms	87.23%	78.72%	65.96%	74.47%
	Legs	61.70%	63.83%	74.47%	72.34%
	Feet	78.72%	78.72%	65.96%	82.98%
	All	89.36%	74.47%	70.21%	70.21%

Table 2. Detailed level of autism spectrum disorder (ASD) recognition of each model including accuracy, true positive rate (TPR), true negative rate (TNR), Cohen's Kappa and PCA featured selected.

Stimuli	Set of Joints	Accuracy	TPR	TNR	Kappa	PCA Features Selected
All	All	70.21%	45.45%	92.00%	0.39	1/20
V	All	89.36%	100.00%	80.00%	0.79	1/14
VA	All	74.47%	59.09%	88.00%	0.48	2/12
VAO	All	70.21%	63.64%	76.00%	0.40	3/12
All	Head	82.98%	100.00%	68.00%	0.67	1/11
All	Trunk	82.98%	63.64%	100.00%	0.65	2/8
All	Arms	74.47%	90.91%	60.00%	0.50	1/15
All	Legs	72.34%	68.18%	76.00%	0.44	3/8
All	Feet	82.98%	81.82%	84.00%	0.66	2/13
V	Head	80.85%	68.18%	92.00%	0.61	1/6
V	Trunk	70.21%	81.82%	60.00%	0.41	1/3
V	Arms	87.23%	72.73%	100.00%	0.74	1/8
V	Legs	61.70%	45.45%	76.00%	0.22	1/5
V	Feet	78.72%	54.55%	100.00%	0.56	2/6
VA	Head	82.98%	63.64%	100.00%	0.65	3/6
VA	Trunk	72.34%	72.73%	72.00%	0.45	1/3
VA	Arms	78.72%	95.45%	64.00%	0.58	1/8
VA	Legs	63.83%	45.45%	80.00%	0.26	1/4
VA	Feet	78.72%	72.73%	84.00%	0.57	2/6
VAO	Head	89.36%	77.27%	100.00%	0.78	2/6
VAO	Trunk	76.60%	68.18%	84.00%	0.53	2/3
VAO	Arms	65.96%	50.00%	80.00%	0.30	2/7
VAO	Legs	74.47%	68.18%	80.00%	0.48	1/5
VAO	Feet	65.96%	45.45%	84.00%	0.30	2/7

Regarding the influence of the virtual stimuli conditions, the V presented the highest accuracy in the study (89.36%), showing that it is the most relevant stimuli of the experiment. In the VA stimuli, the accuracy decrease to 74.47%, and in VAO to 70.21%. Furthermore, the head joints showed the most consistent performance along with the stimuli, from 80.85% in V to 89.36% in VAO, suggesting that it is the most important part of the body to discriminate ASD population. The trunk joints present also a consistent accuracy, from 70.21% in V to 76.60% in VAO, but the discriminate performance is considerably lower than using the head. All the models used three features or less after applying the automatic feature selection procedure.

4. Discussion

ASD is diagnosed according to qualitative clinician judgments, based on symptoms, through semi-structured observations and interviews (ADOS; ADI-R). Given the qualitative nature of the traditional tools, researchers have focused on improving methods of diagnosis and assessment, pointing out the predictive value of behavioral biomarkers, as more objective and quantitative measures. This study aimed, first, to compare tracked body movements data during a multimodal VR stimulation between ASD and TD children. Second, it was verified which body areas might be relevant for the discrimination between the two populations. Third, the study investigated which virtual stimuli condition better discriminate body areas between the two populations. To reach these aims, we applied a machine learning procedure [70] to body movements' analysis of a multimodal VR experience, composed of three stimuli conditions: visual, visual-auditive, and visual-auditive-olfactory.

The study included a preliminary analysis of the frequency distribution of body movements to investigate the differences between groups and a broad set of supervised ML models combining body parameters and stimuli conditions to evaluate the discriminability between ASD and TD children using movement. Results can be discussed on four points: (1) The significant differences between the two groups on body movements; (2) machine learning methods on body movements and features used; (3) the influence of stimuli conditions; and (4) limitations and future studies.

4.1. *Body Movement Parameters' Differences between Groups*

The first aim was to identify differences in terms of body movements between children with ASD and TD children. Figure 4 showed significant differences in15 body joints and 13 of them have showed that ASD children present more body movements than TD children. In particular, 4 legs' joints, 2 head's joints and 1 trunk's joint in V condition, 1 legs' joints and 2 head's joints in VA condition, and 4 head's joints in VAO condition showed higher movements, suggesting that ASD children have performed more head and legs' movements than TD children during the imitation tasks. Previous studies that showed that head tilting, legs flapping, as well as bilateral repetitive movements involving legs walking represent two or more movements features related to ASD children confirm the presence of larger body movements' in ASD than in TD children [8,10]. However, only one joint in the head showed higher movement in TD children than ASD children during the baselines of VA and VAO. This result is partially in opposition to the scientific literature but as mentioned in the introduction, common and complex body movements are also present in TD children. To improve the quantitative methods to discriminate ASD from TD children using body movements' frequencies, we applied machine-learning techniques developing 24 models, combining body joint parts and virtual stimuli conditions. In the next section, we deeply discuss the results.

4.2. *Machine Learning Methods on Body Movements and Features Used*

Concerning the recognition using different parts of the body, the best classification accuracy reached 82.98% for the head parameter by using only one feature selection method, and the same accuracy was achieved for body and foot parameters by using two features' selection method, independently by the specific stimuli condition. Interesting results have also resulted from the model including arms and legs that achieved a classification accuracy of 74.47% and 72.34%, respectively. The results are consistent with the scientific literature that has identified head spinning and banging, body rocking, and stamping the feet, three of the main stereotypies and repetitive movements are related to ASD [8]. Furthermore, these results showed that ML could provide an effective solution to best describe body movements' differences of participant groups' classification during imitation tasks, while the traditional statistical methods (e.g., mean age comparisons) could fail to deal with such complex tasks. To our knowledge, only two previous studies have investigated the predictive value to discriminate between children with and without ASD using an imitation task [70,71]. Both studies focused on the analysis of arm and hand movements during a simple reach-to-drop imitation task, reaching a maximum classification accuracy of 96.7% and 93.8%, respectively. Our study focused on a more complex real-simulated imitation task, composed of three imitation subtasks, waving, dancing, and eating and tracking all body movements.

Thus, the present findings show the feasibility and applicability of a ML method for correctly classifying preschool children with ASD based on real-simulated imitation tasks. In the standard diagnosis of toddlers it is particularly difficult to evaluate repetitive and stereotyped behaviors. The application of technologies, such as cameras and sensors, might have potential clinical applications to support diagnosis providing accurate quantitative methods along with the qualitative traditional methods. Finally, the use of cameras and sensors are more convenient, less expensive, and less invasive technologies than fMRI and EEG to implement in clinical settings.

4.3. The Influence of Stimuli Conditions

Regarding the virtual stimuli conditions, head showed to be the core body movement in the groups' classification during the three stimuli conditions, achieving the best classifications' accuracy of 89.36% in VAO condition, 82.98% in VA condition, and 80.85% in V condition. These results suggest that the greater the sensory stimulation, the greater the stereotypies and repetitive movements, allowing to discriminate children with ASD from TD children. The different classification accuracy among the three stimuli conditions is consistent with previous studies on the sensory sensitivity overload of ASD patients to multimodality stimuli [116–119]. Specifically, ASD patients have shown lower-functioning abilities to filter process and integrate simultaneous information compared to TD subjects [116]. For example, during multiple auditory tones, tasks matched with single visual-flash stimulus ASD patients perceived more flashes than those are presented [117]. Furthermore, EEG studies on ASD patients showed that the amplitude is higher and the latency in the response is delayed than TD subjects [118,119]. Other multimodal sensory stimulations achieved a good accuracy classification between the two groups, resulting in stereotypes and repetitive movements of the trunk (VAO: 76.60%), legs (VAO: 74.47%), arms and feet (VA: 78.72%). Finally, arms and feet movements showed a high accuracy of 87.23% and 78.72 respectively in the classification between groups during the unimodal visual condition.

In general, V condition including all the body achieved the best accuracy (89.36%), including a 100% true positive rate and using only 1 feature of PCA, in contrast to VA (74.47%) and VAO (70.21%). These results, on one hand, highlight that real-simulated imitation activities that can occur in daily life, such as waving (V), dancing (VA), and eating (VAO) allow evaluating body movements discriminating ASD and TD children. Previous studies on discriminating ASD and TD children using imitation tasks have used simple reach-to-grasp and drop arm movement tasks [70] or a hand movement task to target in laboratory settings [71] and our study aimed to investigate whole-body movements in more complex real-simulated scenarios and tasks.

On the other hand, the predominance of the visual influence can depend on the fact that V stimuli was the first condition and could have generated a wow-effect in the subjects. Finally, the model that includes all the data achieved an accuracy of 70.21% with a 45.45% of true positive rate, showing that the feature selection procedures have a critical role to achieve good performance in biomarkers development. This result could suggest that the implemented virtual tasks could fail in detecting RB behaviors.

4.4. Limitations and Future Studies

Despite the promising results, some methodological limitations of the present exploratory study should be reported. The main limitation is the limited sample sizes of participants for each group. Future studies on larger sample sizes could allow validating the ML method, providing also the possibility to test the model. As ASD is a heterogeneous condition, the possibility of training the model with larger groups of ASD and children with typical neurodevelopment would be useful to improve the generalization of the model to a wide condition range of ASD. Also, other comparisons studies, including other neurodevelopment disorders with movement impairments, as the attention deficit hyperactivity disorder, could be valuable by ML for understanding if these groups present similar body movements that are distinct for the different neurodevelopment conditions (e.g., intellectual disability [120]. Indeed, taking also into account different neurodevelopment conditions could improve the specificity of the classifiers for ASD rather than for neurodevelopment disorders in general.

Furthermore, the experimental groups were not matched on measures related to the intelligence quotient performance, cognitive abilities, and motor comorbidities (e.g., dyspraxia), limiting the confidence that the experimental differences observed in the experiment were due to a diagnosis of ASD, and not to differences in other cognitive or non-cognitive factors. Future studies will consider matching these factors in order to improve the reliability and validity of the model results.

Finally, regarding the stimuli conditions, the order of presentation (V-VA-VAO) was not counterbalanced because of the hyper-sensitiveness of ASD children to multiple stimuli [105–108]. Future studies including counterbalanced conditions following high and low children functioning are needed.

5. Conclusions

The present study represents, to our knowledge, the first attempt to discriminate ASD children from children with typical neurodevelopment using body movements parameters of an imitation VR task and machine learning. The significant predictive values of our classification approach might be valuable to support ASD diagnosis, as well as the use of more objective methods and ecological tasks VR-aided along with traditional assessment.

Author Contributions: All authors have contributed to the manuscript as described below: M.A.R. and L.A. designed the study, and M.A.R., L.A., and I.A.C.G. supervised the whole study. Movements' data processing was conducted by J.M.-M. as well as the statistical analyses. The manuscript was originally written by I.A.C.G., M.E.M., G.T.G., and J.M.-M. and the final manuscript was revised by M.A.R. and I.A.C.G. All authors assisted in the revision process. All authors have read and agreed to the published version of the manuscript.

Acknowledgments: We thank Zayda Ferrer Lluch for the development of virtual reality environments.

References

1. American Psychiatric Association. *Diagnostic and Statistical Manual of Mental Disorders (DSM-5®)*; American Psychiatric Pub: Washington, DC, USA, 2013.
2. World Health Organization. Available online: https://www.who.int/news-room/fact-sheets/detail/autism-spectrum-disorders (accessed on 20 November 2019).
3. Anagnostou, E.; Zwaigenbaum, L.; Szatmari, P.; Fombonne, E.; Fernandez, B.A.; Woodbury-Smith, M.; Buchanan, J.A. Autism spectrum disorder: Advances in evidence-based practice. *Cmaj* **2014**, *186*, 509–519. [CrossRef] [PubMed]
4. Lord, C.; Risi, S.; DiLavore, P.S.; Shulman, C.; Thurm, A.; Pickles, A. Autism from 2 to 9 years of age. *Arch. Gen. Psychiatry* **2006**, *63*, 694–701. [CrossRef] [PubMed]
5. Schmidt, L.; Kirchner, J.; Strunz, S.; Broźus, J.; Ritter, K.; Roepke, S.; Dziobek, I. Psychosocial functioning and life satisfaction in adults with autism spectrum disorder without intellectual impairment. *J. Clin. Psychol.* **2015**, *71*, 1259–1268. [CrossRef]
6. Turner, M. Annotation: Repetitive behaviour in autism: A review of psychological research. *J. Child Psychol. Psychiatry Allied Discip.* **1999**, *40*, 839–849. [CrossRef]
7. Lewis, M.H.; Bodfish, J.W. Repetitive behavior disorders in autism. *Ment. Retard. Dev. Disabil. Res. Rev.* **1998**, *4*, 80–89. [CrossRef]
8. Ghanizadeh, A. Clinical approach to motor stereotypies in autistic children. *Iran. J. Pediatr.* **2010**, *20*, 149.
9. Mahone, E.M.; Bridges, D.; Prahme, C.; Singer, H.S. Repetitive arm and hand movements (complex motor stereotypies) in children. *J. Pediatr.* **2004**, *145*, 391–395. [CrossRef] [PubMed]
10. MacDonald, R.; Green, G.; Mansfield, R.; Geckeler, A.; Gardenier, N.; Anderson, J.; Sanchez, J. Stereotypy in young children with autism and typically developing children. *Res. Dev. Disabil.* **2007**, *28*, 266–277. [CrossRef] [PubMed]
11. Singer, H.S. Motor stereotypies. *Semin. Pediatr. Neurol.* **2009**, *16*, 77–81. [CrossRef]
12. Lidstone, J.; Uljarević, M.; Sullivan, J.; Rodgers, J.; McConachie, H.; Freeston, M.; Leekam, S. Relations among restricted and repetitive behaviors, anxiety and sensory features in children with autism spectrum disorders. *Res. Autism Spectr. Disord.* **2014**, *8*, 82–92. [CrossRef]

13. Bodfish, J.W.; Symons, F.J.; Parker, D.E.; Lewis, M.H. Varieties of repetitive behavior in autism: Comparisons to mental retardation. *J. Autism Dev. Disord.* **2000**, *30*, 237–243. [CrossRef] [PubMed]
14. Campbell, M.; Locascio, J.J.; Choroco, M.C.; Spencer, E.K.; Malone, R.P.; Kafantaris, V.; Overall, J.E. Stereotypies and tardive dyskinesia: Abnormal movements in autistic children. *Psychopharmacol. Bull.* **1990**, *26*, 260–266. [PubMed]
15. Goldman, S.; Wang, C.; Salgado, M.W.; Greene, P.E.; Kim, M.; Rapin, I. Motor stereotypies in children with autism and other developmental disorders. *Dev. Med. Child Neurol.* **2009**, *51*, 30–38. [CrossRef] [PubMed]
16. Lord, C.; Rutter, M.; DiLavore, P.C.; Risi, S.A. *Diagnostic Observation Schedule-WPS (ADOS-WPS)*; Western Psychological Services: Los Angeles, CA, USA, 1999.
17. Lord, C.; Rutter, M.; Le Couteur, A. Autism Diagnostic Interview-Revised: A revised version of a diagnostic interview for caregivers of individuals with possible pervasive developmental disorders. *J. Autism Dev. Disord.* **1994**, *24*, 659–685. [CrossRef]
18. Goldstein, S.; Naglieri, J.A.; Ozonoff, S. *Assessment of Autism Spectrum Disorder*; The Guilford Press: New York, NY, USA, 2009.
19. Gonçalves, N.; Rodrigues, J.L.; Costa, S.; Soares, F. Preliminary study on determining stereotypical motor movements. In Proceedings of the 2012 Annual International Conference of the IEEE Engineering in Medicine and Biology Society, San Diego, CA, USA, 28 August–1 September 2012; pp. 1598–1601.
20. Volkmar, F.R.; State, M.; Klin, A. Autism and autism spectrum disorders: Diagnostic issues for the coming decade. *J. Child Psychol. Psychiatry* **2009**, *50*, 108–115. [CrossRef]
21. Lord, C.; Rutter, M.; DiLavore, P.C.; Risi, S. *Autism Diagnostic Observation Schedule*; Western Psychological Services: Los Angeles, CA, USA, 2001.
22. Reaven, J.A.; Hepburn, S.L.; Ross, R.G. Use of the ADOS and ADI-R in children with psychosis: Importance of clinical judgment. *Clin. Child Psychol. Psychiatry* **2008**, *13*, 81–94. [CrossRef]
23. Torres, E.B.; Brincker, M.; Isenhower, R.W., III; Yanovich, P.; Stigler, K.A.; Nurnberger, J.I., Jr.; José, J.V. Autism: The micro-movement perspective. *Front. Integr. Neurosci.* **2013**, *7*, 32. [CrossRef]
24. Paulhus, D.L. Measurement and Control of Response Bias. In *Measures of Social Psychological Attitudes, Volume 1. Measures of Personality and Social Psychological Attitudes*; Robinson, J.P., Shaver, P.R., Wrightsman, L.S., Eds.; Academic Press: San Diego, CA, USA, 1991; pp. 17–59.
25. Edwards, A.L. *The Social Desirability Variable in Personality Assessment and Research*; Dryden Press: Dryden, ON, Canada, 1957.
26. Möricke, E.; Buitelaar, J.K.; Rommelse, N.N. Do we need multiple informants when assessing autistic traits? The degree of report bias on offspring, self, and spouse ratings. *J. Autism Dev. Disord.* **2016**, *46*, 164–175. [CrossRef]
27. Chaytor, N.; Schmitter-Edgecombe, M.; Burr, R. Improving the ecological validity of executive functioning assessment. *Arch. Clin. Neuropsychol.* **2006**, *21*, 217–227. [CrossRef]
28. Franzen, M.D.; Wilhelm, K.L. Conceptual Foundations of Ecological Validity in Neuropsychological Assessment. In *Ecological Validity of Neuropsychological Testing*; Sbordone, R.J., Long, C.J., Eds.; Gr Press/St Lucie Press Inc.: Delray Beach, FL, USA, 1996; pp. 91–112.
29. Brunswick, E. Symposium of the probability approach in psychology: Representative design and probabilistic theory in a functional psychology. *Psychol. Rev.* **1955**, *62*, 193–217. [CrossRef]
30. Gillberg, C.; Rasmussen, P. Brief report: Four case histories and a literature review of Williams syndrome and autistic behavior. *J. Autism Dev. Disord.* **1994**, *24*, 381–393. [CrossRef] [PubMed]
31. Parsons, S. Authenticity in Virtual Reality for assessment and intervention in autism: A conceptual review. *Educ. Res. Rev.* **2016**, *19*, 138–157. [CrossRef]
32. Francis, K. Autism interventions: A critical update. *Dev. Med. Child Neurol.* **2005**, *47*, 493–499. [CrossRef] [PubMed]
33. Albinali, F.; Goodwin, M.S.; Intille, S.S. Recognizing stereotypical motor movements in the laboratory and classroom: A case study with children on the autism spectrum. In Proceedings of the 11th International Conference on Ubiquitous Computing, Orlando, FL, USA, 30 September–3 October 2009; ACM: New York, NY, USA, 2009; pp. 71–80. [CrossRef]
34. Pyles, D.A.; Riordan, M.M.; Bailey, J.S. The stereotypy analysis: An instrument for examining environmental variables associated with differential rates of stereotypic behavior. *Res. Dev. Disabil.* **1997**, *18*, 11–38. [CrossRef]

35. Min, C.H.; Tewfik, A.H. Novel pattern detection in children with autism spectrum disorder using iterative subspace identification. In Proceedings of the 2010 IEEE International Conference on Acoustics, Speech and Signal Processing, Dallas, TX, USA, 14–19 March 2010; pp. 2266–2269.
36. Min, C.H.; Tewfik, A.H. Automatic characterization and detection of behavioral patterns using linear predictive coding of accelerometer sensor data. In Proceedings of the 2010 Annual International Conference of the IEEE Engineering in Medicine and Biology, Buenos Aires, Argentina, 31 August–4 September 2010; pp. 220–223.
37. Nosek, B.A.; Hawkins, C.B.; Frazier, R.S. Implicit social cognition: From measures to mechanisms. *Trends Cogn. Sci.* **2011**, *15*, 152–159. [CrossRef] [PubMed]
38. Lieberman, M.D. Social cognitive neuroscience. In *Handbook of Social Psychology*; Fiske, S.T., Gilbert, D.T., Lindzey, G., Eds.; John Wiley & Sons Inc.: Hoboken, NJ, USA, 2010; pp. 143–193.
39. Forscher, P.S.; Lai, C.K.; Axt, J.R.; Ebersole, C.R.; Herman, M.; Devine, P.G.; Nosek, B.A. A meta-analysis of procedures to change implicit measures. *J. Pers. Soc. Psychol.* **2019**, *117*, 522–559. [CrossRef]
40. LeDoux, J.E.; Pine, D.S. Using neuroscience to help understand fear and anxiety: A two-system framework. *Am. J. Psychiatry* **2016**, *173*, 1083–1093. [CrossRef] [PubMed]
41. Fenning, R.M.; Baker, J.K.; Baucom, B.R.; Erath, S.A.; Howland, M.A.; Moffitt, J. Electrodermal variability and symptom severity in children with autism spectrum disorder. *J. Autism Dev. Disord.* **2017**, *47*, 1062–1072. [CrossRef]
42. Walsh, P.; Elsabbagh, M.; Bolton, P.; Singh, I. In search of biomarkers for autism: Scientific, social and ethical challenges. *Nat. Rev. Neurosc.* **2011**, *12*, 603. [CrossRef]
43. Nikula, R. Psychological correlates of nonspecific skin conductance responses. *Psychophysiology* **1991**, *28*, 86–90. [CrossRef]
44. Alcañiz Raya, M.; Chicchi Giglioli, I.A.; Marín-Morales, J.; Higuera-Trujillo, J.L.; Olmos, E.; Minissi, M.E.; Abad, L. Application of Supervised Machine Learning for Behavioral Biomarkers of Autism Spectrum Disorder Based on Electrodermal Activity and Virtual Reality. *Front. Hum. Neurosci.* **2020**, *14*, 90. [CrossRef] [PubMed]
45. Cunningham, W.A.; Raye, C.L.; Johnson, M.K. Implicit and explicit evaluation: fMRI correlates of valence, emotional intensity, and control in the processing of attitudes. *J. Cogn. Neurosci.* **2004**, *16*, 1717–1729. [CrossRef] [PubMed]
46. Kopton, I.M.; Kenning, P. Near-infrared spectroscopy (NIRS) as a new tool for neuroeconomic research. *Front. Hum. Neurosci.* **2014**, *8*, 549. [CrossRef] [PubMed]
47. Knyazev, G.G.; Slobodskaya, H.R.; Wilson, G.D. Personality and Brain Oscillations in the Developmental Perspective. In *Advances in Psychology Research*; Shohov, S.P., Ed.; Nova Science Publishers: Hauppauge, NY, USA, 2004; Volume 29, pp. 3–34.
48. Gwizdka, J. Characterizing relevance with eye-tracking measures. In Proceedings of the 5th Information Interaction in Context Symposium, Regensburg, Germany, 26–29 August 2014; pp. 58–67.
49. Nickel, P.; Nachreiner, F. Sensitivity and diagnosticity of the 0.1-Hz component of heart rate variability as an indicator of mental workload. *Hum. Factors* **2003**, *45*, 575–590. [CrossRef] [PubMed]
50. Di Martino, A.; Yan, C.G.; Li, Q.; Denio, E.; Castellanos, F.X.; Alaerts, K.; Deen, B. The autism brain imaging data exchange: Towards a large-scale evaluation of the intrinsic brain architecture in autism. *Mol. Psychiatry* **2014**, *19*, 659. [CrossRef] [PubMed]
51. Van Hecke, A.V.; Lebow, J.; Bal, E.; Lamb, D.; Harden, E.; Kramer, A.; Porges, S.W. Electroencephalogram and heart rate regulation to familiar and unfamiliar people in children with autism spectrum disorders. *Child Dev.* **2009**, *80*, 1118–1133. [CrossRef]
52. Alcañiz, M.L.; Olmos-raya, E.; Abad, L. Uso de entornos virtuales para trastornos del neurodesarrollo: Una revisión del estado del arte y agenda futura. *Medicina (Buenos Aires)* **2019**, *79*, 77–81.
53. Amiri, A.; Peltier, N.; Goldberg, C.; Sun, Y.; Nathan, A.; Hiremath, S.; Mankodiya, K. WearSense: Detecting autism stereotypic behaviors through smartwatches. *Healthcare* **2017**, *5*, 11. [CrossRef]
54. Coronato, A.; De Pietro, G.; Paragliola, G. A situation-aware system for the detection of motion disorders of patients with autism spectrum disorders. *Expert Syst. Appl.* **2014**, *41*, 7868–7877. [CrossRef]
55. Goodwin, M.S.; Intille, S.S.; Velicer, W.F.; Groden, J. Sensor-enabled detection of stereotypical motor movements in persons with autism spectrum disorder. In Proceedings of the 7th International Conference on Interaction Design and Children, Chicago, IL, USA, 11–13 June 2008; pp. 109–112.

56. Goodwin, M.S.; Intille, S.S.; Albinali, F.; Velicer, W.F. Automated detection of stereotypical motor movements. *J. Autism Dev. Disord.* **2011**, *41*, 770–782. [CrossRef]
57. Paragliola, G.; Coronato, A. Intelligent monitoring of stereotyped motion disorders in case of children with autism. In Proceedings of the 2013 9th International Conference on Intelligent Environments, Athens, Greece, 16–17 July 2013; pp. 258–261.
58. Rodrigues, J.L.; Gonçalves, N.; Costa, S.; Soares, F. Stereotyped movement recognition in children with ASD. *Sens. Actuators A Phys.* **2013**, *202*, 162–169. [CrossRef]
59. Madsen, M.; El Kaliouby, R.; Goodwin, M.; Picard, R. Technology for just-in-time in-situ learning of facial affect for persons diagnosed with an autism spectrum disorder. In Proceedings of the 10th International ACM SIGACCESS Conference on Computers and Accessibility, Halifax, NS, Canada, 13–15 October 2008; pp. 19–26.
60. Min, C.H.; Tewfik, A.H.; Kim, Y.; Menard, R. Optimal sensor location for body sensor network to detect self-stimulatory behaviors of children with autism spectrum disorder. In Proceedings of the 2009 Annual International Conference of the IEEE Engineering in Medicine and Biology Society, Minneapolis, MN, USA, 2–6 September 2009; pp. 3489–3492.
61. Westeyn, T.; Vadas, K.; Bian, X.; Starner, T.; Abowd, G.D. Recognizing mimicked autistic self-stimulatory behaviors using hmms. In Proceedings of the Ninth IEEE International Symposium on Wearable Computers (ISWC'05), Osaka, Japan, 11–14 October 2005; pp. 164–167.
62. Simonyan, K.; Zisserman, A. Very deep convolutional networks for large-scale image recognition. *arXiv* **2014**, arXiv:1409.1556.
63. Andriluka, M.; Pishchulin, L.; Gehler, P.; Schiele, B. 2D human pose estimation: New benchmark and state of the art analysis. In Proceedings of the IEEE Conference on Computer Vision and Pattern Recognition, Columbus, OH, USA, 23–28 June 2014; pp. 3686–3693.
64. Lin, T.Y.; Maire, M.; Belongie, S.; Hays, J.; Perona, P.; Ramanan, D.; Zitnick, C.L. Microsoft coco: Common objects in context. In Proceedings of the European Conference on Computer Vision, Zurich, Switzerland, 6–12 September 2014; Springer: Cham, Switzerland, 2014; pp. 740–755.
65. Carreira, J.; Agrawal, P.; Fragkiadaki, K.; Malik, J. Human pose estimation with iterative error feedback. In Proceedings of the IEEE Conference on Computer Vision and Pattern Recognition, Las Vegas, NV, USA, 27–30 June 2016; pp. 4733–4742.
66. Iqbal, U.; Garbade, M.; Gall, J. Pose for action-action for pose. In Proceedings of the 2017 12th IEEE International Conference on Automatic Face & Gesture Recognition (FG 2017), Washington, DC, USA, 30 May–3 June 2017; pp. 438–445.
67. Pfister, T.; Charles, J.; Zisserman, A. Flowing convnets for human pose estimation in videos. In Proceedings of the IEEE International Conference on Computer Vision, Santiago, Chile, 7–13 December 2015; pp. 1913–1921.
68. Toshev, A.; Szegedy, C. Deeppose: Human pose estimation via deep neural networks. In Proceedings of the IEEE Conference on Computer Vision and Pattern Recognition, Columbus, OH, USA, 23–28 June 2014; pp. 1653–1660.
69. Wei, S.E.; Ramakrishna, V.; Kanade, T.; Sheikh, Y. Convolutional pose machines. In Proceedings of the IEEE Conference on Computer Vision and Pattern Recognition, Las Vegas, NV, USA, 27–30 June 2016; pp. 4724–4732.
70. Crippa, A.; Salvatore, C.; Perego, P.; Forti, S.; Nobile, M.; Molteni, M.; Castiglioni, I. Use of machine learning to identify children with autism and their motor abnormalities. *J. Autism Dev. Disord.* **2015**, *45*, 2146–2156. [CrossRef]
71. Wedyan, M.; Al-Jumaily, A.; Crippa, A. Using machine learning to perform early diagnosis of autism spectrum disorder based on simple upper limb movements. *Int. J. Hybrid Intell. Syst.* **2019**, *15*, 195–206. [CrossRef]
72. Burdea, G.C.; Coiffet, P. *Virtual Reality Technology*; John Wiley & Sons: Hoboken, NJ, USA, 2003.
73. Fuchs, H.; Bishop, G. *Research Directions in Virtual Environments*; University of North Carolina at Chapel Hill: Chapel Hill, NC, USA, 1992.
74. Parsons, S.; Mitchell, P.; Leonard, A. The use and understanding of virtual environments by adolescents with autistic spectrum disorders. *J. Autism Dev. Disord.* **2004**, *34*, 449–466. [CrossRef]
75. Parsons, T.D.; Rizzo, A.A.; Rogers, S.; York, P. Virtual reality in paediatric rehabilitation: A review. *Dev. Neurorehabil.* **2009**, *12*, 224–238. [CrossRef] [PubMed]

76. Parsons, T.D. Neuropsychological assessment using virtual environments: Enhanced assessment technology for improved ecological validity. In *Advanced Computational Intelligence Paradigms in Healthcare 6. Virtual Reality in Psychotherapy, Rehabilitation, and Assessment*; Springer: Heidelberg/Berlin, Germany, 2011; pp. 271–289.
77. Bowman, D.A.; Gabbard, J.L.; Hix, D. A survey of usability evaluation in virtual environments: Classification and comparison of methods. *Presence Teleoperators Virtual Environ.* **2002**, *11*, 404–424. [CrossRef]
78. Pastorelli, E.; Herrmann, H. A small-scale, low-budget semi-immersive virtual environment for scientific visualization and research. *Procedia Comput. Sci.* **2013**, *25*, 14–22. [CrossRef]
79. Cobb, S.V.; Nichols, S.; Ramsey, A.; Wilson, J.R. Virtual reality-induced symptoms and effects (VRISE). *Presence Teleoperators Virtual Environ.* **1999**, *8*, 169–186. [CrossRef]
80. Guazzaroni, G. (Ed.) *Virtual and Augmented Reality in Mental Health Treatment*; IGI Global: Hershey, PA, USA, 2018.
81. Wallace, S.; Parsons, S.; Westbury, A.; White, K.; White, K.; Bailey, A. Sense of presence and atypical social judgments in immersive virtual environments: Responses of adolescents with Autism Spectrum Disorders. *Autism* **2010**, *14*, 199–213. [CrossRef]
82. Lorenzo, G.; Lledó, A.; Arráez-Vera, G.; Lorenzo-Lledó, A. The application of immersive virtual reality for students with ASD: A review between 1990–2017. *Educ. Inf. Technol.* **2019**, *24*, 127–151. [CrossRef]
83. Bailenson, J.N.; Yee, N.; Merget, D.; Schroeder, R. The effect of behavioral realism and form realism of real-time avatar faces on verbal disclosure, nonverbal disclosure, emotion recognition, and copresence in dyadic interaction. *Presence* **2006**, *15*, 359–372. [CrossRef]
84. Biocca, F.; Harms, C.; Gregg, J. The networked minds measure of social presence: Pilot test of the factor structure and concurrent validity. In Proceedings of the 4th Annual International Workshop on Presence, Philadelphia, PA, USA, 21–23 May 2001; pp. 1–9.
85. Cipresso, P.; Chicchi Giglioli, I.A.; Alcañiz Raya, M.; Riva, G. The past, present, and future of virtual and augmented reality research: A network and cluster analysis of the literature. *Front. Psychol.* **2018**, *9*, 2086. [CrossRef] [PubMed]
86. Cummings, J.J.; Bailenson, J.N. How immersive is enough? A meta-analysis of the effect of immersive technology on user presence. *Media Psychol.* **2016**, *19*, 272–309. [CrossRef]
87. Skalski, P.; Tamborini, R. The role of social presence in interactive agent-based persuasion. *Media Psychol.* **2007**, *10*, 385–413. [CrossRef]
88. Slater, M. Place illusion and plausibility can lead to realistic behaviour in immersive virtual environments. *Philos. Trans. R. Soc. B Biol. Sci.* **2009**, *364*, 3549–3557. [CrossRef]
89. Sundar, S.S.; Xu, Q.; Bellur, S. Designing interactivity in media interfaces: A communications perspective. In Proceedings of the SIGCHI Conference on Human Factors in Computing Systems, Atlanta, GA, USA, 10–15 April 2010; ACM: New York, NY, USA, 2010; pp. 2247–2256.
90. Baños, R.M.; Botella, C.; Garcia-Palacios, A.; Villa, H.; Perpiñá, C.; Alcaniz, M. Presence and reality judgment in virtual environments: A unitary construct? *Cyber Psychol. Behav.* **2000**, *3*, 327–335. [CrossRef]
91. Baños, R.; Botella, C.; Garcia-Palacios, A.; Villa, H.; Perpiñá, C.; Gallardo, M. Psychological variables and reality judgment in virtual environments: The roles of absorption and dissociation. *Cyber Psychol. Behav.* **2009**, *2*, 143–148. [CrossRef]
92. Bente, G.; Rüggenberg, S.; Krämer, N.C.; Eschenburg, F. Avatar-mediated networking: Increasing social presence and interpersonal trust in net-based collaborations. *Hum. Commun. Res.* **2008**, *34*, 287–318. [CrossRef]
93. Heeter, C. Being there: The subjective experience of presence. *Presence Teleoperators Virtual Environ.* **1992**, *1*, 262–271. [CrossRef]
94. Sanchez-Vives, M.V.; Slater, M. From presence to consciousness through virtual reality. *Nat. Rev. Neurosci.* **2005**, *6*, 332. [CrossRef] [PubMed]
95. Alcorn, A.; Pain, H.; Rajendran, G.; Smith, T.; Lemon, O.; Porayska-Pomsta, K.; Bernardini, S. Social communication between virtual characters and children with autism. In Proceedings of the International Conference on Artificial Intelligence in Education, Auckland, New Zealand, 28 June–1 July 2011; Springer: Berlin, Heidelberg, 2011; pp. 7–14.
96. Mohr, D.C.; Burns, M.N.; Schueller, S.M.; Clarke, G.; Klinkman, M. Behavioral intervention technologies: Evidence review and recommendations for future research in mental health. *Gen. Hosp. Psychiatry* **2013**, *35*, 332–338. [CrossRef] [PubMed]

97. Neguț, A.; Matu, S.A.; Sava, F.A.; David, D. Virtual reality measures in neuropsychological assessment: A meta-analytic review. *Clin. Neuropsychol.* **2016**, *30*, 165–184. [CrossRef]
98. Riva, G. Virtual reality in psychotherapy. *Cyber Psychol. Behav.* **2005**, *8*, 220–230. [CrossRef] [PubMed]
99. Valmaggia, L.R.; Latif, L.; Kempton, M.J.; Rus-Calafell, M. Virtual reality in the psychological treatment for mental health problems: An systematic review of recent evidence. *Psychiatry Res.* **2016**, *236*, 189–195. [CrossRef] [PubMed]
100. Mesa-Gresa, P.; Gil-Gómez, H.; Lozano-Quilis, J.A.; Gil-Gómez, J.A. Effectiveness of virtual reality for children and adolescents with autism spectrum disorder: An evidence-based systematic review. *Sensors* **2018**, *18*, 2486. [CrossRef] [PubMed]
101. Cheng, Y.; Ye, J. Exploring the social competence of students with autism spectrum conditions in a collaborative virtual learning environment—The pilot study. *Comput. Educ.* **2010**, *54*, 1068–1077. [CrossRef]
102. Jarrold, W.; Mundy, P.; Gwaltney, M.; Bailenson, J.; Hatt, N.; McIntyre, N.; Swain, L. Social attention in a virtual public speaking task in higher functioning children with autism. *Autism Res.* **2013**, *6*, 393–410. [CrossRef]
103. d'Arc, B.F.; Ramus, F.; Lefebvre, A.; Brottier, D.; Zalla, T.; Moukawane, S.; Leboyer, M. Atypical social judgment and sensitivity to perceptual cues in autism spectrum disorders. *J. Autism Dev. Disord.* **2016**, *46*, 1574–1581. [CrossRef]
104. Hopkins, I.M.; Gower, M.W.; Perez, T.A.; Smith, D.S.; Amthor, F.R.; Wimsatt, F.C.; Biasini, F.J. Avatar assistant: Improving social skills in students with an ASD through a computer-based intervention. *J. Autism Dev. Disord.* **2011**, *41*, 1543–1555. [CrossRef]
105. Maskey, M.; Lowry, J.; Rodgers, J.; McConachie, H.; Parr, J.R. Reducing specific phobia/fear in young people with autism spectrum disorders (ASDs) through a virtual reality environment intervention. *PLoS ONE* **2014**, *9*, e100374. [CrossRef]
106. Baron-Cohen, S.; Ashwin, E.; Ashwin, C.; Tavassoli, T.; Chakrabarti, B. Talent in autism: Hyper-systemizing, hyper-attention to detail and sensory hypersensitivity. *Philos. Trans. R. Soc. B Biol. Sci.* **2009**, *364*, 1377–1383. [CrossRef] [PubMed]
107. Tomchek, S.D.; Huebner, R.A.; Dunn, W. Patterns of sensory processing in children with an autism spectrum disorder. *Res. Autism Spectr. Disord.* **2014**, *8*, 1214–1224. [CrossRef]
108. Ashwin, C.; Chapman, E.; Howells, J.; Rhydderch, D.; Walker, I.; Baron-Cohen, S. Enhanced olfactory sensitivity in autism spectrum conditions. *Mol. Autism* **2014**, *5*, 53. [CrossRef] [PubMed]
109. Dudova, I.; Vodicka, J.; Havlovicova, M.; Sedlacek, Z.; Urbanek, T.; Hrdlicka, M. Odor detection threshold, but not odor identification, is impaired in children with autism. *Eur. Child Adolesc. Psychiatry* **2011**, *20*, 333–340. [CrossRef] [PubMed]
110. Boyd, B.A.; Baranek, G.T.; Sideris, J.; Poe, M.D.; Watson, L.R.; Patten, E.; Miller, H. Sensory features and repetitive behaviors in children with autism and developmental delays. *Autism Res.* **2010**, *3*, 78–87. [CrossRef] [PubMed]
111. Gabriels, R.L.; Agnew, J.A.; Miller, L.J.; Gralla, J.; Pan, Z.; Goldson, E.; Hooks, E. Is there a relationship between restricted, repetitive, stereotyped behaviors and interests and abnormal sensory response in children with autism spectrum disorders? *Res. Autism Spectr. Disord.* **2008**, *2*, 660–670. [CrossRef]
112. Cao, Z.; Hidalgo, G.; Simon, T.; Wei, S.E.; Sheikh, Y. OpenPose: Realtime multi-person 2D pose estimation using Part Affinity Fields. *arXiv* **2018**, arXiv:1812.08008. [CrossRef]
113. Schöllkopf, B.; Smola, A.J.; Williamson, R.C.; Bartlett, P.L. New support vector algorithms. *Neural Comput.* **2000**, *12*, 1207–1245. [CrossRef]
114. Yan, K.; Zhang, D. Feature selection and analysis on correlated gas sensor data with recursive feature elimination. *Sens. Actuators B Chem.* **2015**, *212*, 353–363. [CrossRef]
115. Chang, C.-C.; Lin, C.-J. Libsvm: A Library for Support Vector Machines. *ACM Trans. Intell. Syst. Technol.* **2011**, *2*, 1–27. [CrossRef]
116. O'Neill, M.; Jones, R.S. Sensory-perceptual abnormalities in autism: A case for more research? *J. Autism Dev. Disord.* **1997**, *27*, 283–293. [CrossRef] [PubMed]
117. Foss-Feig, J.H.; Kwakye, L.D.; Cascio, C.J.; Burnette, C.P.; Kadivar, H.; Stone, W.L.; Wallace, M.T. An extended multisensory temporal binding window in autism spectrum disorders. *Exp. Brain Res.* **2010**, *203*, 381–389. [CrossRef] [PubMed]

118. Courchesne, E.; Lincoln, A.J.; Kilman, B.A.; Galambos, R. Event-related brain potential correlates of the processing of novel visual and auditory information in autism. *J. Autism Dev. Disord.* **1985**, *15*, 55–76. [CrossRef] [PubMed]
119. Russo, N.; Foxe, J.J.; Brandwein, A.B.; Altschuler, T.; Gomes, H.; Molholm, S. Multisensory processing in children with autism: High-density electrical mapping of auditory–somatosensory integration. *Autism Res.* **2010**, *3*, 253–267. [CrossRef] [PubMed]
120. Ament, K.; Mejia, A.; Buhlman, R.; Erklin, S.; Caffo, B.; Mostofsky, S.; Wodka, E. Evidence for specificity of motor impairments in catching and balance in children with autism. *J. Autism Dev. Disord.* **2015**, *45*, 742–751. [CrossRef]

12

Why Uptake of Blended Internet-Based Interventions for Depression Is Challenging: A Qualitative Study on Therapists' Perspectives

Mayke Mol [1,2,*], Claire van Genugten [1,2], Els Dozeman [1,2], Digna J. F. van Schaik [1,2], Stasja Draisma [1,2], Heleen Riper [1,2,3,4] and Jan H. Smit [1,2]

1 Department of Research and Innovation, GGZ inGeest, Specialized Mental Health Care, 1081 Amsterdam, The Netherlands; c.genugten@ggzingeest.nl (C.v.G.); e.dozeman@ggzingeest.nl (E.D.); a.schaik@ggzingeest.nl (D.J.F.v.S.); s.draisma@ggzingeest.nl (S.D.); h.riper@vu.nl (H.R.); jh.smit@ggzingeest.nl (J.H.S.)

2 Department of Psychiatry, Amsterdam Public Health Research Institute, VU University Medical Center, 1081 Amsterdam, The Netherlands

3 Department of Clinical, Neuro and Developmental Psychology, Clinical Psychology Section, Vrije Universiteit Amsterdam and the Amsterdam Public Health Research Institute, 1081 Amsterdam, The Netherlands

4 Telepsychiatry and E-Mental Health, Department of Clinical Research, University of Southern Denmark, 5000 Odense, Denmark

* Correspondence: m.mol@ggzingeest.nl

Abstract: (1) Background: Blended cognitive behavioral therapy (bCBT; online and face-to-face sessions) seems a promising alternative alongside regular face-to-face CBT depression treatment in specialized mental health care organizations. Therapists are key in the uptake of bCBT. This study focuses on therapists' perspectives on usability, satisfaction, and factors that promote or hinder the use of bCBT in routine practice; (2) Methods: Three focus groups ($n = 8$, $n = 7$, $n = 6$) and semi-structured in-depth interviews ($n = 15$) were held throughout the Netherlands. Beforehand, the participating therapists ($n = 36$) completed online questionnaires on usability and satisfaction. Interviews were analyzed by thematic analysis; (3) Results: Therapists found the usability sufficient and were generally satisfied with providing bCBT. The thematic analysis showed three main themes on promoting and hindering factors: (1) therapists' needs regarding bCBT uptake, (2) therapists' role in motivating patients for bCBT, and (3) therapists' experiences with bCBT; (4) Conclusions: Overall, therapists were positive; bCBT can be offered by all CBT-trained therapists and future higher uptake is expected. Especially the pre-set structure of bCBT was found beneficial for both therapists and patients. Nevertheless, therapists did not experience promised time-savings—rather, the opposite. Besides, there are still teething problems and therapeutic shortcomings that need improvement in order to motivate therapists to use bCBT.

Keywords: cognitive behavioral therapy; blended treatment; depressive disorder; implementation; therapists' perspective; routine care

---

1. Background

Face-to-face (FtF) cognitive behavioral therapy (CBT) is an evidence-based treatment for depression [1]. According to international guidelines, CBT is a standard option for treating patients with depression in specialized mental health care [2]. Unfortunately, patient access to CBT is hindered by several barriers such as perceived personal stigma, costs, long waiting lists, and limited availability of licensed therapists [3,4]. It seems therefore promising to offer CBT with the support of technology and without the FtF sessions, thereby potentially reducing therapists' time and costs due to increased involvement of patients themselves. In Internet-based cognitive behavioral therapy (iCBT), treatment access can be improved to offer CBT on an online platform. This would help reduce stigma, waiting lists, and costs, since patients can work through sessions at their own pace, in their own time, and therapist time is lessened. It has been shown that iCBT, especially with online therapist guidance, has good clinical effects for patients with depression [5,6].

In geographically dispersed countries like Canada and Australia, online clinics have successfully reached many patients through iCBT (e.g., Mindspot Clinic, Online Therapy Unit) [7]. In the Netherlands, iCBT, with guidance at a distance, has been offered by Interapy for more than two decades (www.interapy.nl). This mental health care organization (MHO) was founded as an online therapy center and provides specialized online evidenced-based care for among other thing depression, trauma and panic disorder. Other MHO's, where face-to-face treatments are the standard, also are implementing iCBT to improve patient access and make treatments more cost-efficient. However, iCBT uptake in MHOs is limited. This might be partly because therapists perceive iCBT to be limited in crisis situations, ineligible for severe depressive symptoms, and having a one-size fits all approach [8,9]. In addition, given the relatively high density of mental health services, the need for iCBT in the Netherlands may differ from elsewhere.

Blended CBT, a new format of iCBT, which has been recently adopted by MHOs in routine care systems in the Netherlands, could address the limitations since online sessions are combined with FtF sessions in a single, integrated, standardized CBT treatment protocol [10]. bCBT aims to improve both quality of care and cost-efficacy by replacing a portion of the FtF sessions with online sessions [11,12]. Through reducing the number of FtF sessions, therapists' time is saved, they can potentially treat more patients, and waiting lists can be shortened. In addition, within the online platform, therapist contact is extended beyond the FtF sessions by online communication. A number of studies have shown that bCBT can be effective in treating patients with depression [13–15]. However, similarly to iCBT in MHOs, the uptake of bCBT by therapists and patients is limited as it has not yet been implemented across the board in MHOs in the Netherlands and elsewhere [16].

The gap between promising research findings and the limited iCBT and bCBT uptake in routine practice was one of the reasons behind the European MasterMind project, designed to increase and evaluate uptake and implementation of Internet-based interventions in ten European countries (www.mastermind-project.eu) [17]. In MasterMind there was a specific focus on therapists' perspectives, as they play a substantial role in the uptake of iCBT and bCBT. And besides, studies concerning therapists' perspectives in routine practice are scarce [18].

In a qualitative study in Germany, several barriers and facilitators were identified based on the perspectives of therapists ($n = 5$) providing bCBT alongside a randomized controlled study [19]. Key issues varied from problematic platform technology to an unclear concept of embedding bCBT in the mental health care system. Despite the barriers, therapists viewed bCBT as an adequate treatment option for patients with depression. To build on this, more in-depth knowledge on therapists' perspectives in specialized routine care could contribute to optimizing uptake of bCBT, as the therapists' workflow and patient-related factors are more complex in daily practice than in research settings.

The objective of this qualitative study was to investigate therapists' perspectives in routine care when transitioning to using bCBT as an alternative alongside CBT for patients with depression within outpatient specialized mental health care settings in the Netherlands. To increase insight into the factors that influence uptake of bCBT in routine care, the following questions were answered using data triangulation [20] in the context of questionnaires, focus groups, and semi-structured interviews with therapists:

- What are the therapist perspectives on bCBT usability (e.g., perceived ease of use of the platform)?

- How satisfied are therapists with offering bCBT (e.g., overall satisfaction with bCBT)?
- What are the therapist perspectives on factors that promote or hinder the use of bCBT in daily practice (e.g., training, patient eligibility, safety)?

2. Methods

2.1. Therapists

Therapists were (CBT trained) psychologists, mental health nurses, or psychiatrists working at seven MHOs where bCBT had been implemented. To be included in the study, therapists had to be trained in the use of the online platform prior to or during the study period.

The therapists were employed at small (200 registrations for depression per year) to large private-non-profit MHOs (5000 depression registrations per year) spread across the Netherlands. All organizations had bCBT available on a platform from the same large commercial provider (Minddistrict; www.minddistrict.com)—most since 2014. MHOs provided bCBT training to (all or a part of) their therapists either 'in-house' or externally by the provider, or via online training. The estimated duration of the training varied from four hours to two days. MHO's stimulated therapists in different ways for bCBT (e.g., by setting bCBT targets or by special blended consultation hours), however therapists could make their own decision about the treatment of choice.

2.2. Recruitment

Through other users of the Minddistrict platform and personal contacts of the authors, 10 MHOs were invited to be part of the study because they implemented an online platform into routine care. One MHO withdrew because it ceased to exist, another MHO was too busy with ongoing other projects and trials, and one MHO switched to a different platform provider and needed time to explore other providers. In total, seven MHOs participated.

Therapists were identified through team managers, and other specially members of different teams, appointed by the manager of the MHOs. Therapists for focus groups or in-depth interviews were purposively sampled to cover diversity of use and experience with bCBT, age, professional background, and geographic region. First, therapists from two MHOs were invited to participate in a focus group. The focus groups were held within the context of the European implementation project MasterMind. The MasterMind project ran from March 2014 to February 2017. For a more detailed description, see the study protocol of the MasterMind study in the Netherlands [18]. In total, 3 focus groups were held with 21 participants.

Second, to add more depth to the topics discussed in the focus groups, complementary semi-structured individual interviews were held with therapists (who had not participated in the focus groups) from seven MHOs. After 15 interviews, no new information or themes were brought up and data saturation was reached. Two weeks prior to the focus group and interviews, all participating therapists received an informed consent form and questionnaires were used to gather information on therapist demographics, satisfaction, and usability of bCBT via a secure online survey tool (Survalyzer; www.survalyzer.com). Figure 1 provides an outline of the study.

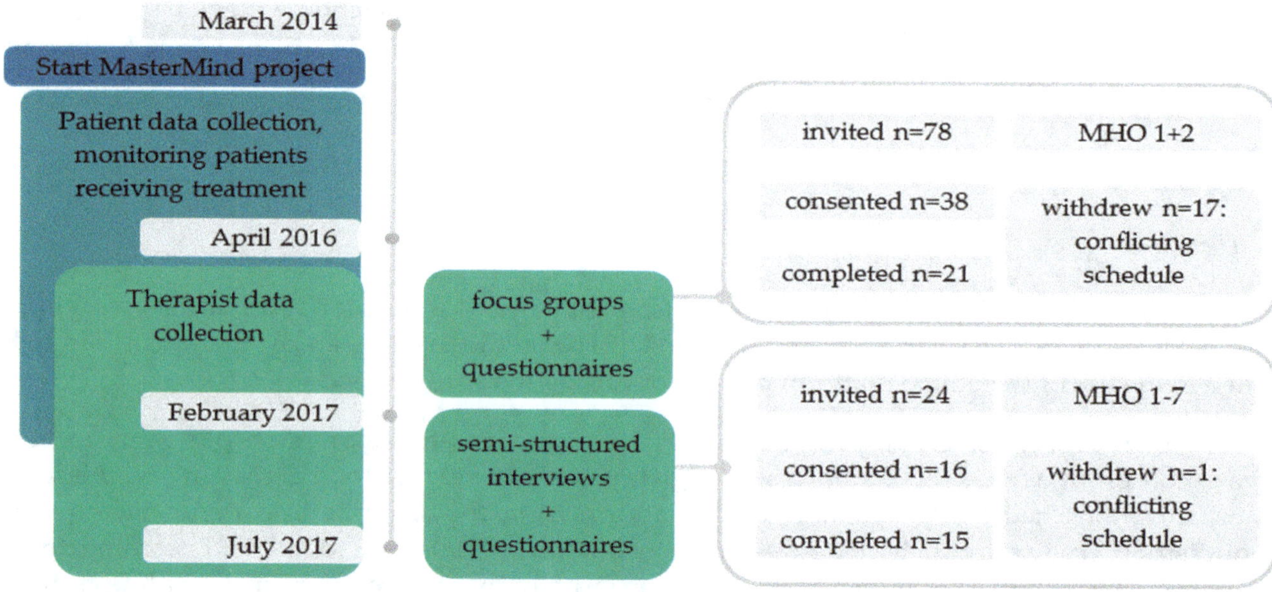

Figure 1. Study outline.

2.3. Intervention

Therapists worked with an integrated bCBT protocol in which FtF and online sessions were alternated. The blended protocol for depression mostly consisted of 10 online sessions. These were supported by FtF sessions (for mild or moderate depression 5 FtF sessions every two weeks; and for (very) severe depression 10 to 11 weekly FtF-sessions). bCBT started and ended with a FtF session. Therapists could individualize the protocol to the patient's needs by repeating and/or skipping online sessions. More detailed information about the protocol can be found elsewhere [21].

Patients could be offered bCBT if (1) they were aged 18 years or older; (2) had a mild, moderate, or severe depression as a primary diagnosis according to the therapist; and (3) were indicated for cognitive behavioral treatment for depression following routine secondary mental health care procedures. Exclusion criteria were (1) not having a valid email address and a computer with Internet access and (2) not having adequate Dutch language skills (both verbal and written).

Therapists had access to the (Minddistrict) platform through a dashboard, which showed treatment sessions, including homework assignments, and had optional functions for a patient diary and depressive symptom questionnaires. The role of the therapists was to monitor the patients' online progress and to provide patients with personalized written feedback to homework assignments after each completed online session. Therapists could additionally communicate through a message function on the platform about practical issues (e.g., upcoming appointments, reminders, or questions about assignments). The safety of the platform was guaranteed by meeting the European requirements for certified data security [22].

2.4. Data Collection

2.4.1. Questionnaires

The 10 items of the System Usability Scale measured perceived usability (SUS) [23]. The SUS is a validated questionnaire for evaluating usability of Internet-based interventions as perceived by therapists and showed a good reliability (omega coefficient = 0.91) [24]. It is unofficially translated in Dutch [25]. The score for the total score range from 0 to 100. A score above the cut-off of 68 is considered to be above average [26]. The Client Satisfaction Questionnaire-3 measured satisfaction with bCBT (CSQ-3), is officially translated to Dutch [27] and was adapted to therapists (e.g., CSQ1 = To what extent has the bCBT intervention met your needs in treating depressed patients?). The CSQ showed good reliability (McDonald omega = 0.95) and validity in a sample of Internet-based depression intervention users [28].

2.4.2. Focus Group Interviews

To identify relevant therapist factors in bCBT uptake, dimensions of the RE-AIM framework (Reach, Effectiveness, Adoption, Implementation, Maintenance) [29], the MAST framework (Model for assessment of telemedicine) [30], and the normalization process theory [31] were used to build and structure the focus group topic list (see File S1 in Supplementary Materials). The main predetermined themes were: patient and therapist factors, barriers and facilitators, satisfaction and usability. The focus group was pilot tested with a moderator and three participants who acted as therapists to refine the topic list and time management. Key questions were presented on a PowerPoint presentation during the therapist focus groups. Via a mobile voting system (Sendsteps; www.sendsteps.com), participants could give their opinion on certain questions and statements in order to stimulate discussion. Discussions were moderated by senior researcher and co-author S.D. with experience in conducting focus groups. They were assisted by researcher and first-author M.M. The focus groups were audio-recorded. The duration of the focus groups was 100–115 min and they took place at the participating MHOs. To increase validity, a transcript of each focus group was sent to each participant for feedback.

2.4.3. Semi-Structured In-Depth Interviews

In semi-structured interviews, therapists were asked individually to reflect on the same topics as in the focus groups to further explore personal experiences. In addition, questions were added based on interview guides from previous research [19,32,33] as well as outcomes of the focus groups; there were slightly different questions for therapists with and without experience in providing bCBT for depression (see File S2 and S3 for the topic lists in Supplementary Materials). After 10 interviews, 3 additional topics were added since these seemed relevant to therapists (e.g., experience with writing online feedback, preferred ratio of online versus FtF sessions and preferred starting point for introduction of online platform). Interviews were conducted by two researchers (M.M. and C.v.G.). The interviews lasted 35–90 min. Most interviews were held at the MHOs (n = 10); five were conducted by telephone for practical reasons. The interviews were audio-recorded. An interview transcript was sent to each participant for respondent validation.

2.5. Data Analyses

Descriptive analyses (frequencies, means, and percentages) of the quantitative data (demographics of therapists, perceived satisfaction, and usability) were performed with SPSS, version 22.0 (IBM Corp. Armonk, NY, USA). Atlas-ti.7 software was used for qualitative analysis (version 7 and 8, Scientific Software Development GmbH. Berlin, Germany).

Focus groups and semi-structured in-depth interview transcripts were concurrently analyzed with thematic analysis techniques guided by the following steps [34]: (1) familiarization with the data; (re-)reading of the transcripts and field notes; (2) generating initial codes; developing a codebook; (3) searching for (sub)themes; identifying broad topics; refining codebook; (4) reviewing the (sub)themes; (5) defining and naming (sub)themes; and (6) reporting. Anonymity was assured by using code numbers instead of names. Each sentence in the transcripts could contain multiple codes, and concurrent sentences of the same thematic code could be conjoined into one unit.

In the results section, therapist' quotes were selected to illustrate the essence of a (sub)theme. The statements reflected perspectives from both focus groups and interviews. We chose to pool these sources as similar topics were discussed and no overlap existed between the therapists who participated in the focus groups and interviews. Both contributed to a more comprehensive understanding of therapists' perspectives. When a perspective concerned a minority of therapists, patients, or other therapists within the participating organizations, this is explicitly mentioned.

To ensure reliability, agreement on codes and concepts between members of the research team was sought. Researchers M.M., C.v.G., and S.D. coded 4 interviews together until acceptable agreement (Fleiss kappa >0.50) was reached [35]. The remaining interviews were divided equally between researchers M.M. and C.v.G. Data collection process, data analysis, and any interim findings, as well as quality and methodological aspects, were discussed in the research group continuously.

2.6. Ethical Issues

The study was approved by the Medical Ethics Committee of the VU medical center, Amsterdam. They confirmed that the Medical Research Involving Human Subjects Act does not apply (registration number 2014.580) because therapists in this study were not required to follow certain procedures on behalf of the research (no randomization), and routine practice was followed. An internal scientific research committee approved the research proposal.

3. Results

Table 1 presents therapist demographics and experience. With respect to distribution of experience with bCBT for depression, 42% of the therapists had considerable bCBT experience (providing bCBT 5 to 20 times or more), 42% had little experience (providing bCBT 1 to 4 times), and 17% had no experience.

Table 1. Therapist demographics and experience.

Therapist Demographics	n = 36
Gender, female, *n* (%)	29 (81)
Age in years, mean (SD; range)	38 (9.5; 24–60)
Professional background, *n* (%)	
Licensed psychologists	20 (56)
Psychologists in training under supervision for health care psychologists	5 (14)
Mental health nurses	5 (14)
Other (e.g., psychiatrists, prevention workers)	6 (16)
Professional experience, *n* (%)	
0–2 years	3 (8)
3–4 years	8 (22)
5–9 years	10 (27)
10 years or more	15 (42)
bCBT depression treatment experience, *n* (%)	
0 times	6 (17)
1–4 times	15 (42)
5–9 times	8 (22)
10–19 times	2 (6)
20 or more times	5 (14)

3.1. bCBT Usability

The mean SUS total score was 69.5 (SD 11.1; range 42.5–90.0). This score indicates sufficient usability of the bCBT platform. In the focus groups and interviews, therapists indicated that the usability had evolved over time. However, the current technical status still needs further improvement. For some, platform usability was a barrier to providing bCBT because many extra actions were required (e.g., logging in, finding the module, setting up the sessions). In addition, there was no integration with other (administrative) computer systems that therapists frequently use (e.g., electronic medical records). Moreover, therapists felt hampered by the lack of knowhow and of a clear overview of all the functions and were unsure how to adapt the protocol. For example, it was unclear to them how to add sessions focused on panic attacks. Some therapists felt the platform usability was complicated and not intuitive. Unexpected updates by the provider did not improve this. For therapists with little bCBT experience, the concern that they would be unable to assist patients with technical problems was also a major barrier. In addition, therapists had negative experiences with contacting the helpdesk (e.g., lack of expertise): "I trained myself to not contact the helpdesk anymore" (T23, experienced).

3.2. *bCBT Satisfaction*

On the CSQ-3, 77% of therapists stated that bCBT met all or almost all their needs; 94% were overall very or mostly satisfied with bCBT; and 97% would recommend bCBT in the future to their patients. Interestingly, in the focus groups and interviews, the opinions of other therapists about satisfaction were divided: some thought that most therapists were generally satisfied, others said: "I also think that therapists are rather dissatisfied. bCBT isn't used on a large scale. This means they must be dissatisfied, otherwise they would use it" (T28, no/little experience).

Most of the therapists indicated that they would like to use bCBT in the future, but this depended on several preconditions that needed to be addressed: platform usability, their current work routine, and more guidelines on how to use bCBT.

3.3. *Factors That Promote or Hinder Uptake of bCBT*

Regardless of the amount of bCBT experience, therapists were in favor of bCBT. Their views on the factors that promoted or hindered the use of bCBT in daily practice were structured along main themes identified in thematic analysis: (1) therapists' needs regarding bCBT uptake, (2) therapists' role in motivating patients for bCBT, and (3) therapists' experiences with bCBT (See Table 2 for main and subthemes).

Table 2. Therapists' blended cognitive behavioral therapy (bCBT) uptake in routine practice, main themes, and subthemes.

Theme (1) Therapists' Needs Regarding bCBT Uptake	Theme (2) Therapists' Role in Motivating Patients for bCBT	Theme (3) Therapists' Experiences with bCBT
Therapist training Therapist motivation Therapist readiness for uptake	Informing patients Patient eligibility Patient resistance	Effectiveness for depression Positive effects Negative effects Treatment protocol Therapeutic relationship Online feedback skills Drop-out and safety

3.3.1. Theme (1) Therapists' Needs Regarding bCBT Uptake

This theme addresses factors related to therapists' needs in providing bCBT to patients with depression. The identified subthemes were: therapist training, therapist motivation, and therapist readiness for uptake (Table 3).

Table 3. Theme (1) Therapists' needs regarding bCBT uptake, subthemes, influencing factors, and illustrative quotes.

Subtheme	Influencing Factors	Illustrative Quotes
Therapist training	(+) sufficient to learn the technical aspects	*"It is nice to have learned beforehand where all the buttons are and what the possibilities are."* (T11, no/little experience)
	(−) lack of therapeutic content and guidelines in the training	*"I miss therapeutic content in the training and the qualifications for the therapists to work with it."* (T25, experience)
	(−) training alone is not enough for uptake in daily practice	*"There is one training and then you're released with the notion: 'now you can manage everything'."* (T7, experience)

Table 3. *Cont.*

Subtheme	Influencing Factors	Illustrative Quotes
	(−) lack of ongoing support	*"There is a lack of time to delve into it, it should be facilitated better and not end with a single training."* (T14, no/little experience)
Therapist motivation	(−) demotivated therapists	*"What bothers me most when it comes to blended is that it has been made mandatory, mainly because we've to meet a certain percentage of blended treatments."* (T34, experience)
	(+) motivated therapists	*"If you are a psychologist, and you are interested in your profession, you should just use it."* (T9, experience)
	(−/+) undecided therapists	*"You have to get out of your comfort zone to discover what the added value of blended is."* (T31, no/little experience)
Therapist readiness for uptake	(−) small select group uses bCBT on a regular basis	*"When I look at my team, it seems only one person is trained, I don't really hear others talk about it."* (T36, experience)
	(+) expected to grow in future	*"I'd like to use blended in the future, but first I'd like more ideas on how to use it* (T6, no/little experience)
	(−/+) making bCBT mandatory	*"I once heard that you need a certain percentage of online contacts—that would work for me."* (T2, experience)

Note. (−) factor that influenced the bCBT uptake negatively, (+) factor that influenced the bCBT uptake positively, (−/+) factor that influenced the bCBT uptake positively and negatively.

Therapist Training

Most therapists found the training formats sufficient for providing bCBT. The focus in the training formats was primarily targeted at technical aspects and less at therapeutic content. The therapists reported that they needed more guidelines and tools for providing online feedback, to keep patients engaged and to prevent them from deviating from the protocol. The training formats in their current form were probably sufficient for the 'early adopters' but less suited for therapists with limited computer skills, the older generation, or new graduates.

Moreover, undergoing training alone was not enough. Therapists found it difficult to familiarize themselves with the platform, and integrate bCBT into existing systems and into their daily workflow. Time constraints were the most frequently cited barrier for uptake of bCBT. This was mainly due to a high caseload. Plus, therapists felt that the implementation ceased after the training was provided, and that the training was fragmented and was introduced too suddenly. Consequently, some organizations offered therapists a special consultation hour or extra training day. Yet, only a select group of motivated therapists turned up at these events. In order to integrate bCBT into their work routine, therapists needed more ongoing technical and content support in the form of supervision or peer review.

Above all, every qualified therapist was considered able to provide blended treatment, mostly because bCBT was perceived as being very similar to regular CBT. However, they also believed that therapist qualifications and professional background have so far been overlooked. They felt sufficient knowledge and professional experience of CBT should be a criterion for being trained in bCBT.

Therapist Motivation

Therapists in this study were motivated for bCBT. Their colleagues could roughly be divided into three groups based on their motivation: demotivated therapists, motivated therapists, and an inexperienced group that needed more motivation.

Therapists estimated that about half of their therapist colleagues were not motivated for bCBT. They thought that perceived pressure from the MHOs and health care insurance companies worked counterproductively. Other reasons were varied. Some thought that a number of colleagues tended to resist every innovation implemented by the organization. For others, the reasons were fear-based:

(1) fear that technology will eventually take over, (2) fear of losing contact when a patient is inactive on the platform, (3) fear of not offering patients the amount of help they need, and/or (4) fear that they would do something wrong or would come across as unprofessional towards patients. A specific group of therapists, who were enthusiastic at the start but due to negative experiences with (other/outdated/unguided) Internet-based interventions, lost interest or became sceptical about the clinical effects of bCBT. This was mainly due to technical issues and higher patient drop-out rates.

Motivated therapists were described as being younger, having affinity with technology, and being interested in innovations in their field. Not every therapist was open to the idea of bCBT in the beginning, but some adjusted their view based on (positive) experiences.

Non-experienced therapists were mainly profiled as lacking computer skills, having technical skills insecurities, and belonging to an older generation with a traditional view on therapy. Interestingly, it was stated multiple times that many therapists were open to bCBT and also were capable of delivering it, but had reservations that first needed to be addressed. On top of a strong preference for FtF treatment over bCBT, there are thought to be many therapists to whom the possibilities of bCBT were unknown or remained unclear. They were often unaware of its added value or of research findings. For them, the need for blended did not come from within. However, even though there might be many reasons not to provide bCBT, therapists believed that only a small proportion are truly resistant to it.

Therapist Readiness for Uptake

Though most therapists received training on the back of an organization-wide roll-out, a number observed that only a select group used bCBT on a daily base. To some, this was related to readiness for uptake: the implementation of bCBT in routine care is considered to be at an early, transitional stage. Although it might be too innovative for therapists and patients, they believed that a change in perception toward bCBT will take place, and that readiness would increase as more patients start asking for bCBT.

There was disagreement with respect to making bCBT obligatory or not. For some, it would feed resistance toward bCBT and fuel the suspicion that bCBT was solely implemented for financial reasons. Others believed that every therapist should 'just use it' or at least try it. It was also felt that treatment should be 'blended, unless a therapist has limited computer skills, or a different therapeutic background or interest'. Most therapists stressed that for them, the precondition that blended stays blended is of great importance, because of the fear that MHOs in the future might gradually transition to online CBT.

3.3.2. Theme (2) Therapists' Role in Motivating Patients for bCBT

The second theme concerns the role of therapists in motivating patients with depression to use bCBT. The identified subthemes were: informing patients, patient eligibility, and patient resistance (Table 4).

Table 4. Theme (2) Therapists' role in motivating patients for bCBT, subthemes, influencing factors, and illustrative quotes.

Subtheme	Influencing Factors	Illustrative Quotes
Informing patients	(−) difficult to motivate some patients	*"Sometimes there is so much going on, which leads me to inform patients in an insecure or doubtful way, that makes them say 'no, I don't want that'."* (T35, no/little experience)
	(−) room for improvement	*"I think that therapists should 'sell' or promote bCBT more with patients."* (T15, experience)

Table 4. *Cont.*

Subtheme	Influencing Factors	Illustrative Quotes
Patient eligibility	(−) eligible patient unknown	*"It is difficult to assess for whom it is eligible. Sometimes someone who grew up with computers says, 'oh no, not for me', and then a 65-year old says 'nice, let's do it'."* (T10, experience)
	(−/+) discussion on comorbidity/complexity/ depression severity	*"I imagine that blended is less suitable for more complex cases. But if I consider what I have in my caseload now, I think it should be doable."* (T5, no/little experience)
	(+) eligibility bCBT = eligibility CBT	*"In principle everyone is eligible for bCBT. I rarely think that it's not an option."* (T7, experience)
Patient resistance	(−) unclear image, too demanding, not enough, negative past experiences	*"Patients don't have a good image of bCBT. In their view it's more like an online questionnaire than a complete module, 'I've already answered those questions ... '."* (T9, experience)
	(+) patient demand expected to increase in the future	*"I think it will make an essential difference if patients ask for it. That's just a matter of time'."* (T1, no/little experience)

Note. (−) factor that influenced the bCBT uptake negatively, (+) factor that influenced the bCBT uptake positively, (−/+) factor that influenced the bCBT uptake positively and negatively.

Informing Patients

Many therapists had difficulties informing patients about bCBT for various reasons. Reasons given included the following: they were convinced that patients preferred FtF contact; blended was considered too demanding for patients; or they thought that patients would not need bCBT. Therapists thought that more effort could be put into convincing patients since the manner in which bCBT is offered could influence patients' reactions.

Therapists found it a disadvantage that patients did not ask for bCBT or lacked a clear idea of what blended entails. Therefore, therapists believed it could be facilitating to offer it with enthusiasm, to explain the added value: 'patients can do more in their own time, there is more information to their disposal, and they have more opportunities to practice, all in a secure environment'. It was indicated that there is a lot of room for improvement when it comes to informing patients. It helped, for example, if patients knew that it is their own therapist who communicates with them on the platform. In addition, to increase uptake, therapists should not offer it as a treatment option, but as the standard approach to treating depression. Some therapists offered blended as something extra, whereas others showed patients the platform during intake to facilitate the switch to the platform at a later point during treatment.

Patient Eligibility

Experienced therapists mentioned that the criteria for bCBT were very similar to the criteria for CBT. No specific patient bCBT profile or type existed; eligibility was found to be person specific, not predictable and sometimes even very surprising. Therapists with little or no bCBT experience gave many different criteria for patient eligibility, which were predominantly based on perceptions.

A contributing factor to difficulties with informing patients was the unknown typology of the eligible bCBT patient. Stated criteria for perceived non-eligibility were extensive: lack of computer skills, preference for FtF treatment, fear of failure, lack of illness insight, low cognitive capacities, limited language skills, insecure home environment, psychotic symptoms, suicidal ideation, personality disorder, trauma, and complex or severe depressive symptoms. Perceived eligible patient criteria were less elaborate: young age, having children, being employed, and mild to moderate depressive symptoms.

Two interesting discussions took place about patient eligibility. Therapists disagreed about patients who, besides depression, had autism, avoidance issues, limited social contacts, poor concentration skills, or had undergone CBT for depression in the past. Some therapists observed that these factors prevented patients from engaging with bCBT, whereas others experienced that these factors made bCBT explicitly eligible for these patients as well. Another point of discussion was the severity of the depressive symptoms. Some therapists thought that bCBT was suitable for patients with complex, severe problems, while others did not: it would be harder to activate them than patients with less complex and more moderate symptoms. They would need more tools and explanations than bCBT can possibly offer them.

Patient Resistance

Several reasons for patient resistance toward bCBT were observed: unclear bCBT image, misfit with the traditional image of therapy among patients who had CBT in the past, fear of not receiving the right amount of help, and thinking that the online component was too demanding. Therapists' found that some patients were more difficult to motivate because they were inclined to generalize negative experiences with previous Internet-based treatments (often unguided treatments in primary care) to all other Internet-based interventions. However, most therapists, especially the experienced ones, thought the vast majority of patients were positive about bCBT when offered. Most therapists agreed that patient demand will increase in the future.

3.3.3. Theme (3) Therapists' Experiences with bCBT

Within this theme, experiences with providing bCBT in routine care are discussed. The identified subthemes were: effectiveness for depression, positive effects, negative effects, treatment format, therapeutic relationship, online feedback skills, drop-out, and safety (see Table 5).

Table 5. Theme (3) Therapists' experiences with bCBT, subthemes, influencing factors, and illustrative quotes.

Subtheme	Influencing Factors	Illustrative Quotes
Effectiveness for depression	(+) effectiveness bCBT = effectiveness of CBT	*"It is CBT in another format, it's not suddenly a different treatment."* (T29, experience)
Positive effects	(+) containing therapist drift	*"I don't skip things. With bCBT, I think that I am much more thorough than without."* (T29, experience)
	(+) making other diagnosis or problems more easily visible	*"You notice much sooner if a patient has difficulties adhering to therapy, whether or not they are doing the work. This becomes clearer faster than in a FtF session."* (T1, no/little experience)
	(+) helps to remember information more easily	*"In a FtF session you say a lot, but afterwards patients also forget quickly. Now they can review what they've learned as many times as they want."* (T10, experience)
	(+) reducing travel time	*"In other countries, factors such as distances and climate play a role, but of course in the middle of the country we have traffic jams. bCBT is very nice for this."* (T9, experience)
	(+) more contact with patient	*"Throughout the treatment you have more frequent short contact moments, which are actually very good."* (T10, experience)
	(+) sharing content with system	*"For the patient you remove the treatment from therapist's office to their own home."* (T12, no/little experience).
	(+) effect of writing	*"Patients have to write, this is for many a very good instrument to order things and gain new insights. I find the writing a very positive addition to the verbal component."* (T15, experience)
	(+) monitoring homework	*"I find it very attractive that there is more control over the homework that they have or haven't done."* (T2, experience)
	(+) facilitating patient self-efficacy	*"In the online part a degree of independence makes patients themselves engage with the treatment. I think that they attribute treatment success to themselves, more than with FtF treatment."* (T22, experience)
Negative effects	(−) no gain in time, costs more	*"I find it takes more time than I expected. Especially if you're still unfamiliar with the module."* (T7, no/little experience)
	(−) unsuitable content	*"I had a traumatized patient, because she couldn't have children. The first example on the platform was 'I have children and I want to be a good mother...'."* (T27, no/little experience)
Treatment format	(−/+) discussion on structure protocol	*"I find it difficult to be flexible in the protocol and not to become a sort of CBT machine."* (T21, no/little experience)
	(−/+) discussion on freedom in protocol to explore depression	*"Usually, when I start without the platform, I think 'never mind'. But also, when the patient isn't ready for it initially, you can say 'Later on, we will start with the online platform'."* (T31, no/little experience)
	(−/+) discussion on 'what is blended'	*"I don't think it's 50/50. The main focus is more on the FtF sessions. I notice that the conversations and the modules do not always run parallel to each other."* (T14, no/little experience)

Table 5. *Cont.*

Subtheme	Influencing Factors	Illustrative Quotes
	(−/+) discussion on introduction platform	*"Whether you start treatment with an online module, right at the outset or only when a basis has been formed, is dependent on the therapist. I think am very comfortable with starting right away."* (T1, no/little experience)
Therapeutic relationship	(−/+) discussion on quality therapeutic relationship	*"It's possible to build a therapeutic relationship, but sometimes it isn't. Yet I think that this isn't dependent on bCBT. Also, with FtF therapy it's possible to succeed in building a therapeutic relationship and sometimes not."* (T15, experience)
Online feedback skills	(−) time providing feedback (−) permanent character of online feedback	*"I reflect more on what I want to write, that is perhaps the reason why it takes more time."* (T7, no/little experience) *"It's difficult to assess whether someone has understood something in the way you intended. If this happens in FtF contact you can talk around it, look friendly and explain. In black and white this is not possible."* (T5, no/little experience)
	(+) connection online feedback and FtF conversations	*"I notice that patients like to come back to a point during the conversations, to go through the exercises together."* (T12, no/little experience)
Dropout & safety	(−/+) discussion on safety risks	*"In the meantime, I experienced that it's okay if the patient also comes to the FtF sessions. You've to make this clear at the start. The risk you lose contact is lower than I expected."* (T9, experience)
	(+) bCBT has no extra risks with regards to suicidal ideation	*"I thought that if you see someone less that it'd be more difficult to assess the suicide risk. But it can just as well lower the threshold to say something online more easily than to discuss FtF."* (T31, no/little experience)
	(+) drop-out bCBT = drop-out CBT	*"I don't have one type of patient that drops out of blended. It's very unpredictable who completes it."* (T30, experience)
	(+) sufficient patient data safety	*"I understood that the online platform is very safe, safer than email."* (T33, experience)

Note. (−) factor that influenced the bCBT uptake negatively, (+) factor that influenced the bCBT uptake positively, (−/+) factor that influenced the bCBT uptake positively and negatively.

Effectiveness for Depression

Therapists agreed that bCBT offered a good foundation for treating patients with depression. Nevertheless, they also found that the therapeutic content of the online sessions needed improvement, especially for patients with severe depressive symptoms who were characterized by more inactivity, complex problems, and longer treatment history. Whether 'the blended' treatment format exists, remained a question. Not based on research findings, but based on their experience, therapists uniformly thought that bCBT and FtF CBT could be equally effective. bCBT mainly helped to structure treatment and both patient and therapist to remain focused.

Positive Effects

The most cited positive effect was containing therapist drift; platform functionalities facilitated therapist (and patient) focus and protocol adherence more than in regular CBT because of the pre-set structure of bCBT. Therapists found it easier to control homework assignments and patients knew what was scheduled next. It was believed that all this positively impacted the quality of the treatment. An additional effect was that other diagnoses besides depression (e.g., autism) or certain problems (e.g., suicidal ideation, non-adherence, low cognitive capacities) were made more visible to the therapists at an earlier treatment stage. This was due to a discrepancy between online symptom monitoring, patients' online expressions, and what was said and shown in FtF sessions. Plus, for therapists, it was more noticeable from the patients' writing skills what the cognitive abilities were.

In the therapists' experience, patients found it easier to remember what was discussed in FtF sessions with bCBT. The information on the platform supported therapists—they had more information available, not only about depression but on other treatment options as well (e.g., sleep, self-image). In addition, because patients with depression often have concentration problems, the unlimited and easy access to treatment information and psychoeducation was very useful.

Reducing travel-time was mentioned as being very convenient for patients, not only for practical reasons (e.g., having children, employment), but also for therapists. bCBT provided an extra tool to stay connected with patients, especially in cases of no-show. Therapists discovered that patients shared the platform content with their immediate circle more easily (e.g., partner, family, or friends). Plus, the effect of writing on the online platform was a big advantage to patients. Patients wrote down their problems, came to new insights, and shared shameful problems more easily because of the distance effect and having time for reflection. bCBT offered patients greater responsibility. As for self-efficacy, some therapists thought that patients tended to attribute the treatment success to themselves more than in FtF treatment.

Negative Effects

Most therapists questioned whether bCBT could shorten treatments and solve waiting list problems. First, therapists spent a lot of time getting to know the platform and secondly, providing therapy via the online environment was time-consuming in contrast to expectations. Perhaps it might be timesaving in the future. However, the common thought was that bCBT is 'just another way of doing the same thing'. Some felt that there is a long way to go before blended interventions are considered equally effective as regular CBT by therapists in general.

Some judged the content on the platform to be too textual, too complex, or too superficial, thus requiring repeat sessions and extra clarification. Moreover, sometimes patients did not recognize themselves in the text and video examples; some found the content pejorative, overly directive, or too intense, resulting in drop-out or even worsening of their mood. Therefore, some therapists felt a strong need for personalization of the content to adapt to the patients' preferences and background.

Treatment Format

While experienced therapists unanimously stated that the pre-set structure of the blended protocol was very beneficial, for therapists with less experience, this was not the case. For them, the protocol was too structured and therefore inflexible. Experienced therapists, who had a better overview of all the functionalities, mentioned that bCBT was very similar to FtF CBT, in which you also adapt to the protocol when needed.

Therapists had different views on the ratio of FtF versus online sessions within bCBT. Some regarded and used bCBT as an addition to the regular number of FtF sessions. Moreover, for some the question 'what is blended?' remained. Therapists had different views on degrees of 'blendedness'. Repeatedly, it was seen as an interchange of FtF sessions with the functionalities of the online platform. For some patients 50%–50% was considered beneficial, for others 90% FtF and 10% online was more appropriate.

Another issue was the time point at which the online platform was introduced. Some therapists preferred to start with weekly FtF sessions and introduced the platform at a later date. For them, it felt unnatural and too distracting for patients to meet every two weeks instead of weekly in the first phase of treatment. They wanted more time to establish a foundation, especially for patients who lacked insight into their depression. Other therapists, who thought it would be better to start with the online platform at once, reasoned that the threshold (for patients and therapists) may be higher when the platform is introduced at a later stage. These therapists also imagined that it motivated patients to be focused from the beginning with the support of the platform.

Therapeutic Relationship

Regarding the quality of a therapeutic relationship in bCBT, therapists' opinions were divided. In the beginning, some doubted whether it was possible to develop a therapeutic relationship because they would see patients less FtF, but changed their opinion later on. In some therapists' experience, it was challenging to build a therapeutic relationship compared to regular CBT; when a patient experienced difficulties with the online platform and asked more attention from the therapist, this frustrated the contact because it was at the expense of the time they had FtF. Nevertheless, others experienced that the relationship in bCBT was similar or even better compared to FtF treatment. bCBT reinforced the relationship, since there was more frequent contact throughout. In addition, the treatment course was more visible to therapists because of online monitoring and this also positively influenced the relationship. Importantly, as in every treatment, the relationship was mainly perceived as more dependent on patient motivation and activation than other factors such as online contact.

Online Feedback Skills

Therapists agreed that every therapist is able to provide online feedback. However, learning how to provide feedback took time and for many, felt like 'a job in its own right'. They were needed for tips, tools, and examples; how to address something negative, how to handle or prevent miscommunication, how to write in a concise manner, how to make feedback personalized and adapt to different patient types. In contrast to FtF sessions, where therapists are able to correct themselves, everything that is written online, has a permanent character: for some, online feedback thus felt uncomfortable.

Therapists stressed the importance of connecting to the language of the patient. They found they had to be careful not to use difficult terminology or be too distant in their language. Most of all, they had to plan sufficient time to write feedback. Therapists noticed that writing online feedback became faster with more experience. Connecting online feedback and topics in FtF sessions and vice versa, was experienced as helpful and was done quite frequently.

Drop-Out and Safety

Two safety risks cited predominantly by inexperienced therapists were the suggestion of 24/7 accessibility to patients and not being able to see how patients reacted to therapist feedback or other online information. Experienced therapists did not mention this or had learned that this was not an issue.

Regarding a much-discussed risk of suicidal ideation, therapists experienced that when there was a clear agreement with patients on not expressing crisis situations on the platform, bCBT had no extra risks compared to FtF treatment. Importantly, it even gave therapists more rapid awareness of whether patients were losing contact. In addition, bCBT provided therapists with an extra preventive communication tool.

Furthermore, experienced therapists reported that there was no specific type of patient that dropped out. Sometimes therapists saw patients who started enthusiastically, but dropped out easily. Importantly, they thought this was no different than with regular CBT: patients dropped out because of certain patient characteristics or other problems than for bCBT-related issues.

Overall, therapists expressed that safety of patient data on the online platform is guaranteed sufficiently. Sharing patient data with, for example, a helpdesk, is still something that therapists were reluctant to do and prevented them from contacting the helpdesk when technical issues occurred. They often then tried to solve their issues with colleagues, but often also broke off the online sessions. Some patients seemed too lax when it came to their data safety, and some were distrustful. Therapists emphasized that it is their responsibility to explain how safe the online platform is, but that this was not clear to all therapists.

4. Discussion

In this study, therapists expressed overall satisfaction with providing bCBT to patients with depression. The perceived usability of the online platform was sufficient. This was also found by other studies exploring patients' perspectives on usability and satisfaction [21,36]. This study showed that therapists see room for improvement with regard to platform usability (e.g., lack of integration with other administrative systems), therapists' work routines, and guideline use on bCBT. From interviews in this study, it became clear that there are specific barriers that prevented therapists from providing bCBT to patients with depression, such as a lack of ongoing support for technical and clinical issues with bCBT. In addition, therapists reported several practical and therapeutic challenges in routine care such as not experiencing timesaving. Nevertheless, there have been factors that might have influenced the uptake positively as well.

4.1. Barriers to bCBT Uptake

Less experienced bCBT therapists felt several barriers prevented them from providing bCBT. First, they found that the training was not sufficient to enable them to adopt bCBT into their work routine. This was partly because the training mainly covered technical aspects and did not provide sufficient guidance on how to work in a blended way with the protocol and how to communicate online. In addition, after undergoing training, ongoing support and attention for bCBT was limited or absent. This was also a reported therapist barrier by Folker et al. [37] who identified implementation challenges perceived by therapists and managers of iCBT in routine care settings in five European countries. Moreover, inexperienced therapists were unsure about the indication for bCBT and the eligibility of the patients. A third issue was that some therapists experienced low patient demand for bCBT. A fourth hindering factor was that for a number of the therapists, the added value of bCBT in terms of clinical effectiveness remained unclear; for others, fear (e.g., of doing something wrong) or distrust (e.g., regarding the intentions of health insurance companies) stood in the way of considering bCBT.

4.2. Challenges with bCBT

Once therapists started working with bCBT, they experienced several challenges. They had difficulty integrating bCBT into their daily workflow. Not only because of technical disconnections with existing IT-systems for patients' administration, but also because of uncertainties regarding the bCBT protocol and logistic integration into their daily therapeutic and administrative schedules. Besides, therapists lacked the conviction that bCBT saved time; for some, it even generated a higher workload, especially in the beginning, and providing online feedback is considered time-consuming as well. It can be estimated, that on average per feedback message, 30 min of therapist time is needed [13]. Internal helpdesks were unable to support therapists sufficiently which even discouraged some from further providing bCBT.

Moreover, therapists displayed different interpretations of the protocol which partly resulted for some in using the online platform on top of the FtF treatment instead of replacing a portion of the FtF sessions. This was previously reported in a naturalistic study on bCBT uptake in routine care as well [38], making the implementation more costly than intended. Kenter et al. [38] argued that their therapists may have needed more extensive training to master specific bCBT skills (e.g., providing online feedback) and that clear guidelines on how to use bCBT in routine practice by the MHO would have helped the therapist to provide bCBT more efficiently. Plus, using the online platform on top of the FtF treatment may result in patient dissatisfaction. A study on patients' experiences with bCBT showed that a diminished interplay between the online and FtF sessions was unsatisfactory for patients, as therapists were less aware of patient activity on the online platform and limited time was made available to discuss the online activity in the FtF sessions [39].

4.3. Advantages of bCBT

One of the main reported advantages of bCBT was the focus and pre-set structure that made therapists and their patients more adherent to the protocol and contained therapist drift. This was also experienced by several therapists who worked with bCBT [14,19] or blended group therapy [40] for depression. Although content improvement (e.g., online patient examples) for severely depressed patients was considered necessary, therapists agreed that bCBT is a good treatment format for the (complex) patient group therapists see in daily practice. They found that bCBT was in many ways similar to FtF CBT when it comes to patient eligibility, effectiveness, therapeutic relationship, and drop-out: 'it is CBT in another format'. Many believed that the implementation phase is still in its infancy; it might be a long way to go before all therapists accept blended interventions as being equally effective to FtF therapy. This idea is also partly justified since the first studies on clinical effects on blended interventions show that it is at least as effective [12,13]. Nonetheless, it is thought that bCBT will eventually be included in care pathways in the future because of the perceived benefits for patients and therapists (e.g., pre-set structure, number of flexible contact moments on demand, information access); an important precondition is to continue to be combined with FtF contact, as providing stand-alone guided iCBT might not yet be realistic for most therapists in routine practice, where FtF treatment is the norm.

4.4. Level of Experience

In our study, therapists with bCBT experience reported different views on safety, flexibility and personalization of the protocol, patient eligibility, and therapeutic relationship than therapists who lacked experience. For example, non-experienced therapists assumed that there were many reasons why patients would be ineligible for bCBT, such as severe depressive symptoms, or found this difficult to assess. By contrast, more experienced therapists stated that it was impossible to predict eligibility; in principle, any patient could be offered bCBT. This may indicate that with experience, perceptions on these important clinical factors of bCBT will change and that when promoting uptake, therapists' needs can shift. This is consistent with Feijt et al. [41] who showed that there are different barriers and facilitators depending on the level of therapist experience with online services, and that potentially, the experience level has unique requirements to be addressed when it comes to the uptake of Internet-based interventions.

4.5. Limitations and Strengths

Although some therapists in this study were skeptical about the effectiveness of bCBT or had negative experiences, all were quite open-minded toward bCBT. Selection bias in our sample is possible, as untrained therapists or those not interested in participating in the study were not reached and therapists were identified through their team managers, and other specially appointed members of different teams. This could have diminished the positive view on bCBT.

Another point is the limited transferability of our findings to other national contexts. In the Netherlands, the digital infrastructure is quite good and MHO's and therapists have the experience that every patient has proper equipment. Moreover, bCBT is covered by health care insurance companies in the same way as face-to-face CBT. Compared to other countries, the Netherlands and others, including Sweden and the United Kingdom, can be considered a frontrunner in implementing bCBT within routine practice [16]. On the other hand, our findings can be taken into account by the 'followers' in the earlier stages of developing, testing, and implementing bCBT.

A strength of this study is the usage of data triangulation to record the perspective of a diverse group of therapists, with different professional backgrounds, differences in experiences with bCBT for depression, and exposure to various implementation strategies from a number of mental health care organizations.

4.6. Future Uptake of bCBT

To speed up bCBT uptake, it is important to identify how barriers can be overcome, challenges solved, and how successes in routine care can be strengthened. From the field of implementation research, it is known that implementation strategies for innovations in mental health care need 'to address multiple levels and barriers to change, (and) are interwoven and packaged as a protocolized or branded implementation intervention' [42]. Based on this and on the findings of this study, the following strategies can be considered in practice and in research to move forward in the implementation of bCBT:

1. Dissemination strategies: to change the focus of cost-effectiveness of bCBT towards personalization, adherence, and treatment quality improvement in disseminating information to therapists and patients. Within organizations, the uptake might gain from informing and motivating therapists and subsequently patients as well. There is a lot of room for improvement when it comes to sufficient knowledge about bCBT. Outside the organizations, patient demand can be stimulated by general practitioners and health insurance companies. Further, although evidence-based knowledge on bCBT is slowly becoming more available, this should be more widespread among patients, therapists, MHOs, and health insurance companies.
2. Top down strategies: bCBT must be embedded top-down from start to finish overcoming its mere project status in many of the MHOs. This could be achieved by intensifying and extending training beyond technical aspects, and by facilitating the integration of ongoing support into existing consultation structures, (instead of creating special consultation options), in order to exchange knowledge and experience with bCBT. It would also help to remind therapists to offer bCBT to patients and to solve technical disconnections with administration- and other IT-systems within a well-equipped help desk. Whether imposing minimum usage norms (e.g., that 25% of the treatments must be blended in the Netherlands) could have a promoting effect is unclear, as this causes resistance for some, but motivated others.
3. Bottom-up strategies: Fragmented use and individual uptake of the blended protocol can create a risk of it being costlier and of leading to a protocolled manner of working. Therapists' need

to personalize modules might be a result of uncertainty and their limited knowledge of all functionalities within the module and platform. Thus, besides a top-down approach, therapists might be more motivated and skilled if uptake is stimulated on a bottom-up basis, through discussing it on the work floor: For instance, it could help to start implementation with a small rollout with a motivated team of therapists, focusing on content development, enhancing online feedback skills and protocol use; to let the therapists be (co-) creators of modules; to construct a place and time within MHOs where therapists can think of ways to further develop bCBT; to experiment; to keep lines with the technical innovations on the platform within reach; including recurring evaluation in order to adapt strategies on the level of therapist experience and updates of the platform.

4.7. Future Research

Testing strategies for uptake would be a fruitful area for further research. The European project, ImpleMentAll (www.implementall.eu), will hopefully provide routine practice with more knowledge as this is uncharted territory for Internet interventions in mental health care [43]. In ImpleMentAll, personalized implementation strategies will be tested to facilitate the use of Internet-based and blended interventions in routine care in several different countries.

In addition, it would support uptake of bCBT to further investigate the ratio and integration of online and FtF sessions. So far, research has focused on an equal distribution. However, it is reasonable to think that depending on the severity of the symptoms, the proportion of blended could be adapted. Moreover, it would be interesting for future studies to also look at the patient perspectives on blended care, preferably done using dyad interviews with their therapists to generate a rich, deeper understanding of the relevant factors in bCBT uptake.

5. Conclusions

Overall, the therapists in this study were satisfied with providing bCBT to patients with depression. That said, a large group of therapists is still wondering how much FtF contact should be included in blended. Plus, important preconditions for implementation were unmet and the technical infrastructure is not free from teething problems. It cannot be expected from therapists that uptake happens spontaneously. It can be considered positive that having bCBT experience can be a possible key to change a therapist's view on important factors such as eligibility and drop-out. Therapists found that there is a good base that can be further developed in terms of ongoing technical support, therapeutic support from their peers and supervisors, while at the same time strategically implementing bCBT on an organizational level to facilitate therapists in the transition of integrating bCBT into their daily practice.

Author Contributions: All authors have contributed substantially to the work reported. All authors critically revised the paper. Conceptualization, M.M., E.D., D.J.F.v.S., H.R. and J.H.S.; Data curation, M.M.; Formal analysis, M.M., C.v.G. and S.D.; Funding acquisition, H.R. and J.H.S.; Investigation, M.M., C.v.G. and S.D.; Methodology, M.M., E.D., D.J.F.v.S., S.D., H.R. and J.H.S.; Software, M.M.; Supervision, H.R. and J.H.S.; Validation, M.M., C.v.G. and S.D.; Visualization, M.M.; Writing—original draft, M.M.; Writing—review & editing, M.M., C.v.G., E.D., D.J.F.v.S., S.D., H.R. and J.H.S. All authors have read and agreed to the published version of the manuscript.

Acknowledgments: The authors would like to thank several people for their contributions: Thuur Smet (data extraction), Nanda Mooij, Bep Verkerk (data management), Martine de Meijer (transcribing interviews). We also would like to thank the therapists and the participating mental health care organizations for their time and effort.

References

1. Cuijpers, P.; Noma, H.; Karyotaki, E.; Cipriani, A.; Furukawa, T.A. Effectiveness and Acceptability of Cognitive Behavior Therapy Delivery Formats in Adults with Depression: A Network Meta-analysis. *JAMA Psychiatry* **2019**, *76*, 700–707. [CrossRef] [PubMed]
2. National Institute for Clinical Excellence. Depression: The treatment and management of depression in adults. In *Clinical Guideline 90*; NICE: London, UK, 2009.

3. World Health Organization. Depression and Other Common Mental Disorders: Global Health Estimates. In *World Health Organization Report*; World Health Organization: Geneva, Switzerland, 2017; pp. 1–24.
4. Boerema, A.M.; Kleiboer, A.; Beekman, A.T.F.; van Zoonen, K.; Dijkshoorn, H.; Cuijpers, P. Determinants of help-seeking behavior in depression: A cross-sectional study. *BMC Psychiatry* **2016**, *16*. [CrossRef] [PubMed]
5. Andrews, G.; Basu, A.; Cuijpers, P.; Craske, M.G.; McEvoy, P.; English, C.L.; Newby, J.M. Computer therapy for the anxiety and depression disorders is effective, acceptable and practical health care: An updated meta-analysis. *J. Anxiety Disord.* **2018**, *55*, 70–78. [CrossRef] [PubMed]
6. Karyotaki, E.; Riper, H.; Twisk, J.; Hoogendoorn, A.; Kleiboer, A.; Mira, A.; MacKinnon, A.; Meyer, B.; Botella, C.; Littlewood, E.; et al. Efficacy of self-guided internet-based cognitive behavioral therapy in the treatment of depressive symptoms a meta-analysis of individual participant data. *JAMA Psychiatry* **2017**, *74*, 351–359. [CrossRef] [PubMed]
7. Titov, N.; Dear, B.; Nielssen, O.; Staples, L.; Hadjistavropoulos, H.; Nugent, M.; Adlam, K.; Nordgreen, T.; Bruvik, K.H.; Hovland, A.; et al. ICBT in routine care: A descriptive analysis of successful clinics in five countries. *Internet Interv.* **2018**, *13*, 108–115. [CrossRef]
8. Erbe, D.; Psych, D.; Eichert, H.C.; Riper, H.; Ebert, D.D. Blending face-to-face and internet-based interventions for the treatment of mental disorders in adults: Systematic review. *J. Med. Internet Res.* **2017**, *19*. [CrossRef]
9. Hadjistavropoulos, H.D.; Nugent, M.M.; Dirkse, D.; Pugh, N. Implementation of internet-delivered cognitive behavior therapy within community mental health clinics: A process evaluation using the consolidated framework for implementation research. *BMC Psychiatry* **2017**, *17*. [CrossRef]
10. Definition Blended Treatment Heleen Riper. Triple-E Website. Available online: https://www.triple-ehealth.nl/en/projects-cat/depressie/ and http://www.webcitation.org/6wZFBY9pX (accessed on 18 January 2018).
11. Kleiboer, A.; Smit, J.; Bosmans, J.; Ruwaard, J.; Andersson, G.; Topooco, N.; Berger, T.; Krieger, T.; Botella, C.; Baños, R.; et al. European COMPARative Effectiveness research on blended Depression treatment versus treatment-as-usual (E-COMPARED): Study protocol for a randomized controlled, non-inferiority trial in eight European countries. *Trials* **2016**, *17*. [CrossRef]
12. Romijn, G.; Batelaan, N.; Koning, J.; van Balkom, A.; de Leeuw, A.; Benning, F.; Hakkaart-van Roijen, L.; Riper, H. Effectiveness and cost-effectiveness of blended cognitive-behavioural therapy for anxiety disorders in specialised mental health care: A 15-week randomised controlled trial with 1-year follow-up. 2019; accepted.
13. Kooistra, L.C.; Wiersma, J.E.; Ruwaard, J.J.; Neijenhuijs, K.; Lokkerbol, J.; Smit, F.; van Oppen, P.; Riper, H. Costs and effectiveness of blended versus standard cognitive behavioral therapy for depressed outpatients in routine specialized mental healthcare: A pilot randomized controlled trial. *J. Med. Internet Res.* **2019**, *21*. [CrossRef]
14. Mansson, K.N.; Skagius Ruiz, E.; Gervind, E.; Dahlin, M.; Andersson, G. Development and initial evaluation of an Internet-based support system for face-to-face cognitive behavior therapy: A proof of concept study. *J. Med. Internet Res.* **2013**, *15*, e280. [CrossRef] [PubMed]
15. Thase, M.E.; Wright, J.H.; Eells, T.D.; Barrett, M.S.; Wisniewski, S.R.; Balasubramani, G.K.; McCrone, P.; Brown, G.K. Improving the Efficiency of Psychotherapy for Depression: Computer-Assisted Versus Standard CBT. *Am. J. Psychiatry* **2017**, *175*. [CrossRef] [PubMed]
16. Topooco, N.; Riper, H.; Araya, R.; Berking, M.; Brunn, M.; Chevreul, K.; Cieslak, R.; Ebert, D.D.; Etchmendy, E.; Herrero, R.; et al. Attitudes towards digital treatment for depression: A European stakeholder survey. *Internet Interv.* **2017**, *8*, 1–9. [CrossRef]
17. Vis, C.; Kleiboer, A.; Prior, R.; Bønes, E.; Cavallo, M.; Clark, S.A.; Dozeman, E.; Ebert, D.; Etzelmueller, A.; Favaretto, G.; et al. Implementing and up-scaling evidence-based eMental health in Europe: The study protocol for the MasterMind project. *Internet Interv.* **2015**, *2*. [CrossRef]
18. Mol, M.; Dozeman, E.; van Schaik, D.J.F.; Vis, C.P.C.D.; Riper, H.; Smit, J.H. The therapist's role in the implementation of internet-based cognitive behavioural therapy for patients with depression: Study protocol. *BMC Psychiatry* **2016**, *16*, 338. [CrossRef]
19. Titzler, I.; Saruhanjan, K.; Berking, M.; Riper, H.; Ebert, D.D. Barriers and facilitators for the implementation of blended psychotherapy for depression: A qualitative pilot study of therapists' perspective. *Internet Interv.* **2018**, *12*, 150–164. [CrossRef]
20. Denzin, N.K. Triangulation 2.0 *. *J. Mix. Methods Res.* **2012**, *6*, 80–88. [CrossRef]

21. Kooistra, L.C.; Ruwaard, J.; Wiersma, J.E.; van Oppen, P.; van der Vaart, R.; van Gemert-Pijnen, J.E.W.C.; Riper, H. Development and initial evaluation of blended cognitive behavioural treatment for major depression in routine specialized mental health care. *Internet Interv.* **2016**, *4*, 61–71. [CrossRef]
22. Regulation (EU) 2016/679 of the European Parliament and of the Council of 27 April 2016 on the Protection of Natural Persons with Regard to the Processing of Personal Data and on the Free Movement of Such Data, and Repealing Directive 95/46/EC (General Data Protection Regulation). Official Journal of the European Union L 119/1. Available online: http://data.europa.eu/eli/reg/2016/679/oj (accessed on 10 December 2019).
23. Brooke, J. SUS-A quick and dirty usability scale. *Usability Eval. Ind.* **1996**, *189*, 4–7.
24. Mol, M.; van Schaik, A.; Dozeman, E.; Ruwaard, J.; Vis, C.; Ebert, D.D.; Etzelmueller, A.; Mathiasen, K.; Moles, B.; Mora, T.; et al. Dimensionality of System Usability Scale among professionals using internet-based interventions for depression: A confirmatory factor analysis. 2019; accepted.
25. Sauro, J. *A Practical Guide to the System Usability Scale: Background, Benchmarks & Best Practices*; Measuring Usability LLC: Denver, CO, USA, 2011.
26. Sauro, J.; Lewis, J.R. Quantifying user research. In *Quantifying the User Experience*; Elsevier: Amsterdam, The Netherlands, 2016; pp. 9–18. [CrossRef]
27. Attkisson, C.C.; Greenfield, T.K. *The Client Satisfaction Questionnaire (CSQ) Scales. Outcome Assessment in Clinical Practice*; Williams & Wilkins: Baltimore, MD, USA, 1995.
28. Boß, L.; Lehr, D.; Reis, D.; Vis, C.; Riper, H.; Berking, M.; Ebert, D.D. Reliability and validity of assessing user satisfaction with web-based health interventions. *J. Med. Internet Res.* **2016**, *18*, e234. [CrossRef]
29. Glasgow, R.E.; Vogt, T.M.; Boles, S.M. Evaluating the public health impact of health promotion interventions: The RE-AIM framework. *Am. J. Public Health* **1999**, *89*, 1322–1327. [CrossRef]
30. Kidholm, K.; Ekeland, A.G.; Jensen, L.K.; Rasmussen, J.; Pedersen, C.D.; Bowes, A.; Flottorp, S.A.; Bech, M. A model for assessment of telemedicine applications: Mast. *Int. J. Technol. Assess. Health Care* **2012**, *28*, 44–51. [CrossRef] [PubMed]
31. May, C.R.; Mair, F.; Finch, T.; MacFarlane, A.; Dowrick, C.; Treweek, S.; Rapley, T.; Ballini, L.; Ong, B.N.; Rogers, A.; et al. Development of a theory of implementation and integration: Normalization Process Theory. *Implement. Sci.* **2009**, *4*. [CrossRef] [PubMed]
32. Kivi, M.; Eriksson, M.C.M.; Hange, D.; Petersson, E.L.; Björkelund, C.; Johansson, B. Experiences and attitudes of primary care therapists in the implementation and use of internet-based treatment in Swedish primary care settings. *Internet Interv.* **2015**, *2*, 248–256. [CrossRef]
33. Wilhelmsen, M.; Hoifodt, R.S.; Kolstrup, N.; Waterloo, K.; Eisemann, M.; Chenhall, R.; Risor, M.B. Norwegian general practitioners' perspectives on implementation of a guided web-based cognitive behavioral therapy for depression: A qualitative study. *J. Med. Internet Res.* **2014**, *16*, e208. [CrossRef]
34. Braun, V.; Clarke, V. Using thematic analysis in psychology. *Qual. Res. Psychol.* **2006**, *3*, 77–101. [CrossRef]
35. Fleiss, L.; Levin, B.; Paik, M.C. The measurement of interrater agreement. In *Statistical Methods for Rates and Proportions*, 3rd ed.; John Wiley & Sons, Inc.: Hoboken, NJ, USA, 2003.
36. Etzelmueller, A.; Radkovsky, A.; Hannig, W.; Berking, M.; Ebert, D.D. Patient's experience with blended video- and internet based cognitive behavioural therapy service in routine care. *Internet Interv.* **2018**, *12*, 165–175. [CrossRef]
37. Folker, A.P.; Mathiasen, K.; Lauridsen, S.M.; Stenderup, E.; Dozeman, E.; Folker, M.P. Implementing internet-delivered cognitive behavior therapy for common mental health disorders: A comparative case study of implementation challenges perceived by therapists and managers in five European internet services. *Internet Interv.* **2018**, *11*, 60–70. [CrossRef]
38. Kenter, R.M.F.; van de Ven, P.M.; Cuijpers, P.; Koole, G.; Niamat, S.; Gerrits, R.S.; Willems, M.; van Straten, A. Costs and effects of Internet cognitive behavioral treatment blended with face-to-face treatment: Results from a naturalistic study. *Internet Interv.* **2015**, *2*, 77–83. [CrossRef]
39. Urech, A.; Krieger, T.; Möseneder, L.; Biaggi, A.; Vincent, A.; Poppe, C.; Meyer, B.; Riper, H.; Berger, T. A patient post hoc perspective on advantages and disadvantages of blended cognitive behaviour therapy for depression: A qualitative content analysis. *Psychother. Res.* **2018**, *29*, 986–998. [CrossRef]
40. Schuster, R.; Sigl, S.; Berger, T.; Laireiter, A.R. Patients' Experiences of Web- and Mobile-Assisted Group Therapy for Depression and Implications of the Group Setting: Qualitative Follow-Up Study. *JMIR Ment. Health* **2018**, *5*, e49. [CrossRef] [PubMed]

41. Feijt, M.A.; De Kort, Y.A.W.; Bongers, I.M.B.; IJsselsteijn, W.A. Perceived drivers and barriers to the adoption of eMental health by psychologists: The construction of the levels of adoption of eMental health model. *J. Med. Internet Res.* **2018**, *20*. [CrossRef] [PubMed]
42. Powell, B.J.; McMillen, J.C.; Proctor, E.K.; Carpenter, C.R.; Griffey, R.T.; Bunger, A.C.; Glass, J.E.; York, J.L. A compilation of strategies for implementing clinical innovations in health and mental health. *Med. Care Res. Rev.* **2012**, *69*, 123–157. [CrossRef] [PubMed]
43. Bührmann, L.; Schuurmans, J.; Ruwaard, J. Tailored Implementation of Internet-based Cognitive Behavioural Therapy in the Multinational Context of the ImpleMentAll Project: A Study Protocol for a Stepped Wedge Cluster Randomized Trial. under review.

Permissions

All chapters in this book were first published by MDPI; hereby published with permission under the Creative Commons Attribution License or equivalent. Every chapter published in this book has been scrutinized by our experts. Their significance has been extensively debated. The topics covered herein carry significant findings which will fuel the growth of the discipline. They may even be implemented as practical applications or may be referred to as a beginning point for another development.

The contributors of this book come from diverse backgrounds, making this book a truly international effort. This book will bring forth new frontiers with its revolutionizing research information and detailed analysis of the nascent developments around the world.

We would like to thank all the contributing authors for lending their expertise to make the book truly unique. They have played a crucial role in the development of this book. Without their invaluable contributions this book wouldn't have been possible. They have made vital efforts to compile up to date information on the varied aspects of this subject to make this book a valuable addition to the collection of many professionals and students.

This book was conceptualized with the vision of imparting up-to-date information and advanced data in this field. To ensure the same, a matchless editorial board was set up. Every individual on the board went through rigorous rounds of assessment to prove their worth. After which they invested a large part of their time researching and compiling the most relevant data for our readers.

The editorial board has been involved in producing this book since its inception. They have spent rigorous hours researching and exploring the diverse topics which have resulted in the successful publishing of this book. They have passed on their knowledge of decades through this book. To expedite this challenging task, the publisher supported the team at every step. A small team of assistant editors was also appointed to further simplify the editing procedure and attain best results for the readers.

Apart from the editorial board, the designing team has also invested a significant amount of their time in understanding the subject and creating the most relevant covers. They scrutinized every image to scout for the most suitable representation of the subject and create an appropriate cover for the book.

The publishing team has been an ardent support to the editorial, designing and production team. Their endless efforts to recruit the best for this project, has resulted in the accomplishment of this book. They are a veteran in the field of academics and their pool of knowledge is as vast as their experience in printing. Their expertise and guidance has proved useful at every step. Their uncompromising quality standards have made this book an exceptional effort. Their encouragement from time to time has been an inspiration for everyone.

The publisher and the editorial board hope that this book will prove to be a valuable piece of knowledge for researchers, students, practitioners and scholars across the globe.

List of Contributors

Alba Quilez-Orden
Department of Psychology and Sociology, University of Zaragoza, 44003 Teruel, Spain
Health Research Institute of Aragón, 50009 Zaragoza, Spain

Jorge Osma
Department of Psychology and Sociology, University of Zaragoza, 44003 Teruel, Spain
Health Research Institute of Aragón, 50009 Zaragoza, Spain
Department of Psychology and Sociology, Universidad de Zaragoza and Instituto de Investigación Sanitaria de Aragón, Ciudad Escolar s/n, 44003 Teruel, Spain

Vanesa Ferreres-Galán
Mental Health Unit of the Regional Hospital of Vinaròs, 12500 Castellón, Spain

Bonifacio Sandín, Julia García-Escalera, Rosa M. Valiente, Victoria Espinosa and Paloma Chorot
Facultad de Psicología, Universidad Nacional de Educación a Distancia (UNED), 20040 Madrid, Spain

Monia Cabinio, Federica Rossetto, Sara Isernia, Francesca Lea Saibene, Monica Di Cesare, Francesca Borgnis, Margherita Alberoni, Valeria Blasi and Francesca Baglio
IRCCS Fondazione Don Carlo Gnocchi ONLUS, via Capecelatro 66, 20148 Milan, Italy

Stefania Pazzi and Tommaso Migliazza
Consorzio di Bioingegneria e Informatica medica (CBIM), 27100 Pavia, Italy

Yonatan Stern
Psychology Department, University of Haifa, Haifa 3498838, Israel
Gonda Brain Research Center, Bar-Ilan University, Ramat Gan 5290002, Israel

Danny Koren
Psychology Department, University of Haifa, Haifa 3498838, Israel

Renana Moebus, Gabriella Panishev and Roy Salomon
Gonda Brain Research Center, Bar-Ilan University, Ramat Gan 5290002, Israel

Cosimo Tuena
ATN-P Lab, Department of Psychology, IRCSS Auxologico Italiano, Via Magnasco 2, 20149 Milano, Italy

Silvia Serino
MySpace Lab, Department of Clinical Neurosciences, University Hospital Lausanne-CHUV, CH-1011 Lausanne, Switzerland

Pietro Cipresso and Giuseppe Riva
ATN-P Lab, Department of Psychology, IRCSS Auxologico Italiano, Via Magnasco 2, 20149 Milano, Italy
Department of Psychology, Catholic University of the Sacred Heart, Largo Gemelli, 1, 20100 Milan, Italy

Fabiana Monteiro, Marco Pereira, Maria Cristina Canavarro and Ana Fonseca
Center for Research in Neuropsychology and Cognitive Behavioral Intervention (CINEICC), Faculty of Psychology and Educational Sciences, the University of Coimbra Rua do Colégio Novo, 3000-315 Coimbra, Portugal

Patricia Gual-Montolio, Verónica Martínez-Borba, Juana María Bretón-López and Carlos Suso-Ribera
Department of Basic and Clinical Psychology and Psychobiology, Jaume I University, Avda. Vicent Sos Baynat s/n, 12071 Castellon de la Plana, Spain

Jessica Isbely Montana, Marta Matamala-Gomez, Marta Maisto, Petar Aleksandrov Mavrodiev, Barbara Diana, Fabrizia Mantovani and Olivia Realdon
Department of Human Sciences for Education, University of Milano-Bicocca, Piazza dell'Ateneo Nuovo 1, 20126 Milano, Italy

Cesare Massimo Cavalera
Department of Psychology, Catholic University of the Sacred Heart, Largo Gemelli 1, 20100 Milan, Italy

Ángel Castro and Juan Ramón Barrada
Facultad de Ciencias Sociales y Humanas. Universidad de Zaragoza. Calle Atarazanas, 4. 44003 Teruel, Spain

Pedro J. Ramos-Villagrasa and Elena Fernández-del-Río
Facultad de Ciencias Sociales y del Trabajo. Universidad de Zaragoza. Calle Violante de Hungría, 23. 50009 Zaragoza, Spain

Desirée Colombo
Department of Basic Psychology, Clinic and Psychobiology, Universitat Jaume I, Av. Sos Baynat, s/n, 12071 Castellón, Spain

Javier Fernández-Álvarez
Department of Psychology, Università Cattolica del Sacro Cuore, Largo Gemelli, 1, 20100 Milan, Italy

Andrea Patané and Marta Kwiatkowska
Department of Computer Science, University of Oxford, Wolfson Building, Parks Rd, Oxford OX1 3QD, UK

Michelle Semonella
Applied Technology for Neuro-Psychology Lab, IRCCS Istituto Auxologico Italiano, 20149 Milan, Italy

Azucena García-Palacios and Cristina Botella
Department of Basic Psychology, Clinic and Psychobiology, Universitat Jaume I, Av. Sos Baynat, s/n, 12071 Castellón, Spain
CIBER Fisiopatología Obesidad y Nutrición (CIBERobn), Instituto Salud Carlos III, 28029 Madrid, Spain

Mariano Alcañiz Raya, Javier Marín-Morales, Maria Eleonora Minissi, Gonzalo Teruel Garcia and Irene Alice Chicchi Giglioli
Instituto de Investigación e Innovación en Bioingeniería (i3B), Universitat Politécnica de Valencia, 46022 Valencia, Spain

Luis Abad
Red Cenit, Centros de Desarrollo Cognitivo, 46020 Valencia, Spain

Mayke Mol, Claire van Genugten, Els Dozeman, Digna J. F. van Schaik, Stasja Draisma and Jan H. Smit
Department of Research and Innovation, GGZ inGeest, Specialized Mental Health Care, 1081 Amsterdam, The Netherlands
Department of Psychiatry, Amsterdam Public Health Research Institute, VU University Medical Center, 1081 Amsterdam, The Netherlands

Heleen Riper
Department of Research and Innovation, GGZ inGeest, Specialized Mental Health Care, 1081 Amsterdam, The Netherlands
Department of Psychiatry, Amsterdam Public Health Research Institute, VU University Medical Center, 1081 Amsterdam, The Netherlands
Department of Clinical, Neuro and Developmental Psychology, Clinical Psychology Section, Vrije Universiteit Amsterdam and the Amsterdam Public Health Research Institute, 1081 Amsterdam, The Netherlands
Telepsychiatry and E-Mental Health, Department of Clinical Research, University of Southern Denmark, 5000 Odense, Denmark

Index

www.ingramcontent.com/pod-product-compliance
Lightning Source LLC
LaVergne TN
LVHW060057220926
848484LV00008BA/2114